GENITAL INFECTIONS AND INFERTILITY

Edited by **Atef M. Darwish**

Genital Infections and Infertility
http://dx.doi.org/10.5772/60460
Edited by Atef M. Darwish

Contributors

Hosni Salem, Nourhan Mesbah, Liyun Shi, Huanhuan Wang, Zhe Lu, Wei Wu, Qiuqin Tang, Yiqiu Chen, Hao Gu, Yankai Xia, Jiahao Sha, Xinru Wang, Katiuska Satue Ambrojo, Sanusi Ibrahim, Attilio Di Spiezio Sardo, Poongothai Jayaramasamy, Manonmani Samiappan, Doblin Sandai, Luigi Auletta, Maria Pia Pasolini, Chiara Del Prete, Silvia Fabbri, María Damiani, Agustín Luján, Silvina Fili, Rutvij Dalal, María Del Carmen Colín Ferreyra, Thana Khawcharoenporn, Beverly Sha, Reza Peymani, Alan DeCherney, Atef M.M. Darwish

Published by InTech

Janeza Trdine 9, 51000 Rijeka, Croatia

Publishing Process Manager Sandra Bakic

Technical Editor InTech DTP team

Cover InTech Design team

First published June, 2016

Printed in Croatia

Additional hard copies can be obtained from orders@intechopen.com

Genital Infections and Infertility, Edited by Atef M. Darwish

p. cm.

Print ISBN 978-953-51-2488-7

Online ISBN 978-953-51-2487-0

For EU product safety concerns:
IN TECH d.o.o., Prolaz Marije Krucifikse Kozulić 3, 51000 Rijeka, Croatia,
info@intechopen.com or visit our website at intechopen.com.

Meet the editor

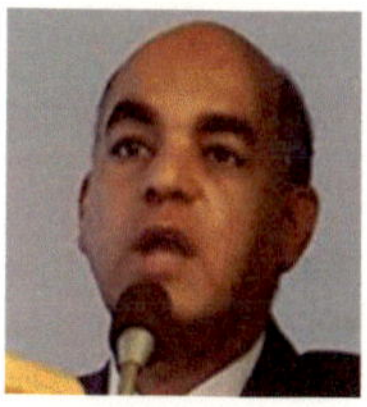

Dr. Atef M. Darwish graduated from Assiut School of Medicine in 1985 with an excellent grade and first-class honors. He completed a residency in Obstetrics and Gynecology at the Department of Obstetrics and Gynecology, Assiut University and Ain Shams University in 1986–1989. He got his master's degree in 1989 with excellent degree. Between 1992 and 1994, he spent 2 years at the endoscopy unit of Ulm University, Germany. Thereafter, he received his medical doctorate in 1995 through a combined program between the University of Ulm, Germany, and the University of Assiut, Egypt, with excellent degree. He joined many centers in the United States and Europe concentrating on the reproductive medicine. Currently, he is a professor of Obstetrics and Gynecology, Faculty of Medicine, Assiut University since July 2005. Moreover, he is a consultant of Obstetrics and Gynecology in 3 hospitals, and a moderator and lecturer of many endoscopic societies. He authored more than 70 papers and edited 5 books, and presented more than 88 presentations in national and international meetings. His special interest has been in the area of gynecologic laparoscopy and hysteroscopy, reproductive medicine, and assisted reproduction. In 2009, he got a PhD degree in Reproductive Medicine at the University of Utrecht, the Netherlands.

Contents

Preface

Despite being frequently diagnosed by human gynecologists, andrologists, and even veterinary gynecologists, genital tract infections didn't gain enough interest in the context of infertility diagnosis and management. This book will focus on the impact of genital tract infections on human and veterinary fertility. It is divided into four sections, namely female genital infections, male genital infections, specific microorganisms causing genital infections, and veterinary genital infections.

Section 1 starts with an overview on the relationship between infection and infertility. This chapter is followed by discussing the hidden as well as overt female genital tract infections in cases with unexplained infertility. More intensive evaluation of the role of chronic endometritis is addressed in a separate chapter. If the woman becomes pregnant, description of causes and management of abnormal vaginal discharge are described in the last chapter of this section.

Section 2 highlights the relationship of male genital tract infections and infertility. The first chapter overviews different male genital tract infections that may cause infertility. The second chapter discusses decreased sperm quality as a result of some genital infections. The last chapter explains definite correlation between infections and male infertility.

Section 3 covers some important issues regarding the common microorganisms that may be implicated in infertility induction or that may result from invasive infertility diagnosis and treatment procedures. You will enjoy reading separate chapters on yeast infections, human immunodeficiency virus (HIV) infection, staphylococcal infection, and *Chlamydia trachomatis* infections. The recent interest in microbiome and infertility is demonstrated in one chapter. The last chapter of this section addresses the genetic influence on infections and risk of infertility.

Incorporation of a special section (4) on the impact of some genital infections on the fertility in males and the association of pregnancy loss with these infections is an interesting positive point of this book. It sends a message to all health-interested physicians that genital infections should be put in mind during evaluation of infertility or recurrent pregnancy loss even in animals.

By this way, the current book puts an updated overview on the impact of genital tract infections on fertility in women, men, and animals. Infertility specialists should promptly manage genital tract infections before proceeding to more sophisticated intensive investigations. Lastly, proper infection control principles should be kept in mind all the time to avoid introducing infection to infertility cases.

Atef M. Darwish
Department of Obstetrics and Gynecology,
Woman's Health University Hospital,
Faculty of Medicine,
Assiut University, Egypt

Section 1

Gynecologic Genital Infections

Chapter 1

Infection and Infertility

Rutvij Dalal

Additional information is available at the end of the chapter

http://dx.doi.org/10.5772/64168

Abstract

About 1/3rd of all women diagnosed with subfertility have a tubo-peritoneal factor contributing to their condition. Most of these alterations in tubo-ovarian function come from post-inflammatory damage inflicted after a pelvic or sexually transmitted infection. Salpingitis occurs in an estimated 15% of reproductive-age women, and 2.5% of all women become infertile as a result of salpingitis by age 35. Predominant organisms today include those from the Chamydia species and the infection causes minimal to no symptoms – leading to chronic infection and consequently more damage. Again, a large proportion of patients suffering from pelvic infection contributing to their subfertility are undiagnosed to be having an infection. Chronic inflammation of the cervix and endometrium, alterations in reproductive tract secretions, induction of immune mediators that interfere with gamete or embryo physiology, and structural disorders such as intrauterine synechiae all contribute to female infertility. Infection is also a major factor in male subfertility, second only to abnormal semen parameters. Epididymal or ductal obstruction, testicular damage from orchitis, development of anti-sperm antibodies, etc are all possible mechanisms by which infection can affect male fertility.

Keywords: Infertility, Infection, pelvic inflammatory disease, salpingitis, epididymo-orchitis, antisperm antibodies

1. Introduction

The association between infection and infertility has been long known. Of all causes of female Infertility, tubal or peritoneal factors amount to about 30-40. The infections that lead to asymptomatic infections are more damaging as lack of symptoms prevents a patient from seeking timely medical intervention and consequently chronic damage to pelvic organs. Indeed, timely management of sexually transmitted or other infections goes a long way in preventing damage, disability, chronic pelvic pain, altered tubo-ovarian relationship and consequently helps in maintaining fertility.

Tubal and peritoneal pathology is among the most common causes of infertility and the primary diagnosis in approximately 30-35% of infertile couples. A history of pelvic inflammatory disease (PID), septic abortion, ruptured appendix, tubal surgery, or ectopic pregnancy suggests the possibility of tubal damage. PID is unquestionably the major cause of tubal factor infertility and ectopic pregnancies. Classic studies in women with PID diagnosed by laparoscopy have revealed that the risk of subsequent tubal infertility increases with the number and severity of pelvic infections; overall, the incidence is approximately 10-12% after one episode, 23-35% after two, and 54-75% after three episodes of acute PID.[1] The most frequent causes for pelvic infections are sexually transmitted pathogens and intrauterine manipulations like curettage, evacuation, etc.

2. Epidemiology

Approximately 35% of women with an infertility problem are afflicted with post-inflammatory changes of the oviduct or surrounding peritoneum that interfere with tubo-ovarian function. Most of these alterations result from infection. Salpingitis occurs in an estimated 15% of reproductive-age women, and 2.5% of all women become infertile as a result of salpingitis by age 35.[2] Because in most cases, especially those caused by *Chlamydia trachomatis*, signs and symptoms are often minimal or non-existent, the actual percentage of women with upper genital tract infections is probably underestimated.

Unfortunately, the impact of infectious sequelae on human reproduction continues to increase as a consequence of sexual promiscuity and the popularity of non-barrier methods of contraception. *C. trachomatis* and gonorrheal infections, as well as mixed anaerobic infections, are the most prevalent causes of upper genital tract infections resulting in pelvic inflammatory disease (PID). Bacterial vaginosis, *Trichomonas vaginalis,* and *Candida albicans* are the most prevalent bacterial, protozoan, and fungal causes of lower genital tract infections. Although gonorrheal infections have been on the decline in the last decade, chlamydial infections of the male and female genital tract continue to be an increasing problem, and *C. trachomatis* is the major cause of tubal factor infertility.[3] *C. trachomatis* is usually recovered three to five times more frequently than *Neisseria gonorrhoeae* from the reproductive tracts of infected individuals.

Women are twice as likely as men to acquire gonorrhea or *Chlamydia* during a single act of unprotected intercourse with an infected partner. Many newly infected women have no symptoms and so do not seek medical intervention and continue to spread the infection to other sexual partners. An estimated 10% to 20% of untreated women with endocervical gonorrhea or chlamydial infection eventually develop salpingitis.[4] Scholes et al[5] recommended routine testing of sexually active women to prevent sequelae like pelvic inflammatory disease and consequently infertility. Despite the current focus on sexually transmitted diseases (STDs), infertility may also follow blood-borne infections such as tuberculosis, mixed aerobic and anaerobic infections of other pelvic sites, inflammatory complications of surgical trauma, post-abortal and puerperal sepsis, and appendicular rupture.

3. Infections and male infertility

Acute and chronic genital tract infections are well-known causes of infertility in men (Table 1). Episodes of acute orchitis or epididymitis may result in permanent damage to the testis or to obstruction in the efferent ejaculatory ducts. *C. trachomatis* causes approximately 50% of epididymitis in sexually active men under age 35. Unilateral epididymal obstruction is seldom diagnosed, and its effect on fertility is largely unknown. However, 80% of men with unilateral ductal obstruction have antibodies to sperm, a potential cause of male infertility.[6] Appropriate assessment of a semen sample including tests like presence of seminal Fructose, neutral alpha-glucosidase and pH go a long way in differentiating between obstructive and non-obstructive azoospermia.

Orchitis	mumps, tuberculosis, syphilis, pancreatitis
Epididymitis	gonorrhea, tuberculosis, chlamydiae, ureaplasmas,*Pseudomonas*, coliform, and other bacterial infections
Seminal vesiculitis	tuberculosis, trichomoniasis, other bacteria
Urethritis	gonorrhea, chlamydiae, ureaplasmas, trichomoniasis

Table 1. Male Genital Tract Infections That May Cause Infertility

Most men do not develop antibodies to their own spermatozoa because the male genital tract is essentially a closed tube, and sperm are isolated from the immune system. Genital tract infections, even those without symptoms, can weaken this barrier, leading to sperm leakage and the influx of immunologically competent cells. Genital tract infections are a major cause of anti-sperm antibody formation in men.[7] Similarly, genital tract infections and anti-sperm antibody formation in men can lead to immune-mediated infertility in women.[8]

Mumps orchitis is a well-known testicular infection resulting in damage to the germinal epithelium. Systemic infections, whether bacterial or viral, may also cause depression of sperm production for variable periods. Between 2 and 6 months may be required for normal seminal cytology to reappear after a severe febrile illness. Urethral stricture is an occasional complication of untreated gonorrhea. Although the stricture does not in itself interfere with sperm motility, it may cause recurring urinary tract infection or prostatitis and epididymitis.

The fertility of a couple may be impaired if the man has a chronic bacterial prostatitis. Chronic prostatitis is presumed to be caused by a pathogenic organism and in most cases is associated with leukocytes in the semen. The prevalence of leukocytospermia among male infertility patients is about 10% to 20%. Although the exact role of WBCs in semen and its importance with respect to fertility is not clearly elucidated, there is some evidence that treating such patients with long term antibiotics does have a favourable impact on the semen parameters.[9] According to a study the presence in semen of counts more than 10,000 colony-forming units/ml had a negative effect on IVF pregnancy rates when *E. coli, Proteus,* or *S. aureus* organisms were isolated.[10] Again, there is some evidence that the occurrence of leucocytes in semen yields abnormal sperm function tests, possibly because of the damaging effects of free radicles of WBCs to the sperms in their journey through the epididymis.[11] There is also substantial evidence that infection contributes to the development of sperm antibodies. Sperm antibodies have been detected in 48% of men with culture-positive asymptomatic infections, 47% of men with a history of urethritis or prostatitis, and in only 5% of men with no infection and a normal semen analysis.

The presence of IgA antibodies was associated with reduced fertility.[12] High concentrations of sperm antibodies can interfere with fertility by several mechanisms. Antibodies on sperm heads or tails may cause sperm to agglutinate. Tail-bound antibodies also interfere with sperm motility. Antibodies anywhere on spermatozoa can lead to sperm phagocytosis through binding to Fc or complement receptors on phagocytic cells. Similarly, antibody-bound sperm react with cervical mucus leading to sperm immobilization and expulsion from the female genital tract. Antibodies on sperm can interfere with sperm binding and penetration of the oocyte.[13] Similar to the situation in women, *C. trachomatis* infection of the male genital tract is often asymptomatic and therefore may persist for a long time. One study using PCR analysis of semen specimens suggested that an asymptomatic unsuspected *C. trachomatis* male genital tract infection may be the cause of previously unexplained infertility.[14] In response to a persistent asymptomatic chlamydial infection and HSP60 production, $\gamma\delta$ T cells may be induced in the male genital tract; $\gamma\delta$ T cells are capable of releasing proinflammatory cytokines and could therefore initiate an antisperm immune response within the genital tract.

4. Infections and female infertility

4.1. Pelvic inflammatory disease

PID is a common but vaguely defined complex of signs and symptoms resulting from the spread of pathogenic microorganisms from the vagina and endocervix to the uterus, body of the endometrium, and fallopian tubes. PID can also follow aseptic induced abortion or as a post-partum infection. *C.Trachomatis* salpingitis can be seen in as many as 15% patients who undergo an induced abortion. PID has reached epidemic proportions and according to the CDC, the cost of PID measured in lost earnings and money spent for health services was estimated at $4.2 billion in 1990.[15] According to a Swedish study[16] tubal infertility occurs in approximately 11% of women who have one episode, in 23% of women who have two episodes, and in 54% of women who have three or more episodes of salpingitis. (Table 2)

As could be seen from Table 2, they found that tubal infertility is directly related to a number of factors present during the initial episode of salpingitis, which include (besides the number of episodes) the initial severity of tubal inflammation, the organisms responsible, and the occurrence of a subsequent ectopic pregnancy. The best predictor of subsequent infertility is the degree of tubal inflammation observed through the laparoscope during the acute phase. Women with a pelvic abscess have had the highest (85% to 90%) rate of subsequent infertility.[17]

Clinical Findings	Tubal Occlusion
Degree of acute inflammation at laparoscopy*	
Mild	6%
Moderate	13%
Severe	30%
Number of episodes of salpingitis*	
One	11%
Two	23%
Three or more	54%
Type of salpingitis†	
Gonococcal	9%
Nongonococccal	16%

* Westrom L: Incidence, prevalence and trends of acute pelvic inflammatory disease and the consequences of industrialized countries. Am J ObstetGynecol 135:880, 1980.

† Westrom L: Effects of acute pelvic inflammatory disease on infertility. Am J ObstetGynecol 121:707, 1975

Table 2. Factors Influencing the Frequency of Tubal Occlusion after Salpingitis

Prompt recognition and vigorous treatment reduce subsequent severe complications of salpingo-oophoritis, such as generalized pelvic peritonitis, abscess formation, and adnexal destruction. However, many patients of PID are often asymptomatic. Approximately 60% to 80% of women with acute salpingitis have a normal temperature or no white blood cell elevation. This finding correlates with the observation that most women with tubal infertility have never been treated for a recognized episode of salpingitis. Epidemiologic studies support the concept of silent PID wherein a strong link exists between serum antibodies to *C. trachomatis* and tubal factor infertility or ectopic pregnancy in patients without a history of clinical PID.[18]

4.1.1. Treatment strategies

Prompt treatment is the key in adequate eradication of the responsible organism(s) and preventing long term sequelae like hydrosalpinx, infertility, ectopic pregnancy, and chronic pelvic pain. If the patients with mild symptoms had only cervicitis or endometritis and not salpingitis, prompt treatment before the onset of salpingitis would have a major impact on preventing tubal occlusion. Failure to use doxycycline or azithromycin to inhibit *C. trachomatis* may contribute to chronic salpingitis.[19] Approximately one half of the women with an ectopic pregnancy have grossly visible tubal damage or a partial occlusion of the tubes. About 7% to 10% of pregnancies that occur after an episode of salpingitis are in an ectopic location, and women with salpingitis have a 10-fold higher rate of ectopic pregnancy than does the general population. Approximately 40% of women who have had an ectopic pregnancy are not able to achieve an intrauterine pregnancy subsequently.[20]

4.1.2. PID and HIV

A population-based study of fertility in women with human immunodeficiency virus type 1 (HIV-1) infection in Uganda demonstrated that fertility is greatly reduced in HIV-1-infected women because of a lower rate of conception and increased rates of miscarriage and stillbirth. Numerous epidemiologic studies have demonstrated that there is a synergy among bacterial and viral STDs. Bacterial STDs have been implicated in the enhancement of HIV transmission. Conversely, the immunosuppression caused by HIV worsens the clinical course of other STDs. The low prevalence and incidence of pregnancy among HIV-infected women could reflect pre-existing tubal factor infertility and higher clinical and subclinical fetal losses resulting from HIV-1 infection.[21]

Pelvic inflammatory disease that is non-tubercular in origin can be divided into gonococcal, chlamydial, and nongonococcal-nonchlamydial disease based on the results of endocervical or peritoneal fluid cultures.

4.2. Gonococcal infection

Gonococcal PID still a major cause of infertility in women in developing Asian and African countries.[22] The bacterium N. Gonorrhea (Figure 1) elicits a pyogenic, inflammatory reaction characterised by purulent exudates. As the organisms replicate, the ensuing local tissue damage diminishes the oxidation-reduction potential of the environment – this explains why it is common to discover co-existing pathogens.The recovery of *N. gonorrhoeae* from tubal or peritoneal fluid in acute salpingitis patients with endocervical gonorrhea ranges from 6% to 70%. Approximately one third of patients have *N. gonorrhoeae* as a sole isolate, one third have *N. gonorrhoeae* plus a mixture of aerobic and anaerobic bacteria, and one third have a mixture of aerobic and anaerobic bacteria in the cul-de-sac only.[23]

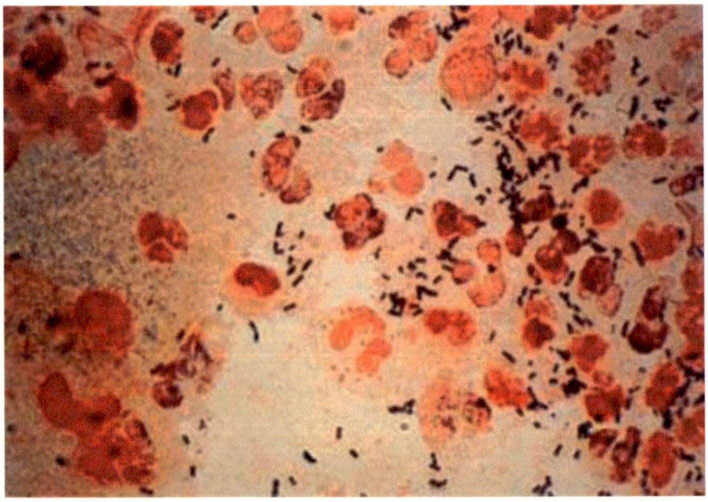

Figure 1. Neisseria Gonorrhea bacteria

http://dx.doi.org/10.5772/64168

N. gonorrhoeae secretes a toxin that can destroy cilia of adjacent cells in the tubal epithelium. Not only is the organism difficult to isolate from pus, but the recovery of *N. gonorrhoeae*depends on the stage of infection. The gonococcus is most frequently isolated within 2 days of the onset of symptoms and is rarely isolated if symptoms are present for 7 or more days.[24] Most symptomatic gonococcal PID cases have their onset during or just after the menses. These observations are consistent with the view that the gonococcus initiates the infection and, if the infection is not promptly treated, sets the stage for a mixed aerobic-anaerobic infection, involving pathogens that originate in the cervix and vagina.

4.3. Chlamydial infection

C. trachomatis is an intracellular bacterium that proliferates in columnar epithelial cells, where it remains protected from host immune defences by a cell membrane. It takes a longer time for *C. trachomatis* to divide (24 to 48 hours) than for classic bacteria (1 to 4 hours). There is a characteristically long time between infection and the onset of symptoms among women with *C. trachomatis*, and only mild symptoms usually occur. Widespread or systemic symptoms are unusual, although infection of the endosalpinx can produce generalized peritonitis by contiguous spread, including perihepatitis (Fitz-Hugh-Curtis syndrome).

Chlamydia appears to be a particularly important organism in infertility. There are multiple published reports in which women with tubal infertility have a 25% to 70% higher incidence of *C. trachomatis* antibody than do infertile women with normal tubes.[25] In many developed countries, *C. trachomatis* infections are now clearly the leading cause of tubal infertility. *C. trachomatis* causes the same spectrum of disease (*e.g.* urethritis, cervicitis, endometritis, salpingitis) as the gonococcus. *C. trachomatis* causes salpingitis more frequently than the gonococcus. Also, the degree of acute tubal damage among women with chlamydial infection equals or exceeds that observed with gonococcal infection. Women with chlamydial infection may have gonorrhea and *vice versa.*

C. trachomatis is inhibited *in vitro* by doxycycline and azithromycin but not by cephalosporins. Women with salpingitis should be treated with tetracyclines or other antibiotics that inhibit *C. trachomatis*, because cephalosporin therapy alone does not eradicate *C. trachomatis*.[26] Lack of symptoms ensures that the undetected *C. trachomatis* are able to ascend from the lower to the upper genital tract, evade the host's immune response and persist for long periods of time.

Figure 2 shows the life cycle of Chlamydia infection. Extracellular *C. trachomatis* elementary bodies (EB) infect epithelial cells. Within the cell, the EBs convert to reticulate bodies (RB), which replicate by binary fission. The RBs then convert back to EBs that are released from the cell and infect other epithelial cells. The presence of extracellular EBs activates the host's immune response, and interferon-γ is released. The interferon blocks RB replication, resulting in the formation of large, aberrant RBs. However, the RBs remain viable, and when the extracellular infection is cleared and interferon-γ is no longer present, normal RB replication resumes. These repeated cycles of replication and immune activation followed by chlamydial persistence in epithelial cells of the fallopian tube eventually lead to scar formation and tubal occlusion.[27] As has been already discussed, Witkin and co-workers found that women

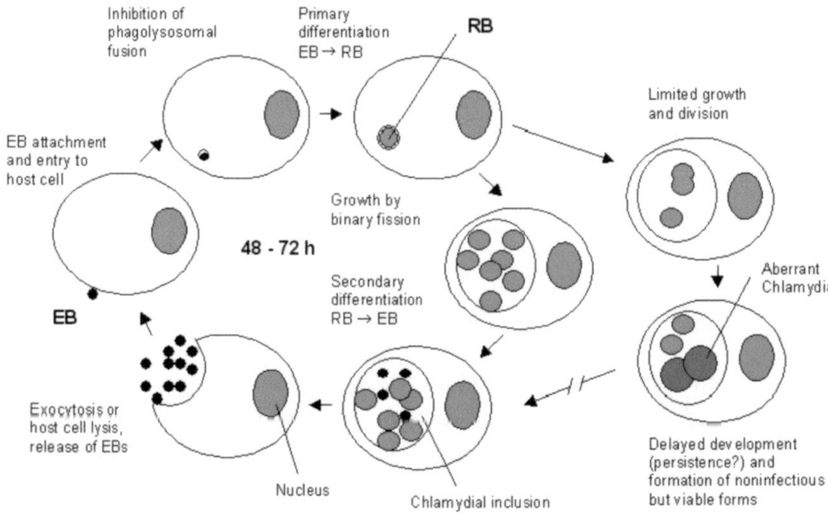

Figure 2. Effect of interferon-γ on the life cycle of *Chlamydia trachomatis*.

previously infected with chlamydia – detected by circulating systemic humoral immunity to HSP 60 had unfavourable outcomes with IVF.[18]

4.4. Nongonococcal-nonchlamydial infection

Approximately 1/4th of women with PID have a nongonococcal-nonchlamydial cause.[28] Patients with nongonococcal PID have the onset of pain distributed evenly throughout the cycle and less frequently associated with menses. There is less fever, vaginal discharge, and liver tenderness than with gonococcal PID. Despite these differences, the clinical presentation does not adequately distinguish between the two, and reliance on culture is necessary. There may be a critical number of organisms needed to breach the normally present protective host defence mechanisms and lead to infection. There is probably a continuum from bacterial vaginosis to endometritis and salpingitis, because women with bacterial vaginosis are significantly more likely to be diagnosed with PID.[29] The substantial isolation rate of bacteria other than gonococci or *C. trachomatis* from tubal fluid of these PID patients has shown that bacterial vaginosis organisms can cause acute salpingitis without antecedent chlamydial or gonococcal infection. Peritoneal or tubal cultures have yielded a mixed aerobic and anaerobic flora in 35% to 50% of patients, anaerobes alone in 15%, and aerobes alone in approximately 30% to 40% of patients. Between 4% and 17% of women with PID have had *M. hominis*, and 2% to 20%, have had *U. urealyticum* recovered from the fallopian tubes.[30]

4.5. Genital mycoplasmas and unexplained infertility

Mycoplasmas share characteristics of bacteria (they reproduce on cell-free media) and viruses (they have no cell wall and are 100 to 300 μm in diameter). Two species of mycoplasmas have been commonly isolated from the female and male reproductive tracts: *M. hominis* and the heterogeneous group known collectively as T mycoplasma (so named for their characteristic "tiny" colonies). A distinctive property of the T strains is their ability to hydrolyze urea, and they have been named *U. urealyticum*. A third species, *Mycoplasma genitalium* has been isolated from the urethra of men and is believed to be a cause of urethritis.

Genital mycoplasmas may be of etiologic importance in nonspecific urethritis, cervicitis, and vaginitis; some cases of acute salpingitis; fever after abortions; chorioamnionitis; and puerperal infections. However, the causal role of genital mycoplasmas in infertility is still unresolved.

4.6. Genital tuberculosis

Tuberculosis continues to be endemic in many poor parts of the world like Latin America and Asia. The incidence of pelvic tuberculosis is difficult to assess as many patients are asymptomatic, therefore the disease often comes to light only incidentally during the course of investigation for a gynecological complaint. Schaefer[31] as early as in 1976 reported that 4-12% of women dying from pulmonary tuberculosis manifest evidence of genital involvement. He further mentioned that 5-10% of infertile women suffer from tuberculosis. The incidence of tuberculosis amongst women with infertility is believed to be higher in the third world countries.

The causative agent is *Mycobacterium tuberculosis* (95%) but in 5% cases it is *Mycobacterium bovis*. Genital tuberculosis almost always occurs secondary to a primary focus elsewhere, the commonest site being the lungs, but rarely from the kidneys, joints, GIT or as a part of a generalized military infection. The mode of spread is hematogenous or lymphatic and rarely from direct contiguity with an intra-abdominal organ or affected peritoneum. The fallopian tubes are affected first followed by subsequent dissemination to other genital organs – this explains the bilateral tendency of the disease. Primary genital tuberculosis is rare and possibly originates from the semen or saliva of a positive sexual partner. Tuberculosis of the cervix is present in about 5% of cases.

The leading presenting complaints in women suffering from genital tuberculosis include infertility, menstrual problems, abdominal pain, vaginal discharge and rarely genital fistulas or mass per abdomen. Sometimes general symptoms of low grade temperature, weight loss and fatigue may raise the suspicion of hitherto unsuspected tuberculosis. Classis feature is failure of fever to subside in spite of broad spectrum antibiotics. Therefore, a clinical course that is refractory to antibiotic therapy for the usual pelvic inflammatory disease should alert the physician to the possibility of tuberculosis. Pelvic examination may reveal findings like thickened adnexa which may be tender. However it may be completely normal.

Infertility is an important presenting symptom. In fact in 35-60% cases it is the only complaint. About 75% present with primary infertility and 25% give history of previous conception. These patients may or may not give a history of contact with a person suffering from pulmonary tuberculosis.

Diagnosing tuberculosis still remains a challenge. This is due to a wide variety of clinical presentation and lack of diagnostic tests with a good positive predictive and negative predictive value. A single, reliable, convenient, economical test that has a good degree of sensitivity and specificity is yet to be discovered. Diagnosis still remains subjective, and is done usually at the time of laparoscopy done for evaluating infertility or chronic pelvic pain. Pathognomic sign of appearance of small tubercles all over the peritoneum that represent caseating granulomas is seen only rarely. Other findings include appearance of tubo-ovarian masses with varying degree of intra-pelvic adhesions, bead like growths or rigid lead-pipe appearance of fallopian tubes, hydrosalpingx and military white tubercles on the serosa of the uterus. Samples can be taken for acid-fast bacilli staining (Figure 3) or culture. However both methods have low sensitivity. Polymerase chain reaction is highly sensitive, but may yield false positives due to contamination of sample from air or water contaminants. Mantoux test has limited utility now.

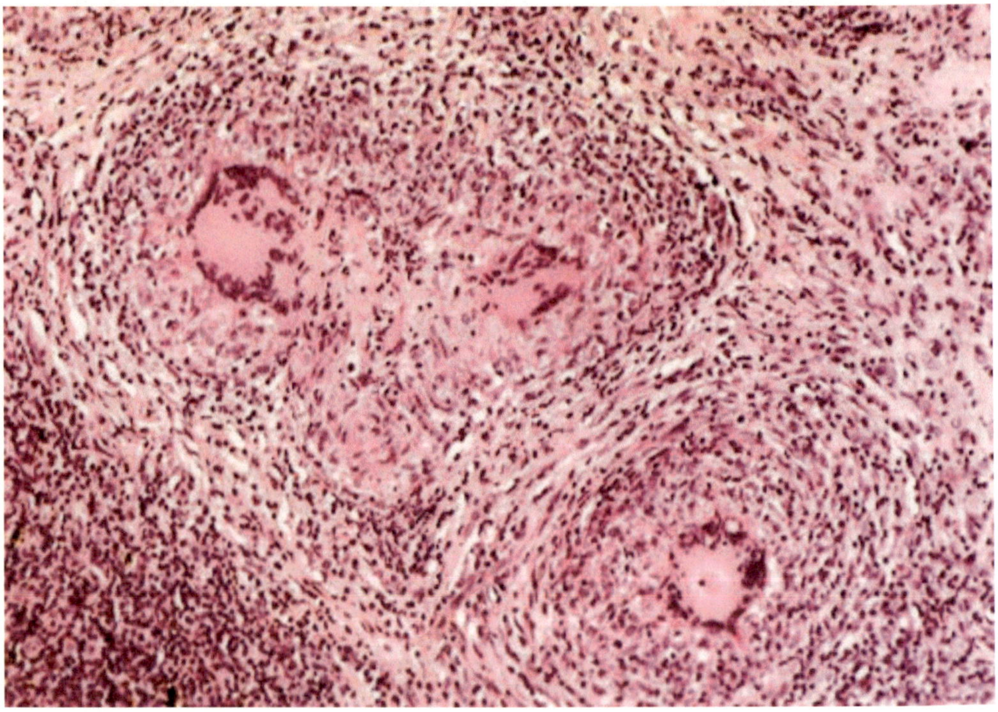

Figure 3. Typical tubercular lesion in histo-pathology

4.6.1. Treatment of tuberculosis

Extra pulmonary tuberculosis usually requires 8 to 10 months of continuous treatment particularly in developing countries to prevent emergence of multi-drug resistant tuberculosis, which is very common if treatment is given for a short period and stopped. Also, premature discontinuation of treatment may render the organisms resistant and lead to re-emergence of infection with much more severity. The therapeutic phase is divided into an intensive phase of about 2 to 4 months and continuation phase of 4 to 6 months. The two drugs used throughout

http://dx.doi.org/10.5772/64168

the treatment period are usually rifampicin (10 mg/kg/day, not exceeding 600 mg/d) and isoniazid (5 mg/kg/day not exceeding 300 mg). In the past the third drug used during the initial 2-4 months was Ethambutol (5-25 mg/kg/day not to exceed 2.5 gm/day) but now pyrazinamide (15-30 mg/kg/day, not to exceed 2.5 gm/day) is preferred because it does not have the ocular toxicity which is seen with ethambutol. Rifampicin is safe in pregnancy.[32] Most of these drugs are hepatotoxic and have various side effects, these have to be watched for. Surgery for the management of tuberculosis is not preferred, and reserved for special situations like persistence of an adnexal mass in spite of anti-tubercular treatment or irresponsiveness of the infection to anti-tubercular therapy.

5. Pathogenesis of PID

In gonococcal and chlamydial salpingitis, the microorganisms ascend by surface extension from the lower genital tract through the cervical canal by way of the endometrium to the fallopian tubes (Figure 4A). There can be adhesion of the mucosal folds, destruction of cilia, occlusion of the infundibulum, and production of a pyosalpinx. The gonococcal infection may spread beyond the endosalpinx, with possible focal abscess formation and perisalpingitis. In some cases of nongonococcal salpingitis, particularly with *M. hominis*,[33] the pathogens may enter through lesions in the cervix or endometrium and spread to the parametria and tubes through lymphatics and blood vessels (Fig. 4B). The inflammatory swelling that affects the parametria and the tubes is more pronounced than in gonococcal salpingitis, but the endosalpinx is usually intact.

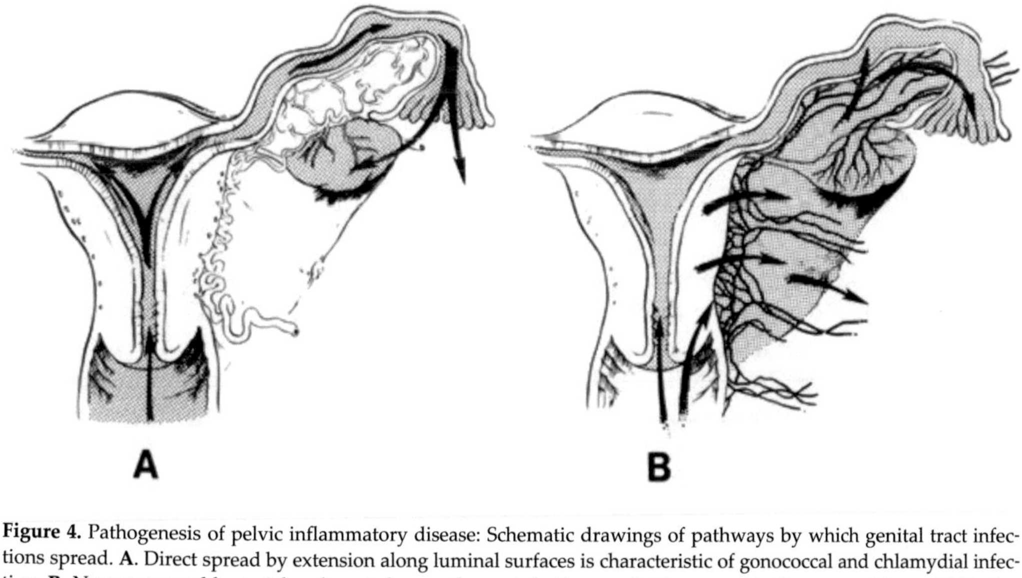

Figure 4. Pathogenesis of pelvic inflammatory disease: Schematic drawings of pathways by which genital tract infections spread. **A.** Direct spread by extension along luminal surfaces is characteristic of gonococcal and chlamydial infection. **B.** Nongonococcal bacterial and genital mycoplasma infections probably spread to the parametria and fallopian tubes primarily through lymphatics and blood vessels.

The sequelae of PID that are responsible for infertility include chronic interstitial salpingitis, hydrosalpinx, salpingitis isthmicanodosa, and periadnexal adhesions. Infertility may also occur because of abnormal secretory, ciliary, and peristaltic function of the fallopian tube. The postulated interrelationships of STDs and endogenous organisms in the pathogenesis of tubal infertility secondary to PID are depicted in Figure 5.[34]

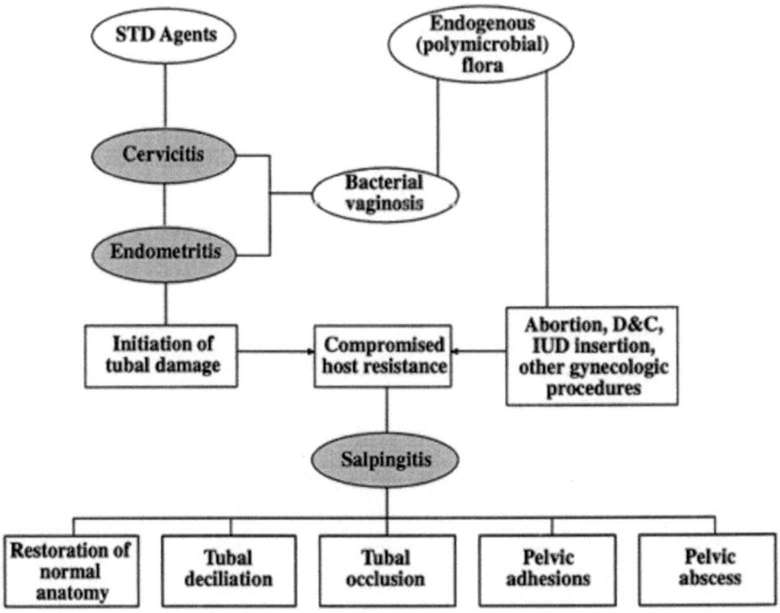

Figure 5. Postulated interactions of sexually transmitted microorganisms with endogenous lower genital tract microflora in the pathogenesis of pelvic inflammatory disease and tubal factor infertility.(Adapted from Sweet RL, Gibbs RS: Infectious Diseases of the Female Genital Tract, p 399. 3rd ed. Baltimore: Williams & Wilkins, 1995.)

6. Treatment of PID

There is controversy over the issue of outpatient versus inpatient treatment of patients with acute salpingitis. For economic and logistical reasons, most women are treated on an outpatient basis. The decision for hospitalization is usually based on the clinical severity of the illness, although criteria vary. It seems reasonable to treat major pathogens such as *N. gonorrhoeae* and *C. trachomatis* in every patient. An antibiotic regimen that takes into account the polymicrobial nature of the cause of acute salpingitis must be used. However, after treatment with different antibiotics, similar infertility rates have been found.[35] Women treated after 3 or more days of symptoms had significantly more infertility than those treated earlier.[36] Better recognition and treatment of cervicitis and endometritis before salpingitis develops is even more important in the prevention of infertility than the treatment of salpingitis *per se.* Recommended treatment schedules for uncomplicated salpingitis are shown as below:

http://dx.doi.org/10.5772/64168

For acute salpingitis

Parenteral Regimen A

Cefotetan 2 g, IV every 12 hours,

or

Cefoxitin, 2 g, IV every 6 hours,

plus

Doxycycline, 100 mg, IV or orally every 12 hours

Parenteral Regimen B

Clindamycin, 900 mg, IV every 8 hours,

plus

Gentamicin loading dose IV or IM (2 mg/kg of body weight), followed by a maintenance dose (1.5 mg/kg) every 8 hours. Single daily dosing may be substituted.

Regimen A

Ofloxacin, 400 mg, orally twice each day for 14 days,

plus

Metronidazole, 500 mg, orally twice each day for 14 days.

Regimen B

Ceftriaxone, 250 mg, IM once,

or

Cefoxitin, 2 g, IM plus Probenecid, 1 g, orally in a single dose concurrently

once,

or

Other parenteral third-generation cephalosporin (e.g., ceftizoxime, cefotaxime),

plus

Doxycycline, 100 mg, orally twice each day for 14 days. (Include this regimen with one of the above regimens.)

(Centers for Disease Control and Prevention: 1998 Guidelines for treatment of sexually transmitted diseases. MMWR Morb Mortal Wkly Rep 1998;47(RR1):82–82.)

Patients with suspected abscesses or severe illness that may indicate the presence of organisms other than gonococci or chlamydiae should be hospitalized. Recommended treatment regimens inhibit not only *N. gonorrhoeae* and *C. trachomatis* but also a wide variety of aerobic and anaerobic bacteria. For instance, parenteral clindamycin is effective against *C. trachomatis* and anaerobes.

The concomitant use of steroids with antibiotics has been thought to reduce the sequelae of salpingitis, but in a prospective study, Falk [77] could show no beneficial effect as judged by hysterosalpingography findings or subsequent laparotomy. Prevention of PID recurrence and its adverse effects on fertility also requires treatment of asymptomatic male sexual partners.In patients with postinflammatory tubal disease, pregnancy outcome has been correlated with the presence or absence of fallopian tube rugaeon hysterosalpingograms. Pregnancy occurred in 61% of patients with moderate to excellent rugal patterns, whereas only 7% of patients with no demonstrable rugae conceived postoperatively.[38]

Today and in the foreseeable future, assisted reproductive technologies (ART), endoscopic surgery, and microsurgery have an important place in the management of infertility that results from tubal disease. There are some tubal causes of infertility for which surgery can offer little or no chance of success, such as after severe bilateral hydrosalpinx, multisite tubal obstruction, or in patients with extensive and dense pelvic adhesions. At the other end of the spectrum are patients who can achieve a 50% to 65% intrauterine pregnancy rate after microsurgical or laparoscopic adhesiolysis when the fimbriae are spared from disease and a male factor is not encountered.[39] In choosing between IVF and tubal surgery, the physician must compare success rates (which can are best defined by the birth of a live baby) and take into account the patient's age, presence of a male subfertility factor, the personal priorities of the couple, and the availability of expertise.

7. Early treatment and fertility preservation

The best prevention is to detect and treat early-stage asymptomatic and symptomatic infections. This can be achieved by the screening of all sexually active reproductive age women and by educating clinicians and patients on the importance of this testing. The importance of practicing safe sex methods cannot be over emphasized in public. Scholes et al found a 60% reduction in salpingitis prevalence rates when the population was screened for *C.trachomatis* infections compared to when they were not.[5]

With the advent of modern DNA amplification tests like Polymerase Chain Reaction (PCR) available very sensitive and specific testing on microbes can be done in a matter of hours. This obviates the need of many organisms as is the case with conventional cultures. Also, the newer tests are also more specific yielding a higher positive predictive value thus avoiding unnecessary treatments. Microbes like *C. trachomatis*[40], *T. vaginalis*[41], and *N. gonorrhoeae*[42] can be detected in samples obtained from the vaginal introitus, and there is no longer a requirement for a speculum examination. There have been efforts to make chlamydial and gonococcal vaccines, but not met much success.

8. Conclusion

The best hope for reducing the incidence of infertility related to infection lies in prevention and early detection and treatment of newly acquired asymptomatic or mildly symptomatic infections. The importance for the preservation of future fertility of avoiding high-risk sexual behaviour and the mandatory use of condoms must be stressed. Concomitantly, there must be an increased awareness by health care providers and consumers of the need for intensive screening using the latest and most effective molecular techniques followed by early effective treatment if positive.

Author details

Rutvij Dalal*

Address all correspondence to: rutvij.dalal@gmail.com

Wings Hospitals, Ahmedabad, India

References

[1] Westrom LV: Sexually transmitted diseases and infertility. Sex Transm Dis 21: 532–537, 1994

[2] Westrom LV: Sexually transmitted diseases and infertility. Sex Transm Dis 21: 532–537, 1994

[3] Cates W Jr, Wasserheit JN: Genital chlamydia infections: Epidemiology and reproductive sequclac. Am J ObstetGynecol 164: 1771, 1991

[4] Eschenbach DA: Infertility caused by infection. ContempObstetGynecol 32: 29– 46, 1987

[5] Scholes D, Stergachis A, Heidrich FE et al: Prevention of pelvic inflammatory disease by screening for cervical chlamydia infection. N Engl J Med 334: 1362– 1366, 1996

[6] Hendry WF, Parslow JM, Stredouska J et al: The diagnosis of unilateral testicular obstruction in subfertile males. Br J Urol 54: 774, 1982

[7] Witkin SS, Toth A: Relationship between genital tract infections, sperm antibodies in seminal fluid and infertility. Fertil Steril 40: 805– 808, 1983

[8] Witkin SS: Production of interferon gamma by lymphocytes exposed to antibody-coated spermatozoa: A mechanism for sperm antibody production in females. Fertil Steril 50: 498– 502, 1988

[9] Grimarellou H, Tympanidis K, Bitos NA et al: Infertility and chronic prostatitis. Andrologia 16: 417– 422, 1984

[10] Shalika S, Dugan K, Smith RD et al: The effect of positive semen bacterial and *Ureaplasma* cultures on in-vitro fertilization success. Hum Reprod 12: 2789– 2792, 1997

[11] Kovalski NN, deLamirandi E, Gagnon C: Reactive oxygen species generated by human neutrophils inhibit sperm motility: Protective effect of seminal plasma and scavengers. Fertil Steril 58: 809– 816, 1992

[12] Clarke GN, Lopata A, McBain JC et al: Effect of sperm antibodies in males on human *in vitro* fertilization (IVF). Am J Reprod Immunol 8: 62, 1985

[13] Witkin SS, Viti D, David SS et al: Relation between antisperm antibodies and the rate of fertilization of human oocytes *in vitro*. J Assist Reprod Gen 9: 9– 13, 1993

[14] Witkin SS, Jeremias J, Grifo JA, Ledger WJ: Detection of *Chlamydia trachomatis* in semen by the polymerase chain reaction in male members of infertile couples. Am J ObstetGynecol 168: 1457, 1993

[15] Washington AE, Katz P: Cost and payment source for pelvic inflammatory disease.Trends and projections 1983 through 2000. JAMA 266: 2565– 2569, 1991

[16] Westrom L: Effects of acute pelvic inflammatory disease on infertility. Am J Obstet-Gynecol 121: 707, 1975

[17] Landers DV, Sweet RL: Tubo-ovarian abscess: Contemporary approach to management. Rev Infect Dis 5: 176, 1983

[18] Witkin SS, Sultan KM, Neal GS et al: Unsuspected *Chlamydia trachomatis* infection and *in vitro* fertilization outcome. Am J ObstetGynecol 171: 1208– 1214, 1994

[19] Grimes DA, Blount JH, Patrick J et al: Antibiotic treatment of pelvic inflammatory disease: Trends among private physicians in the United States: 1966 through 1983. JAMA 256: 3223, 1986

[20] Pisarska MD, Carson SA, Buster JE: Ectopic pregnancy. Lancet 351: 1115– 1120, 1998

[21] Gray RH, Waiver MJ, Serwadda D et al: Population-based study of fertility in women with HIV-1 infection in Uganda. Lancet 351: 98– 103, 1998

[22] Paavonen J: Immunopathogenesis of PID and infertility—What do we know and what shall we do. J Br Fertil Soc 1: 42– 45, 1996

[23] Holmes KK, Eschenbach DA, Knapp JS: Salpingitis: Overview of etiology and epidemiology. Am J ObstetGynecol 138: 893, 1980

[24] Sweet RL: Diagnosis and treatment of acute salpingitis. J Reprod Med 19: 21, 1977

[25] Jones RB, Ardery BR, Jui SL, Cleary RE: Correlation between serum antichlamydial antibodies and tubal factor as a cause of infertility. Fertil Steril 38: 553, 1982

[26] Sweet RL, Schachter J, Robbie MO: Failure of beta-lactam antibiotics to eradicate *Chlamydia trachomatis* in the endometrium despite apparent clinical cure of acute salpingitis. JAMA 250: 2641, 1983

[27] Witkin SS: Immune pathogenesis of asymptomatic *Chlamydia trachomatis* infections in the female genital tract. Infect Dis ObstetGynecol 3: 169, 1995

[28] Eschenbach DA, Buchanan TM, Pollock HM et al: Polymicrobialetiology of acute pelvic inflammatory disease. N Engl J Med 293: 166, 1975

[29] Eschenbach DA, Hillier S, Critchlow C et al: Diagnosis and clinical manifestations of bacterial vaginosis. Am J ObstetGynecol 158: 819– 828, 1988

[30] Sweet SL, Mills J, Hadley WK et al: Use of laparoscopy to determine the microbiologic etiology of acute salpingitis. Am J ObstetGynecol 13: 68, 1979

[31] Schaefer G. Female genital tuberculosis. ClinObstetGynaecol 1976; 19:223

[32] Snider DE, Layde PM, Johnson MW, Lyle HA. Treatment of tuberculosis during pregnancy. Am Rev Respir Dis 1980;122:65-78

[33] Miller BR, Freundt EA, Black FT et al: Experimental infection of the genital tract of female grivet monkeys for *Mycoplasma hominis*. Infect Immunol 20: 248, 1978

[34] Sweet RL, Gibbs RS: Infectious Diseases of the Female Genital Tract, p 399. 3rd ed. Baltimore: Williams & Wilkins, 1995

[35] Westrom L, Iosif S, Svensson L et al: Infertility after acute salpingitis: Results of treatment with different antibiotics. CurrTher Res 26 (Suppl 6): 752, 1979

[36] Hillis SD, Joesoef R, Marchbanks PA et al: Delayed care of pelvic inflammatory disease as a risk factor for impaired fertility. Am J ObstetGynecol 168: 1503– 1509, 1993

[37] Falk V: Treatment of acute non-tuberculous salpingitis with antibiotics alone and in combination with glucocorticoids. ActaObstetGynecolScand 44 (Suppl 6): 5, 1965

[38] Young PE, Egan JE, Barlow JJ et al: Reconstructive surgery for infertility at the Boston Hospital for Women. Am J ObstetGynecol 108: 1092, 1970

[39] Novy MJ: Tubal surgery or IVF: Making the best choice in the 1990s. Int J Fertil 40: 292–297, 1995

[40] Witkin SS, Inglis SR, Polaneczky M: Detection of *Chlamydia trachomatis* and *Trichomatis vaginalis* by polymerase chain reaction in introital specimens from pregnant women. Am J ObstetGynecol 175: 165, 1996

[41] Heine RP, Wiesenfeld HC, Sweet RL, Witkin SS: Polymerase chain reaction analysis of distal vaginal specimens: A less invasive strategy for detection of *Trichomonas vaginalis*. Clin Infect Dis 24: 985, 1997

[42] Hook EW, Ching SF, Stephens J et al: Diagnosis of *Neisseria gonorrhoeae* in women by using the ligase chain reaction on patient-obtained vaginal swabs. J ClinMicrobiol 35: 2129, 1997

Chapter 2

Unexplained Female Infertility Alert Over Overt and Hidden Genital Infections

Atef M. Darwish

Additional information is available at the end of the chapter

http://dx.doi.org/10.5772/64056

Abstract

Female genital tract infections represents a real challenge for the gynecologists. The exact role of these infections in infertility induction is not clear. The impact of uterine infections on implantation is not clearly defined. This chapter will discuss the implication of overt as well as hidden genital tract infection among women with unexplained infertility. Whether these infections cause infertility or induced by infertility diagnostic as well as therapeutic procedures will be addressed. In short, this chapter will attract attention of gynecologists to put the possibility of genital tract infections in every case of infertility particularly cases with unexplained infertility.

Keywords: Unexplained infertility, hidden infections, manifest infections, hysteroscopy, laparoscopy

1. Introduction

1.1. What's unexplained infertility (UI)?

Current definitions of infertility lack uniformity, rendering comparisons in prevalence between countries or over time difficult and inconclusive. The absence of an agreed definitions compromises clinical management and undermines the impact of research findings [1]. Idiopathic or unexplained infertility (UI) term is used whenever the cause remains unclear even after basic infertility work-up which usually includes semen analysis, detection of ovulation and fallopian tubal patency testing. The current diagnostic tools for intrauterine causes of infertility include transvaginal ultrasonograogy, hysterosalpingography (HSG) or saline infusion sonography (SIS) [2]. The levels of investigations to explain infertility are insufficient and require more intensive evaluation. In a previous open access free book chapter published by InTech [3], many explanations of UI utilizing endoscopic evaluation that were missed by many organizations were demonstrated.

2. Position of genital tract infections in infertility work-up

International societies didn't include infections as a definite cause of infertility. Practically, local gynecologic examination should be an essential routine step in infertility evaluation. Both speculum and bimanual examinations can detect or suspect a wide variety of lower or upper genital tract infections. With the extensive routine use of transvaginal ultrasonography (TVS) in all gynecologic clinics, unfortunately many gynecologists miss the five basic steps of gynecologic examination which can detect definite infertility causes (inspection of the external genitalia, palpation of the external genitalia, palpation of the vaginal walls and fornices, bimanual examination and vaginal speculum examination). Moreover, many women don't prefer local gynecologic examination due to fear or inconvenience. Gynecologic examination is a cheap valuable basic step that should not be ignored. Moreover, local examination can detect many vaginal and cervical disorders. For instance, some congenital anomalies like transverse or longitudinal vaginal septae, Gartner's cyst in one of the fornices which occludes the external os or congenital vaginal atresia. Practically and literally, genital tract infection detected by speculum examination can be a direct cause of female subfertility.

3. Manifest (overt) genital tract infections

Overt uterine causes of infertility would include clinically symptomatizing cervical and uterine infections, intrauterine adhesions, polypi or uterine cavity malformations. Gynecologists usually pay little care towards manifest lower and upper genital tract infections among infertile women and rely mainly on ultrasonography and hormonal profile.

4. Increasing rate of lower genital tract infections

Cervicitis as well as vaginitis has been one of the common diseases influencing the health of female genital system. The happening rate of female vaginal and cervical inflammation is increasing rapidly in modern world which may be organism mutations, immunological changes, and poor hygiene in underdeveloped world or liberal sexual behaviors particularly in western countries. Fortunately enough, with the increased medical knowledge, health education, improved diagnosis and aggressive lines of therapy, prompt eradication of these infections is possible.

5. Impact of lower genital tract infection on fertility

In general, cervicitis has a negative impact on pregnancy. When a woman is diagnosed with cervicitis, especially for those who have severe cervicitis, the possibility of infertility is high. When cervicitis occurs, the cervix secretes more discharge with large amount of WBCs and pathogens thus hindering normal vaginal environment. This changes the PH of the vagina and kills semen as if pyospermia exists. The activity of sperms will be limited and their living time will be shortened. Furthermore, WBCs can swallow the sperms. Moreover, because of the thick and purulent discharge, it is more difficult for semen to swim-up into the uterine cavity. Of clinical importance, long standing endocervicitis is usually associated with mucosal proliferation with narrowing of the cervical canal and even inflammatory polyp formation preventing smooth ascend of sperms. In addition, severe untreated longstanding cervicitis can cause infertility by affecting nearby organs. It may cause endometritis, cervical endometriosis, acute or chronic PID, tubal blockage, hydrosalpinx and even more deeper infections like urinary diseases. In such cases, treatment becomes more sophisticated and requires more aggressive lines of management. Lastly, local genital medications would affect sperm quality and adds another fertility obstacle.

6. Prevalence of local genital tract infections among infertile women

Since a long time, many studies clearly demonstrated that genital tract infections would decrease fertility of women. For instance, in a previous study [4], 92 infertile women were compared with 86 pregnant controls regarding rates of isolation of Neisseria gonorrhoeae, Candida albicans, Trichomonas vaginalis and other facultative organisms. They found that the rate of isolation of Neisseria gonorrheae was 17.4% among infertile women compared with 10.5% in the group of pregnant women ($p > 0.05$). There was no significant difference between the groups in the rate of isolation of Candida albicans, Trichomonas vaginalis and other facultative organisms. High rates of isolation of microorganisms were observed in both groups. However, women with secondary infertility had higher rate of carriage of Neisseria gonorrheae, Candida albicans and Staphylococcus aureus as compared with women with primary infertility. Nearly 15% of infertile women had previous episodes of pelvic inflammatory disease and 26% had had induced abortions. A positive history of vaginal discharge was a poor predictor of vagina and endocervical carriage of microorganisms. They concluded that high rates of pathogenic organisms exist in the lower genital tract of infertile women and controls. Women with secondary infertility are more likely to have pathogenic organisms than women with primary infertility and recommended routine screening for this group of infertile women.

7. Vaginal microbiome and female infertility

Vaginal microbiome is a new era under continuous evaluation and research. It is well established that the vagina is colonized by bacteria that serve important roles in homeostasis. Imbalances in the proportion of bacteria may lead to a predisposition to infection or reproductive complications. Molecular-based approaches found high variations within and between women than previously reported. Moreover, the vaginal microbiome may increase or decrease according to the health status, menstrual cycle or menopause with ethnic variations. Dysbiosis and the transmission of sexually transmitted infections are affected by the composition of the microbiome. An understanding of the diversity of the vaginal microbial environment during states of health is essential for the identification of risk factors for disease and the development of appropriate treatment [5]

The effect of known pathogens such as Mycoplasma, tuberculosis, Chlamydia trachomatis, and Neisseria gonorrhoeae is clear, causing subclinical changes thought to be risk factors in subfertility. Colonizing the transfer-catheter tip with Lactobacillus crispatus at the time of embryo transfer may increase the rates of implantation and live birth rate while decreasing the rate of infection [6]. On the other hand, the presence of vaginal–cervical microbial contamination at the time of embryo transfer is associated with significantly decreased pregnancy rates [7]. Nevertheless, the exact implication of microbiome in infertility requires more studies.

8. Role of cervical-vaginal swab in overt lower genital tract infections

8.1. The vaginitis wet mount test

It is the simplest and cheapest test to detect vaginal infection by taking a high vaginal swab to be examined by wet mount microscopy. It may detect vaginal yeast infection, trichomoniasis and bacterial vaginosis. Vaginal bleeding may alter the results. The patient should be instructed to avoid condoms or tampon use or vaginal sex 24 hours before the test. Moreover, vaginal pessaries, creams or douches should not be used during the 2 to 3 days before the test.

The test is very easy where a speculum is inserted inside the vagina while the patient is in the lithotomy position to get a sample fluid from the upper vagina. The sample is then smeared on a glass slide mixed with few drops of saline and examined by wet mount microscopy. Normally, no yeast, trichomonas or clue cells are found on the slide.

8.2. Additional vaginal discharge tests

In a previous study [8], we performed more evaluation of vaginal discharge as a screening for bacterial vaginosis. Sterile cotton tipped swab was inserted in the posterior vaginal fornix, then two swabs were taken. The first swab was rolled on a clean slide, and then a drop of isotonic saline was added and the slide was examined microscopically (¥400) for the presence of clue cells;7 0.1 mL methylene blue was also added to the wet preparation, so that the blue stained bacteria on clue cells could be easily seen. A second swab of secretions was applied to a clean glass slide and allowed to dry in air. This sample was later fixed by flame and Gram staining was performed to visualize clue cells. The slide was examined under oil immersion microscopy (¥1000). After examination of vaginal discharge, the diagnosis of BV was made if three of the four criteria of Amsel and Thomson's criteria were fulfilled: these include thin homogenous vaginal discharge, vaginal pH 4.5, characteristic amine or fishy odor when alkali (10% KOH) is added to the specimen of vaginal secretions, and the presence of clue cells on wet mount examination of vaginal fluid. Clue cells are described as a vaginal epithelial cell with an ill-defined outline that appeared to be granular because of the large number of bacillary *G.*

vaginalis (and other bacteria) attached to their surface. To be significantly indicative of BV, more than 20% of the epithelial cells on the slide should be clue cells.

8.3. Screening for Chlamydial Infection [9]

The primary focus of chlamydia screening efforts should be to detect chlamydia infection, prevent complications and test and treat their partners. Several sequelae can result from *C. trachomatis* infection in women including PID, ectopic pregnancy, and infertility. *C. trachomatis* urogenital infection can be diagnosed in women by testing first-catch urine or collecting swab specimens from the endocervix or vagina. Nucleic acid amplification tests (NAATs) are the most sensitive tests for these specimens and therefore are recommended for detecting *C. trachomatis* infection [10]. NAATs that are FDA-cleared for use with vaginal swab specimens can be collected by a provider or self-collected in a clinical setting. Self-collected vaginal swab specimens are equivalent in sensitivity and specificity to those collected by a clinician using NAATs, and women find this screening strategy highly acceptable [11]. Previous evidence [12] suggests that the liquid-based cytology specimens collected for Pap smears might be acceptable specimens for NAAT testing, although test sensitivity using these specimens might be lower than that associated with use of cervical or vaginal swab specimens; regardless, certain NAATs have been FDA-cleared for use on liquid-based cytology specimens.

8.4. Cervical screening opportunity

Perfect diagnosis utilizing a simple bivalve vaginal speculum is the key of success for proper diagnosis and subsequent treatment of local genital tract infections. Don't ignore to screen for premalignant cervical lesions even if your patient is young. Premalignant cervical lesions usually precede invasive cervical cancer by about 17-25 years. So, your patient's health should have the priority before treating infertility. Screening starts by meticulous naked eye examination of the cervix. It is a very important costless step. In a previous study [13], we tested the reliability of unaided Naked-Eye Examination (UNEE) of the cervix as a sole screening test for cervical premalignant and malignant lesions as compared to the standard cervical cytology. A total of 3,500 non pregnant women aged between 25 and 55 years were included. An unlubricated bivalve speculum was inserted into the vagina under good light to visualize the cervix. A thorough UNEE of the cervix was done to detect any apparent lesions. Cervical smears were obtained using the long tip of Ayre's spatula. An additional endocevical sample was obtained by cytobrush. Woman with abnormal Pap smear or visible cervical lesions by UNEE were scheduled for colposcopic examination. A biopsy was taken in every abnormal colposcopic examination. Preinvasive cervical lesions (CIN 1-3) diagnosed by various diagnostic tools used in the study and confirmed by histopathological examination were 9 / 3500 cases (2.57 %). Invasive cervical lesions were diagnosed in 6 /3500 cases (1.71 %). The sensitivity of UNEE was much more better than Pap smear (80 % vs 60 %) but less than colposcopy (86.7 %). However, specificity of UNEE was lower than Pap smear (91.16 %) vs. 100 %) and better than colposcopy (83.12 %). UNEE had poor positive predictive value (3.75 %) when compared to Pap smear (100 %) and to colposcopy (20 %). The negative predictive values of the three tests were nearly comparable. Whenever access to Pap smear is limited, UNEE performed by general gynecologists and a well-trained nurse is an acceptable alternative for detection of cervical premalignant or malignant lesions especially in low resource settings. Optimally, a Pap smear should be taken routinely from every patient. Any suspicion of premalignant or malignant lesions deserves a colposcopically-guided biopsy.

9. How to manage local cervical inflammatory lesions in women with UI?

If you see an inflammatory cervical polyp, it should be excised in the office utilizing a sterile ring forceps. It should be sent for histopathologic assessment. Any bleeding from its pedicle can be controlled by simple gauze compression or rarely cauterization. Other lesions like ectopy, ectropion or chronic non-specific cervicitis can be treated by an ablative therapy. In a prospective study [14], we tested the efficacy, tolerability and safety of 70% trichloroacetic acid (TCA) painting versus monopolar spray coagulation of the cervix for treating persistent benign cervical lesions that failed to respond to local medications. We included a total of 246 cases with objective evidence of benign cervical lesions that were divided into 2 groups according to the line of management. Group A comprised 126 cases subjected to spray monopolar coagulation while group B comprised 120 cases subjected to trichloroacetic acid application. Cervical smearing and colposcopy with or without cervical biopsy to exclude underling malignant lesions was done. TCA painting or spray monopolar coagulation of the benign cervical lesion(s). Follow-up was performed to assess relief of symptoms and cervical morphology for one month. Main outcome measures include success of management tool, relief of symptoms and normal cervical morphology after one month of therapy. We achieved a statistically significant cure rate of cervical lesions after treatment in both groups without significant difference between both groups. Failure rate was reported more in group B than group A mainly due to hypertrophied ectopy and cervical polyp. Patient in group A reported low satisfaction (26.9%) and poor tolerability rate (44.5%) as compared to patients in group B, who reported high satisfaction (77.5%), and good tolerability rate (77.5%), this difference was statistically significant. We concluded that both topical application of 70% TCA and monopolar spray coagulation offer considerable efficacy, acceptable success rates and minimal complications. Spray coagulation is significantly superior in terms of less persistent or incompletely healed lesions. Nevertheless, topical application of 70% TCA has the advantages of simplicity, higher patient tolerability and safety that can be widely used by gynecologists who have limited experience with surgical procedures. It is highly recommended if the cervical lesion is ectopy or non-specific cervicitis but not hypertrophic lesion like hypertrophic ectopy or polyp.

9.1. Hidden genital tract infections in UI

Hidden uterine factors of infertility may include thin endometrium, poor endometrial receptivity, and immunological incompatibility which have received good interest in modern practice [15]. Literally, little attention has been directed towards asymptomatic hidden intrauterine infections like Mycoplasma, Ureaplasma, Klebsiella and Chlamydia trachomatis particularly among infertile women [16].

http://dx.doi.org/10.5772/64056

9.2. Prevalence of hidden intrauterine infections (IUI) in UI

In an unpublished study, we tried to find out if women with UI have high prevalence of hidden intrauterine infections (IUI). We included 100 women allocated into two groups. A study group included 50 women with UI and control group included 50 fertile women who came for contraceptive advice. Sample size calculation was carried out using Epi Info software version 7 (CDC, 2012). A calculated sample of 82 (41 cases and 41 controls) was needed to detect an effect size of 0.1 between the two groups unexplained infertility and control group, with a p value < 0.05 and 80% power. Inclusion criteria for UI were criteria according to The Practice Committee of the American Society for Reproductive Medicine (ASRM) [17] which includes normal semen analysis at least twice, patent fallopian tubes as seen by hystrosalpingography (HSG) and positive ovulation utilizing ultrasound or serum progesterone in the second half of the cycle.

Exclusion criteria included current or recent use of systemic or local antibiotics, vaginal douches or creams in the preceding month. Inclusion criteria of the control group included new clients attending the family planning outpatient clinic asking for a contraceptive method and not complaining of recent or recurrent abnormal vaginal discharge. In both groups, patients were subjected to a detailed history taking stressing on possible use of vaginal creams or vaginal douches in the preceding month followed by thorough and meticulous vaginal and general examinations. Patients with evidence of overt upper or lower genital tract infection on routine clinical examination were also excluded from this study. In both groups, in lithotomy position, an un-lubricated bivalve vaginal speculum was inserted intravaginally then an endouterine swab was taken utilizing a soft 3 mm pipette. After injection of few milliliters of 0.9% saline, the aspirate was immediately sent to bacteriology department for assessment. The endouterine swab was incubated on Amies transport medium (Himedia), pleuropneumonia-like organism broth (PPLO) (Himedia – Cat. No. M266), and brain heart infusion (BHI) (Himedia – Cat. No. M210), to isolate Mycoplasma hominis. The plates were kept under microaerophilic conditions at 37 °C. Liquid media were examined daily for 10 days for the color change indicating growth. Other media like columbia Agar base (Himedia – Cat. No. M144) and MacConkey Agar (Himedia – Cat. No. MM081), were used to identify other organisms by conventional methods. Vaginalis Agar (Himedia – Cat. No. M1057) medium was used to detect Gardnerella vaginalis. Part of the fluid was fixed on slides, frozen in acetone, and subjected to a direct immunofluorescence assay (IFA) with fluorescence isothiocyanate conjugated anti-chlamydia trachomatis monoclonal antibodies (Imagen TM Chlamydia, Dako Cytomation, UK). Detection of group B streptococci (GBS) was done by specific antiserum on the isolated colonies (HiStrep – Latex test kit – Himedia LK06-50NO). The isolated organisms were confirmed biochemically using API system (20A Biomerrieux RES 20300). All women with unexplained infertility (group A) were subjected to diagnostic laparoscopy using standard double puncture technique. Laparoscopic findings were correlated with bacteriologic findings.

There was a statistically insignificant difference between both groups regarding the age and residence (p value >0.05) and it was highly significant regarding parity (p value <0.001). Hidden IUI were diagnosed by culture and biochemical confirmation in 42 cases (84%) and 10 cases

(20%) in both groups respectively with a high statistically significant difference (P=0.001). The most common organisms detected in the study group were Mycoplasma (24%), klebsiella (20%), Chlamydia (18%) and Proteus (10%). In group A, positive laparoscopic findings were reported in 33 patients (66 %). There was a significant correlation between the positive cases of hidden IUI and the pathological lesions diagnosed by laparoscopy (P Value= 0.0001). The most common laparoscopic abnormalities were hyperemic uterus, peritubal adhesions and chronic salpingitis which were reported in 10 (20%), 6 (12%) and 4 (8%) cases respectively, which demonstrate a highly significant correlation between confirmed hidden IUI and abnormal laparoscopic findings in UI. Laparoscopy revealed upper genital tract pathology in 30 cases (71.4%) of positive cases of hidden infections (42 cases) and it was negative in 3 cases (37.5%) of negative cases of hidden intrauterine infections (P Value= 0.0001). Cases with abnormal laparoscopic findings (33 cases) could be explained by positive culture of hidden intrauterine infection in UI group except 7 cases of endometriosis and 3 cases were culture-free. Abnormal laparoscopic findings were found more in positive cases with Mycoplasma (10 cases), Chlamydia (8 cases), Klebsiella (3 cases) and Proteus (2 cases) respectively.

9.3. Discussion on prevalence of hidden IUI

Hidden IUI may be a possible cause of UI [18]. This can be achieved by alterations in the intraperitoneal environment that may lead to an inflammatory process in the absence of visible abnormalities [19]. In our work, high prevalence of hidden IUI (84%) proved by culture of endouterine discharge in women with UI raise the recommendation that before starting a lengthy and costly list of sophisticated level II investigations of both partners, attention to hidden IUI is a mandatory basic step in UI. It has been found that women with tubal factor were two to three times more likely to have genital tract infections than women with other types of infertility [20]. We think that culture would be accepted as a basic screening tool for hidden IUI due to availability and feasibility in many hospitals. Screening test should not be expensive, time consuming or complicated before being extended to all hospitals particularly in low resource countries with limited resources.

Our work demonstrated a high prevalence of Mycoplasma (24%), klebsiella (20%), Chlamydia (18%) and Proteus (10%) among women with UI. These results of high prevalence compared to fertile women would call for more attention to screening protocols in all infertility units dealing with UI ideally prior to laparoscopic intervention. Due to high prevalence of Chlamydia in infertile women in a previous study, screening for Chlamydia was recommended for cases with all cases with UI [18]. We reported Mycoplasma in about one quarter of positive cases. Likewise, mycoplasma was reported in 32% of infertile cases with a statistically significant difference from fertile group [12]. In this study, proteus infection was reported in 10% of infected cases. This particular organism is commonly noticed in the urinary system infections. Reporting it in the genital tract would requires more studies to define its role in infertility. Unlike others, we reported low prevalence of Ureaplasma in only 4% of cases despite its previous reports of up to 32% infertile cases [18]. This big difference may clarify the variability of frequency of hidden intrauterine infections in different populations and highlights importance of studies on prevalence in each community.

Laparoscopic evaluation of infertility is the cornerstone test for tubal and peritoneal factors of infertility [21]. In this study we documented 33 cases (66%) with abnormal laparoscopic findings among the infertile group. Abnormal laparoscopic findings were reported in about 53 % of infertile women in a previous stud [22]. The most frequent abnormal laparoscopic finding in their study was pelvic adhesions. More frequent abnormal laparoscopic findings in UI up to 87.2% were reported by others [23] who described endometriosis lesions, peritubal adhesions and tubal obstruction. In a previous study, 114 women with UI were examined laparoscopically. Laparoscopy revealed pelvic pathology in 95 patients. Endometriosis, pelvic adhesions and tubal disease were observed and treated in 72, 46 and 24 patients, respectively. They could treat 72 patients of them, and 35 of them conceived using their own tubes. However they concluded that diagnostic laparoscopy should be strongly considered in UI work-up, and tubal efficacy should not be underestimated [24]. In our work, there was a significant correlation between the positive cases of BV and the pathological lesions diagnosed by laparoscopy especially hyperemic uterus, chronic salpingitis and peritubal adhesions (P Value= 0.0001). Subsequently, we recommend meticulous screening of women with these abnormal laparoscopic findings for possibility of hidden intrauterine infections.

Performing laparoscopy for UI is not universally agreed and questionable since it is an invasive procedure with serious morbidities and mortalities. However, in an detailed book chapter, many benefits of performing endoscopic evaluation of cases of UI were well demonstrated [3].

Limitations of this study included small sample size of individual types of hidden intrauterine infections and lake of precise description of a particular abnormal laparoscopic finding for each organism are clear limitations of this study. Due to ethical considerations, both groups were not homogeneous in that the case group had undergone investigations such as ultrasound and HSG, while the controls had not. We could reasonably argue that instrumentation for HSG might cause retrograde infections that were later on detected at laparoscopy. Some of the "positive" laparoscopic findings are questionable and probably too subjective. This study would be a more meaningful study if included the impact of proper treatment on fertility of women with UI.

We concluded that despite being an underestimated cause of female infertility, hidden IUI are frequent and implicated in UI. Laparoscopy is very beneficial in explaining the effect of hidden intrauterine infections on the upper genital tract but it is not a screening tool for IUI. We recommend postoperative screening for hidden IUI in UI cases with abnormal laparoscopic findings. Further studies are required to test the impact of proper treating these infections on subsequent fertility in cases of UI.

10. Similar studies

One hundred seventy infertile women and 45 pregnant women in the third trimester were evaluated in one study for the prevalence of uterine infections [25]. Classical methods and real time PCR were applied to each cervical sample to detect the presence of these sexually transmitted microorganisms; the ELISA method was applied to blood samples to detect C.

trachomatis antibodies (IgA, IgM and IgG). The proportion of C. trachomatis IgG was significantly higher in the infertile group (23.8%) than in the pregnant group (4.4%), $p < 0.05$. For C. trachomatis antigen (Ag) and N. gonorrhoea Ag no differences were observed between the two groups. The prevalence of mycoplasma genital infections was higher in the pregnant group (U. urealyticum - 53.3% and M. hominis - 20%) than in the infertile group (U. urealyticum - 39.7% and M. hominis - 7.3%). Higher rate of co-infection with C. trachomatis and mycoplasma were observed among the infertile women (25.7%) than among the pregnant women (7.7%). This combination could be involved in the appearance of pelvic inflammatory disease (PID) and its sequele, including infertility. C. trachomatis IgG determination still remains the gold standard for the diagnosis of PID and should be used as a screening test for the prediction of tubal damage in infertile women. They concluded that in view of the large number of cases involving the co-existence of genital infections with C. trachomatis, M. hominis and U. urealyticum, it is clearly necessary to perform screening for all three microorganisms among all women of reproductive age but especially those who are infertile.

Another study [26] was constructed to investigate the detection rates of Chlamydia trachomatis, Neisseria gonorrhoeae, Mycoplasma genitalium, Mycoplasma hominis, Ureaplasma urealyticum, Gardnerella vaginalis, Escherichia coli, Streptococcus agalactiae and Enterococcus faecalis, in asymptomatic fertile and infertile women. It encompassed 161 women, including 101 women treated for infertility and 60 fertile women who had already given birth to healthy children. The material for the presence of C. trachomatis, N. gonorrhoeae, M. genitalium, M. hominis and U. urealyticum was collected from the cervical canal and analyzed by PCR. Furthermore, BD Probe Tec ET system was used to detect C. trachomatis infection. Vaginal swabs were collected for classification of bacterial vaginosis and aerobic vaginitis and assessed according to the Nugent score, as well as by traditional culture methods. U. urealyticum was identified in 9% of the infertile women and in 8% of controls. Presence of M. hominis was demonstrated only in the former (4%) and C. trachomatis only in latter (3%). N. gonorrhoeae and M. genitalium were not found in any of the examined women. The frequency of aerobic vaginitis in both groups was estimated at 12%. There were 7% bacterial vaginosis cases in the study group, and none in the control group ($p=0.0096$). They concluded that despite having no symptoms of an ongoing acute inflammation of the reproductive tract, many women may experience permanent or periodic shifts of equilibrium of the vaginal and/or cervical microflora. BV develops more frequently in infertile patients when compared to the fertile women.

11. Infection induced by infertility work-up maneuvers

During the course of infertility work-up, women are subjected to many invasive diagnostic procedures like hysterosalpingography, hysteroscopy, sonohystrography, premenstrual biopsy or laparoscopy. Moreover, some therapeutic procedures are done to treat definite problems like selective salpingography, egg retrieval, operative resectoscopy or hysteroscopy and operative laparoscopy in addition to some minor vaginal maneuvers. All these diagnostic and operative interventions carry the risk of introduction of infection to the genital tract and disruption of the natural protective mechanisms. The gynecologist should pay attention to the possibility of inducing infection and stick to aseptic strict precautions during every step. Lastly, whenever suspicion of introduction of infection is raised, proper broad spectrum antibiotics should be considered.

12. Keynote points

Infertility specialists should not underestimate overt lower or upper genital tract infections. Vaginal including speculum examination is an important basic step during infertility evaluation. Gynecologists should keep asepsis during all steps of examination or investigation of the infertile female. Use of appropriate antibiotics is recommended whenever prolonged or invasive procedure is performed. Prompt and aggressive treatment of any detected upper or lower genital tract infection is mandatory to prevent short and long-term sequel that would compromise the fertility status of the female. Concomitant treatment of the male partner shouldn't be forgotten to avoid relapse or persistence of female infections. Think hidden infection of the genital tract in all cases of UI before performing sophisticated procedures like ART. Uterine microbiome is a recent entry to our armamentarium, however its relevance and treatment is unknown and requires more research.

Author details

Atef M. Darwish*

Address all correspondence to: atef_darwish@yahoo.com

Department of Obstetrics and Gynecology, Woman's Health University Hospital, Faculty of Medicine, Assiut University, Egypt

References

[1] Boivin J, Bunting L, Collins JA, Nygren KG. International estimates of infertility prevalence and treatment-seeking: potential need and demand for infertility medical care. Hum Reprod 2007;22:1506–1512.

[2] Darwish AM, Youssef AA. Screening sonohysterography in infertility. Gynecol Obstet Invest. 1999;48(1):43-7.

[3] Darwish AM. Endoscopic explanation of unexplained infertility. In. Contemporary Gynecologic Practice. Edited by Darwish AM. InTech Pub Com, Feb 2015, Ch1.

[4] Okonofua FE, Ako-Nai KA, Dighitoghi MD. Lower genital tract infections in infertile Nigerian women compared with controls. Genitourin Med. 1995 Jun;71(3):163-8.

[5] Green KA, Zarek SM, Catherino WH. Gynecologic health and disease in relation to the microbiome of the female reproductive tract. Fertil Steril. 2015 Dec;104(6):1351-7.

[6] Sirota I, Zarek SM, Segars JH Potential influence of the microbiome on infertility and assisted reproductive technology. Semin Reprod Med. 2014 Jan;32(1):35-42.

[7] Selman H, Mariani M, Barnocchi N, Mencacci A, Bistoni F,Arena S, Pizzasegale S, Brusco G, Angelini A· Examination of bacterial contamination at the time of embryo transfer, and its impact on the IVF/pregnancy outcome J Assist Reprod Genet. 2007 Sep; 24(9): 395–399.

[8] Darwish AM, Makarem MH, Alnashar EM, Hamadeh SM. Screening for bacterial vaginosis in high-risk pregnancy: the experience of a developing country. Acta Obstet Gynecol Scand. 2005;;84(5):483-5.

[9] Keegan M, Diedrich M, Peipert J. *Chlamydia trachomatis* Infection: Screening and Management. J Clin Outcomes Manag. 2014 Jan; 21(1): 30–38.

[10] Papp J, Schachter J, Gaydos C, Van Der Pol B. Recommendations for the Laboratory-Based Detection of Chlamydia trachomatis and Neisseria gonorrhoeae — 2014 CDC Recommendations and Reports. March 14, 2014 / 63(RR02);1-19

[11] Fang J, Husman C, DeSilva L, Chang R, Peralta L. Evaluation of self-collected vaginal swab, first void urine, and endocervical swab specimens for the detection of Chlamydia trachomatis and Neisseria gonorrhoeae in adolescent females. J Pediatr Adolesc Gynecol. 2008 Dec;21(6):355-60.

[12] Hopwood J, Mallinson H, Hodgson E, Hull L. Liquid based cytology: examination of its potential in a chlamydia screening programme. Sex Transm Infect. 2004 Oct; 80(5): 371–373.

[13] Darwish AM, Abdullah SA, Zahran KM, Abdel-Fattah NA. Reliability of naked eye examination for the diagnosis of benign cervical lesions. J Low Genit Tract Dis. 2013 Apr;17(2):182-6.

[14] Darwish AM, Zahran KM. Trichloroacetic acid application versus spray monopolar diathermy for treating benign cervical lesions: a randomized controlled clinical trial. J Low Genit Tract Dis. 2013 Jul;17(3):248-54.

[15] Choudhury SR, Knapp LA. Human reproductive failure: Immunological factors. Hum Reprod Update 2001; 7(2):113-134.

[16] Cassell GH, Younger JB, Brown MB, Blackwell RE, Davis JK, Marriott P, Stagno S. Microbiologic study of infertile women at the time of diagnostic laparoscopy: Association of Ureaplasma urealyticum with a defined subpopulation. N Engl J Med 1983; 308: 502.

[17] The Practice Committee of the American Society for Reproductive Medicine, authors. Optimal evaluation of the infertile female. Fertil Steril 2006; 86(5 suppl):S264–S267.

[18] Gupta A, Gupta A, Gupta S, Mittal A, Chandra P, Gill AK. Correlation of mycoplasma with unexplained infertility. Arch Gynecol Obstet 2009 Dec; 280(6):981-5.

[19] Hossein Rashidi B, Chamani Tabriz L, Haghollahi F, Jeddi-Tehrani M, Naghizadeh MM, Shariat M, et al. Effects of Chlamydia trachomatis Infection on Fertility; A Case-Control Study. J Reprod Infertil. 2013;14(2):67-72.

[20] Spandorfer SD, Neuer A, Giraldo PC, Rosenwaks Z., Witkin SS. Relationship of abnormal vaginal flora, proinflammatory cytokines and idiopathic infertility in women undergoing IVF. J Reprod Med 2001; 46: 806-10.

[21] Tsuji I, Ami K, Miyazaki A, Hujinami N, Hoshiai H. Benefit of diagnostic laparoscopy for patients with unexplained infertility and normal hysterosalpingography findings. Tohoku J Exp Med. 2009;219(1):39-42.

[22] Gocmen, A. and T. Atak. "Diagnostic laparoscopy findings in unexplained infertility cases." Clin Exp Obstet Gynecol 2012;39(4): 452-453.

[23] Nakagawa, K., S. Ohgi, T. Horikawa, R. Kojima, M. Ito and H. Saito. "Laparoscopy should be strongly considered for women with unexplained infertility." J Obstet Gynaecol Res 2007;33(5): 665-670.

[24] Bonneau C, Chanelles O, Sifer C, Poncelet C. Use of laparoscopy in unexplained infertility. European Journal of Obstetrics & Gynecology and Reproductive Biology 2012; 58-60.

[25] Miron ND, Socolov D, Mareş M, Anton G, Nastasa V, Moraru RF, Virág K, Anghelache-Lupaşcu I, Deák J. Bacteriological agents which play a role in the development of infertility. Acta Microbiol Immunol Hung. 2013 Mar;60(1):41-53.

[26] Tomusiak A, Heczko PB, Janeczko J, Adamski P, Pilarczyk-Zurek M, Strus M. Bacterial infections of the lower genital tract in fertile and infertile women from the south-eastern Poland. Ginekol Pol. 2013 May;84(5):352-8.

Chapter 3

Chronic Endometritis

Attilio Di Spiezio Sardo, Federica Palma, Gloria Calagna, Brunella Zizolfi and Giuseppe Bifulco

Additional information is available at the end of the chapter

http://dx.doi.org/10.5772/63023

Abstract

Chronic endometritis is a persistent inflammation of the inner lining of the uterine cavity. Several studies have demonstrated that it is a condition frequently associated with repeated unexplained implantation failure at in vitro fertilization, recurrent miscarriage, as well as poor obstetric outcomes such as preterm labor.

The aim of this paper is to provide information about diagnosis and treatment of this condition to improve reproductive outcome. In fact, significantly higher rate of successful pregnancies was achieved in those patients in whom antibiotic treatment was able to normalize both hysteroscopic and histologic endometrial pattern compared with women who were not treated or with persistent disease. Hysteroscopy with endometrial biopsy is assumed to be the best method for the detection of chronic endometritis. So, we support the importance of hysteroscopy as a part of the diagnostic workup of infertile women.

Keywords: Infections, chronic endometritis, infertility, hysteroscopy, antibiotic therapy

1. Introduction

1.1. Definition and etiology

Endometritis is defined as inflammation of the endometrium, grouped in various typologies, depending on the underlying causality.

It may present in acute or chronic forms.

The acute form is principally a transitional phase of short duration generally arising due to the persistence of placental or abortive residues, or in combination with pelvic inflammatory disease, or with inflammatory conditions of bacterial/viral etiology elsewhere in the urogenital tract [1–4].

Chronic inflammation may follow the acute stage—which is the most frequently seen—or it may occur more subtly, as chronic inflammation 'ab initio', without passing through an acute stage.

Chronic endometritis can reveal a microbiological origin or a mechanical–chemical origin [5].

In the latter case, the most frequent causative agents are common pyogenic pathogens (streptococci, staphylococci, enterococci, *Escherichia coli*), as well as bacteria such as *Chlamydia trachomatis, Neisseria gonorrhoeae, Mycoplasma,* and *Ureaplasma urealyticum*. It has also been described in cases of postpartum endometritis secondary to herpes simplex virus (HSV) and cytomegalovirus (CMV) infections, particularly in patients with HIV [6–8].

However, although the etiology in most cases is polymicrobial, the results obtained by traditional culture tests are laboratory dependent, and often, given the use of endometrial sampling devices, vaginal and endocervical contamination cannot be excluded.

Also worth mentioning is tubercular endometritis, because in recent years there has been an increased incidence of tuberculosis in Western countries, owing to migration from countries with a high incidence of endemic tuberculosis.

Endometritis of chemical–mechanical origin, on the other hand, is generally caused by the presence of pessaries or intrauterine devices.

2. Clinical appearance

Chronic endometritis is often clinically silent. Therefore, it is impossible to accurately determine its true prevalence in the general population [5].

In some cases, however, it can be associated with *infertility* [9–11].

Endometrial inflammation seems to interfere with the physiological mechanisms of oocyte fertilization and embryonic implantation.

Repeated implantation failure (RIF) is defined as failure to conceive following two or three embryo transfer cycles or cumulative transfer of 10 good quality embryos [12,13].

In a retrospective study reported by Johnston-MacAnanny [14], women with a history of RIF after in vitro fertilization (IVF) were positively diagnosed with chronic endometritis in about 30% of cases and women diagnosed with chronic endometritis had lower implantation rates (11.5%) after IVF cycles.

In contrast, Kasius et al. [15] reported that the clinical implication of chronic endometritis seems minimal because they diagnosed this condition only in 2.8% of asymptomatic infertile patients with a normal transvaginal ultrasound examination (TVS). The same authors reported that the reproductive outcome at conventional In Vitro Fertilization (IVF) or Intra-cytoplasmic sperm injection (ICSI) cycles was not negatively affected by chronic endometritis, but they underlined that the low prevalence and unknown clinical significance of endometritis warrant further study [15, 16].

Cicinelli et al. [12], in a recent pilot research, demonstrated that chronic endometritis was a condition frequently associated with RIF (66.0%). It was about double compared with 30.3% reported by Johnston-MacAnanny et al. [14]. This discrepancy could be explained by the very strict selection criteria employed in this study (for example, in order to rule out any confounding factor and inflammatory conditions, they considered clinical or ultrasonographic evidence of ovarian endometrioma as an exclusion criterion) and by the expertise of their group in hysteroscopic and histological diagnosis of chronic endometritis. In this population study, the most prevalent infectious agents were common bacteria and mycoplasma. In addition, the normalization of the hysteroscopic endometrial pattern was associated with a significant improvement of the reproductive outcome of the IVF cycle performed after antibiotic treatment.

Chronic endometritis is also related to recurrent miscarriage (RM) [17].

RM, defined as three or more miscarriages before 20 weeks of pregnancy, affects about 3% of all couples [4, 18].

In a recent paper, it was demonstrated that in women with repeated abortions, chronic endometritis is a frequent finding (68.3%) and that women who received adequate antibiotic treatment had a significantly higher rate of successful pregnancies compared to women who were not treated or with persistent disease. Also in this population, the most prevalent infectious agents were common bacteria and *Mycoplasma* [12, 18].

In conclusion, untreated chronic endometritis seems to diminish the success rates of both spontaneous conception and IVF cycles, as well as to contribute to adverse obstetrical outcomes, as intrauterine infections, preterm delivery, and postpartum endometritis [2–4, 12, 16, 19–21]. Furthermore, all these results suggest that hysteroscopy should be a part of the diagnostic work-up of infertile women complaining of unexplained RM and with RIF [18, 22].

However, the exact mechanisms by which chronic endometritis can lead to a compromised fertility are not yet fully understood and are still the subject of numerous studies.

Very recently, it was shown that in the endometrial mucosa of infertile patients suffering from chronic endometritis, there is an altered distribution of natural killer cells. In particular, in chronic endometritis, there is a decrease in CD56 lymphocytes and an increase in CD16 lymphocytes, hence, an altered maternal immune tolerance towards the embryo, along with adverse effects on the mechanisms of implantation, and a defective trophoblastic invasion [23].

Other symptoms related to chronic endometritis are as follows [24]:

- *Abnormal uterine bleeding*: such a symptomatology can present in the form of intermenstrual spotting or metrorrhagia; however, to date, the relationship between abnormal uterine bleeding and chronic endometritis is not clear.
- *Dysmenorrhea*: the current hypothesis identifies, as a major cause of dysmenorrhea, the prostaglandins, which are released through the endometrial cell membranes damaged by the inflammatory process.
- *Dyspareunia*.

- *Leucorrhea and urinary symptoms*: occasionally, there is a malodorous, purulent vaginal discharge, with increased urinary frequency and/or symptoms similar to those of cystitis, along with concomitant bladder irritation.
- *Fever*: Elevated in the acute phase; in some cases, a mild fever in the chronic form.

Tubercular endometritis merits special mention; this type of chronic endometrial inflammation virtually always occurs secondary to respiratory or abdominal localization, with a clear predilection for adnexal localization. It is generally limited to young women of childbearing age, being rare in the menopause.

The symptomatology varies from overt forms, in which the inflammatory process has affected the appendages, to completely latent forms. In the presence of tubercular endometritis, changes in menstrual flow may occur, ranging from polymenorrhea to amenorrhea, accompanied by an almost universal history of sterility/infertility.

3. Prehysteroscopic diagnosis

The diagnosis of chronic endometritis by means of two-dimensional transvaginal sonography (TVS) is difficult due to the absence of pathognomonic signs associated with the condition [12].

Indirect sonography signs are as follows:

- hematometra;
- endometrium with hyperechogenic spots;
- intracavitary synechiae;
- increase in endometrial thickness, asynchronous with the phase of the menstrual cycle.

4. Hysteroscopic diagnosis

A hysteroscopy, performed in the proliferative phase of the menstrual cycle, allows to identify the signs of endometrial inflammation.

Under examination with CO2, chronic endometritis typically presents with endometrial areas, which are bright red with white central dots, focally or diffusely distributed over the endometrial surface, assuming an appearance considered to resemble a 'strawberry' pattern, similar to the colposcopic pattern 'punctated with white spots'.

Other findings may be conspicuous due to the presence of friable, white patches that bleed easily on contact. These features are, however, very unspecific, as they may also be related to lesions of the vascular bed in reaction to the intracavitary CO_2 distension medium, or emerging due to immunological disorders, or hypertension, and they may yet be so mild as to evade diagnosis.

Uterine distension with saline has, among other advantages, that of causing no adverse side effects on endometrial microcirculation, thus facilitating the diagnosis of chronic endometritis [25].

The criteria proposed by Cicinelli et al. [26] to establish a hysteroscopic diagnosis of chronic endometritis are as follows (Figures 1–3):

- Hyperemia: The vascular network appears accentuated, especially at periglandular level.
- Stromal edema: The endometrium presents, in the proliferative phase, as both pale and thickened.
- Micropolyps: Manifesting with small pedunculated, vascularized protrusions of the uterine mucosa (<1 mm) covered by endometrium and characterized by an accumulation of inflammatory cells (lymphocytes, plasma cells, and eosinophils) intermingled with normal stromal cells.

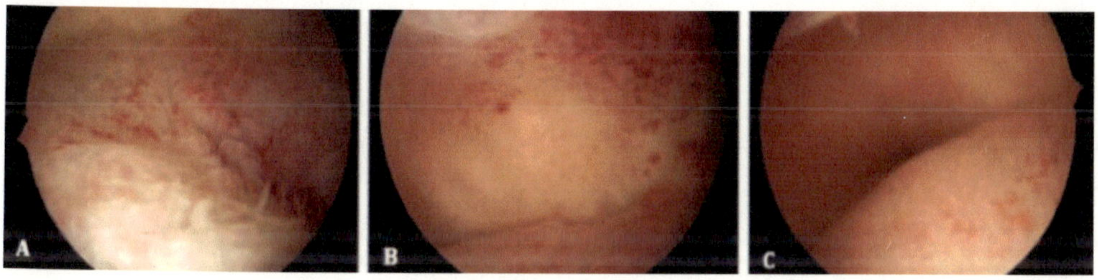

Figure 1. Hysteroscopic view of chronic endometritis in a 30-year-old infertile woman. Saline used as distension medium does not affect endometrial microcirculation, making it easier to identify the characteristic signs of chronic endometritis. Note the micropolyps, which appear as small pedunculated, vascularized protrusions (<1 mm) on the uterine mucosa (A). The close-up view clearly shows a marked accentuation of the vascular network at the level of the uterine fundus (B). To right, an overt stromal edema is evident (C), though the examination was carried out in the early proliferative phase.

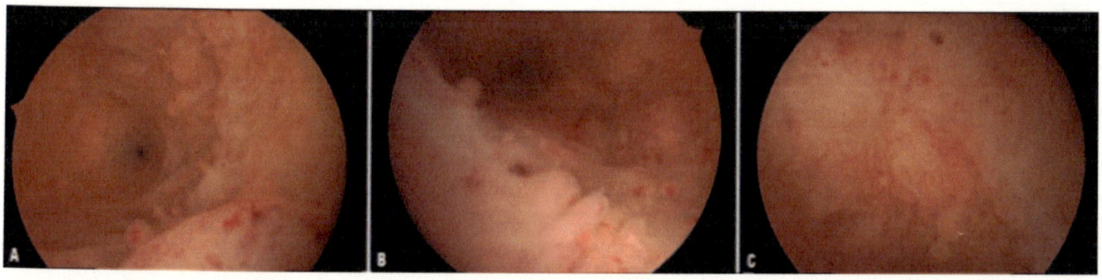

Figure 2. Hysteroscopic view of chronic endometritis in a 34-year-old woman with a positive anamnesis of three early spontaneous abortions (A–C). The stromal edema is clearly evident on the posterior wall (A) and micropolyps are detected on any of the uterine walls (A–C).

A study led by Cicinelli in 2005 [26] showed that the absence of stromal edema and hyperemia —detected at hysteroscopy—has a high negative predictive value (98.8%), i.e., the absence of

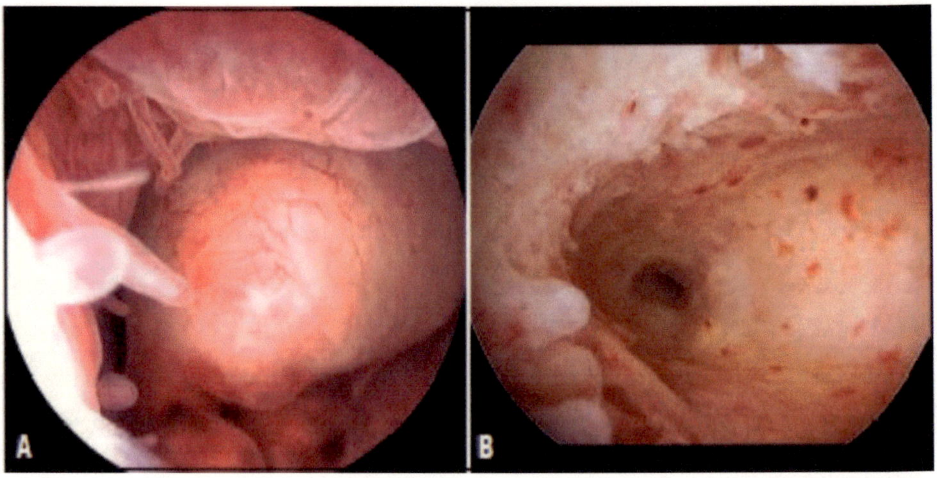

Figure 3. Detail of micropolyps under hysteroscopic examination using a liquid distension medium: the micropolyps, which appear with a varied morphology, are scattered over the uterine wall and may often be encountered with polyps (A) and/or pseudopolyps.

these findings allows the hysteroscopist to rule out, with reasonable certainty, the presence of endometrial inflammation.

Conversely, if micropolyps are found, which is almost always associated with hyperemia or stromal edema, this should be interpreted a reliable sign of inflammation, as corroborated by the high positive predictive value attributed to this finding (98.4%).

The presence of focal hyperemia with isolated micropolyps is associated, histologically, with a mild type of endometrial inflammation; conversely, the findings of generalized hyperemia, diffused micropolyps, or a thickened endometrium with polypoid diffusion are all associated with moderate-to-severe endometrial inflammation [27, 28].

In summary, the presence of hyperemia, edema, and stromal micropolyps has a demonstrated diagnostic accuracy of 93.4%.

The potential development of endometritis, if left untreated, leads to the formation of intrauterine synechiae.

Regarding tuberculous endometritis, certain hysteroscopic signs suggestive of disease have been described, such as the presence of a thin, uneven, and pale endometrium with irregular whitish spots scattered over the uterine walls [29].

It is not uncommon to observe intrauterine adhesions, while a much rarer finding is the presence of classic tubercles in the endometrial mucosa. Differential diagnosis should be established against the presence of granulomatous endometritis (sarcoidosis) and that of the fungal form [30]. Even CMV-related endometritis can manifest itself in the granulomatous form.

Finally, there is a rare form of endometritis that may mimic, at macroscopic level, an endometrial carcinoma [31]. This is xanthogranulomatous endometritis, whose etiology is still

http://dx.doi.org/10.5772/63023

under debate, and which occurs predominantly in elderly women with cervical stenosis and pyometra. Histologically, it is characterized by xanthogranuloma, consisting of lipid-rich histiocytes, giant cells, lymphocytes, neutrophils, and plasma cells.

5. Histological diagnosis

The histological diagnosis of chronic endometritis is based on the presence of a number of criteria that have been widely described in the literature: superficial stromal edema, increased stromal density, and inflammatory stromal infiltration, which is predominated by the presence of lymphocytes and plasma cells [32]. The presence of the latter is considered by some authors as a marker specific to endometritis; according to some, in particular, the presence of a few or even a single stromal level plasma cell is enough to settle the diagnosis on chronic endometritis [33].

However, the majority of authors agree upon a greater importance that an overall view of all histological aspects be established (the coexisting presence of several criteria suggestive of chronic endometritis—rather than focusing on a single diagnostic criterion).

An unusual distribution pattern of leukocytes in the endometrial mass and the presence of an increased number of B lymphocytes may contribute to the diagnosis because the B lymphocytes in the endometrium normally make up less than 1% of the leukocyte count.

6. Treatment

The therapy for chronic endometritis is pharmacological and is based on the administration of broad-spectrum antibiotics [34, 35].

Generally, the drug of choice is doxycycline, administered in doses of 100 mg every 12 hours for 14 days, or alternatively, the administration of cephalosporins, macrolides, or quinolones is possible. It is preferable for the partner to also undergo the same antibiotic treatment.

Where antibiotic therapy fails and/or where the presence of endometritis persists, an endometrial culture with a relative antibiogram should be considered and an appropriate antibiotic treatment must be prescribed.

In particular, according to the Centers for Disease Control guidelines, the therapies recommended are in case of [12]:

- positive for Gram-negative bacteria: Ciprofloxacin 500 mg twice a day for 10 days as first line therapy;
- Gram-positive bacteria: Amoxicillin+clavulanate 1 g twice a day for 8 days;
- *Mycoplasma* and *U. urealyticum* infections: Josamycin 1 g twice a day for 12 days; while, in case of persistence, minocycline 100 mg twice a day for 12 days;

- negative cultures: Ceftriaxone 250 mg IM in a single dose plus doxycycline 100 mg orally twice a day for 14 days with metronidazole 500 mg orally twice a day for 14 days.

In case of persistence of signs of chronic endometritis at subsequent hysteroscopy, the protocol can be repeated up to three times.

In the presence of confirmed tuberculous endometritis, the patient should be given a specific antibiotic therapy for tuberculosis (isoniazid, ethambutol, rifampicin, and pyrazinamide for 2 months, followed by isoniazid and rifampicin for another 4 months).

Author details

Attilio Di Spiezio Sardo[1*], Federica Palma[2], Gloria Calagna[3], Brunella Zizolfi[1] and Giuseppe Bifulco[2]

*Address all correspondence to: cdispie@tin.it, attiliodispiezio@libero.it

1 Unit of Obstetrics and Gynecology, University of Federico II, Naples, Italy

2 Unit of Obstetrics and Gynecology, University of Modena and Reggio Emilia, Italy

3 Unit of Obstetrics and Gynecology, University of Palermo, Italy

References

[1] Taylor S, Frydman R. Hysteroscopy and sperm infection. Contracept Fertil Sex1996; 24: 549–51.

[2] Gravett MG, Hitti J, Hess DL, Eschenbach DA. Intrauterine infection and preterm delivery: evidence for activation of the fetal hypothalamic pituitary-adrenal axis. American Journal of Obstetrics and Gynecology 2000; 182: 1404–13.

[3] Eckert LO, Moore DE, Patton DL, Agnew KJ, Eschenbach DA. Relationship of vaginal bacteria and inflammation with conception and early pregnancy loss following in vitro fertilization. Infectious Diseases in Obstetrics and Gynecology 2003; 11: 11–7.

[4] Romero R, Mazor M. Infection and preterm labor. Clinical of Obstetrics and Gynecology 1988; 31: 553–84.

[5] Farooki MA. Epidemiology and pathology of chronic endometritis. International Surgery 1967; 48: 566–73.

[6] Giraldo-Isaza MA, Jaspan D, Cohen AW. Postpartum endometritis caused by herpes and cytomegaloviruses. Obstetrics and Gynecology 2011; 117: 466–7.

[7] Hollier LM, Laurie Scott L, Murphree SS, Wendel GD. Postpartum endometritis caused by herpes simplex virus. Obstetrics and Gynecology 1997; 89 (5): 836–8.

[8] Remaldi S, Finci V, Ismail A, Zacharie S, Vassilakos P. Herpetic endometritis after pregnancy. Pathology Research and Practice 1995; 191: 31–4.

[9] Kamiyama S, Teruya Y, Nohara M, Kanazawa K. Impact of detection of bacterial endotoxin in menstrual effluent on the pregnancy rate in in vitro fertilization and embryo transfer. Fertility and Sterility 2004; 82: 788–92.

[10] Polisseni F, Bambirra EA, Camargos AF. Detection of chronic endometritis by diagnostic hysteroscopy in asymptomatic infertile patients. Gynecologic and Obstetric Investigation 2003; 55: 205–10.

[11] Salim R, Ben-Shlomo I, Colodner R, Keness Y, Shalev E. Bacterial colonization of the uterine cervix and success rate in assisted reproduction: results of a prospective survey. Human Reproduction 2002; 17: 337–40.

[12] Cicinelli E, Matteo M, Tinelli R, Lepera A, Alfonso R, Indraccolo U, Marrocchella S, et al. Prevalence of chronic endometritis in repeated unexplained implantation failure and the IVF success rate after antibiotic therapy. Human Reproduction. 2015; 30: 323–30.

[13] El-Toukhy T, Taranissi M. Towards better quality research in recurrent implantation failure: standardizing its definition is the first step. Reproductive Biomedicine Online 2006;12:383–5.

[14] Johnston-Mac-Ananny EB, Hartnett J, Engmann LL, Nulsen JC, Sanders MM, Benadiva CA. Chronic endometritis is a frequent finding in women with recurrent implantation failure after in vitro fertilization. Fertility and Sterility 2010; 93: 437–41.

[15] Kasius JC, Fatemi HM, Bourgain C, Sie-Go DM, Eijkemans RJ, Fauser BC, Devroey P, et al. The impact of chronic endometritis on reproductive outcome. Fertility and Sterility 2011; 96(6): 1451–6.

[16] Kasius JC, Broekmans FJM, Sie-Go DM, Bourgain C, Eijkemans MJC, Fauser BC, Devroey P, et al. The reliability of the histological diagnosis of endometritis in asymptomatic IVF cases: a multicenter observer study. Human Reproduction 2012; 27: 153–8.

[17] Kitaya K. Prevalence of chronic endometritis in recurrent miscarriage. Fertility and Sterility 2011; 95: 1156–8.

[18] Cicinelli E, Matteo M, Tinelli R, Pinto V, Marinaccio M, Indraccolo U, De Ziegler D, et al. Chronic endometritis due to common bacteria is prevalent in women with recurrent miscarriage as confirmed by improved pregnancy outcome after antibiotic treatment. Reproductive Sciences. 2014; 21: 640–7.

[19] Feghali J, Bakar J, Mayenga JM, Segard L, Hamou J, Driguez P, Belaish-Allart J. Systematic hysteroscopy prior to in vitro fertilization. Gynecol Obstet Fertil 2003; 31: 127–31.

[20] Espinoza J, Erez O, Romero R. Preconceptional antibiotic treatment to prevent preterm birth in women with a previous preterm delivery. American Journal of Obstetrics and Gynecol 2006; 194: 630–7.

[21] Romero R, Espinoza J, Mazor M. Can endometrial infection/inflammation explain implantation failure, spontaneous abortion, and preterm birth after in vitro fertilization? Fertility and Sterility 2004; 82: 799–804.

[22] Zolghardri J, Momthan M, Aminian K, Ghaffarpasand F, Tavana Z. The value of hysteroscopy in diagnosis of chronic endometritis in paticns with unexplained recurrent spontaneous abortion. European Journal of Obstetrics and Gynecology and Reproductive Biology 2011; 217–20.

[23] Matteo M, Cicinelli E, Greco P, Massenzio F, Baldini D, Falagario T, Rosenberg P, Castellana L, Specchia G, Liso A. Abnormal pattern of lymphocyte subpopulations in the endometrium of infertile women with chronic endometritis. American Journal of Reproductive Immunology 2009; 322–9.

[24] Greenwood SM, Moran JJ. Chronic endometritis: morphologic and clinical observations. Obstetrics and Gynecology 1981; 58: 176–84.

[25] Cicinelli E, Resta L, Nicoletti R, Tartagni M, Marinaccio M, Bulletti C, Tartagni M, Marinaccio M, Bulletti C, Colafiglio G. Detection of chronic endometritis at fluid hysteroscopy. Journal of Minimally Invasive Gynecology 2005; 12: 514–8.

[26] Cicinelli E, Resta L, Nicoletti R, Zappimbulso V, Tartagni M, Saliani N. Endometrial micropolyps at fluid hysteroscopy suggest the existence of chronic endometritis. Human Reproduction 2005; 20: 1386–9.

[27] Cicinelli E, De Ziegler D, Nicoletti R. Chronic endometritis: correlation among hyseroscopic, hystologic and bacteriologic findings in a prospective trial with 2190 consecutive office hysteroscopies. Fertility and Sterility 2008; 89: 677–84.

[28] Cicinelli E, Tinelli R, Lepera A, Pinto V, Fucci M, Resta L. Correspondence between hysteroscopic and hystologic findings in women with chronic endometritis. Acta ObstetGynecol Scand 2010; 89: 1061–5.

[29] Cicinelli E, Tinelli R, Colafiglio G, Saliani N, Pastore A. Tubercular endometritis: a rare condition reliably detectable with fluid hysteroscopy. Journal of Minimally Invasive Gynecology 2008; 15: 752–54.

[30] Sharma JB Roy KK, Pushparaj M, Karmakar D, Kumar S, Singh N. Increased difficult and complications encountered during hysteroscopy in women with genital tuberculosis. Journal of Minimally Invasive Gynecology 2011; 18; 660–65.

[31] Dogan-Ekici AI, Usubütün A, Küçükali T, Ayhan A. Xanthogranulomatous endometritis: a challenging imitator of endometrial carcinoma. Infectious Diseases in Obstetrics and Gynecology 2007; 347–63.

[32] Smith M, Hagerty KA, Skipper B, Bocklage T. Chronic endometritis: a combined histopathologic and clinical review of cases from 2002 to 2007. International Journal of Gynecologic Pathology 2010; 29: 44–50.

[33] Pitsos M, Sturnick J, Heller D. Association of pathologic diagnoses with clinical findings in chronic endometritis. Journal of Reproductive Medicine 2009; 54 (6): 373–7.

[34] Andrews WW, Goldenberg RL, Hauth JC, Cliver SP, Cooper R, Conner M. Interconceptional antibiotics to prevent spontaneous preterm birth: a randomized clinical trial. American Journal Obstetrics and Gynecology 2006; 194: 617–23.

[35] Cravello L, Porcu G, D'Ercole C, D'Ercole C, Roger V, Blanc B. Identification and treatment of endometritis. ContraceptFertil Sex 1997; 25: 585–6.

Chapter 4

Management of Abnormal Vaginal Discharge in Pregnancy

Sanusi Mohammed Ibrahim, Mohammed Bukar and Bala Mohammed Audu

Additional information is available at the end of the chapter

http://dx.doi.org/10.5772/62599

Abstract

Abnormal vaginal discharge in a pregnant woman causes discomfort and increases risk of complications. Management of such patient is difficult as the physician will need to distinguish leucorrhoea of pregnancy from pathological vaginal discharge and also to decide on the drugs to prescribe that are not contraindicated in pregnancy.

The objective of the study is to discuss the prevalence, causes and treatment of abnormal vaginal discharge in pregnant women.

Searches from PubMed and using other scientific search engines were performed. The chapter was supported with findings from the authors' previous study on the same topic. In the study, high vaginal and endocervical swab samples were collected from 400 pregnant women with complaints of abnormal vaginal discharge and another 400 controls.

The result showed that the prevalence of abnormal vaginal discharge in pregnancy was 31.5%. Vulval pruritus, 200 (75%), was a significant feature (χ^2 = 1.011, $P <$ 0.001), and *Candida albicans*, 160 (40%), was the commonest cause.

Although antibiotic sensitivity testing was not done for *Candida albicans, all the microorganisms were sensitive to Augmentin®*

The prevalence of abnormal vaginal discharge in pregnancy was high and *C. albicans* was the commonest cause. Assessment of pregnant woman complaining of vaginal discharge for aetiology is necessary in order to give an appropriate treatment.

Keywords: Vaginal discharge, Pregnancy, Antibiotic treatment, Maiduguri, Nigeria

1. Introduction

Most pregnant women have vaginal discharges that are either physiologic or pathologic. The challenge to the clinician is to separate the vaginal infections with potentially serious input for pregnancy from annoying but not serious secretions, irritation and pruritus [1]. Infectious vaginitis is usually caused by yeast, such as *Trichomonas vaginalis,* bacterial vaginosis, gonorrhoea, *Chlamydia trachomatis, Mycoplasma,* Group B streptococcus or herpes [1]. Normal vaginal secretions consist of water, electrolytes, epithelial cells, microbial organisms, fatty acid and carbohydrate compounds [1, 2].The concentration of anaerobic bacteria is usually five times than that of aerobic organisms. The most prevalent organisms in the vagina are lactobacilli, *Streptococci, Staphylococcus epidermidis, Gadnerella vaginalis* and *Escherichia coli.* Anaerobic species that are frequently isolated include *Peptostreptococci,* anaerobic *lactobacilli* and *bacteroides* [3].

Vaginal pH, glycogen content and amount of secretion influence the quantity and type of organisms present in the vagina. Lactobacilli restrict the growth of other organisms by producing lactic acid, thus maintaining a low pH. These organisms also produce hydrogen peroxide, which is toxic to anaerobes. The normal vaginal bacterial population assists in inhibiting the growth of pathologic vaginal organisms. If the normal vaginal ecosystem is altered, there is a greater chance of proliferation of pathogenic organisms. The challenge of treating vaginitis in pregnancy is the necessity of making accurate diagnosis and treating correctly [2]. True infections (some of which can have dangerous effect on gestation) must be separated and distinguished from the exaggeration of physiologic discharge by pregnancy. Infection with bacterial vaginosis, *Chlamydia trichomonas* or Group B Streptococcus has been associated with septic abortion, premature rupture of membranes and premature delivery [2, 4].

2. Management of common causes of abnormal vaginal discharge in pregnancy

2.1. Vulvovaginal candidiasis

Vulvovaginal candidiasis (VVC) is a common cause of vaginal discharge worldwide [5, 6]. It is estimated that approximately 75% of women will experience an episode of VVC [7]. Candidiasis is caused by the fungus, *Candida* species. *Candida* species include *Candida albicans, Candida tropicalis, Candida pseudotropicalis, Candida krusei* and *Candida stellaloidea.* Other strains are *torulopsis, glabrata* and *rhodotromla. C. albicans* accounts for 60–80% of vaginal fungal infection [5–7], *Candida glabrata* accounts for 20% and *C. tropicalis* accounts for 6–23% [5]. Predisposing factors to VVC include pregnancy, diabetes mellitus, immunosuppressive therapy (cytotoxic drugs, steroids, etc.), antibiotics, oral contraceptives, immunodeficient conditions (HIV, cancer, chronic illness) and tight fitting and nylon undergarments [5]. Heat and moisture favour the growth of *Candida* species [8]. VVC can be sexually transmitted, and several studies reported an association between candidiasis and orogenital sex [7, 9].

http://dx.doi.org/10.5772/62599

C. albicans can be identified by culture from the vagina during pregnancy in approximately 25% of women [10]. While the prevalence of VVC in pregnancy in Zabrze of Poland is 42% [11], few studies in Africa reported the prevalence of 65% [12], 42% [13] and 23% [14] in Benin City of Nigeria, Addis Ababa of Ethiopia and Papua of New Guinea, respectively. Similarly, studies in India reported incidences ranging from 45% to 61% [15, 16].

Most patients with VVC will complain of vaginal discharge [5]. Dyspareunia, vulval pruritus and burning are the main symptoms [17]. Patients commonly complain of pruritus and burning after intercourse or upon urination. Erythema and oedema of the labia majora and minora and rashes on the perineum and thighs may be seen on physical examination, and a whitish, thick and curd-like vaginal discharge is usually present [17]. Recurrence requiring repeated treatment during pregnancy is likely [18].

The diagnosis is made on both clinical examination and laboratory identification of *Candida* by positive wet-mount test or potassium hydroxide (KOH) preparation [17]. In the wet-mount test, the spores and *Candida* are seen when vaginal discharge or scrapings from vulval lesions are mixed with normal saline and viewed under high-power magnifications. The presence of yeast blastospores or pseudohyphae can be detected in approximately 30–50% of patients with symptomatic VVC [17]. The addition of 10% KOH to the solution lyses white blood cells, red blood cells and vaginal epithelial cells, making the alkali-resistant branching budding hyphae of *Candida* easier to see[17]. Because vaginal pH usually remains normal in VVC, positive results from these two tests in combination with a normal vaginal pH are helpful in confirming the diagnosis. Most studies demonstrate that most of vaginal isolates are *C. albicans* [17]. Therefore, fungal cultures have not been used by most clinicians as part of the initial evaluation [17].

Various drug formulations are effective in treating both uncomplicated and complicated infections [10]. Both intravaginal and oral agents are available [10, 19]. Uncomplicated VVC includes sporadic or infrequent VVC, mild-to-moderate VVC, VVC with likely infecting agent being *C. albicans*, and non-immunocompromised patient. Complicated VVC is recurrent candidal infection or severe infection or non-albicans candidiasis (*C. tropicalis, C. glabrata*, etc.), VVC in uncontrolled diabetes mellitus, VVC with associated immunosuppression, VVC with debilitation or VVC in pregnancy [10]. Women who have four or more candidal infections during a year are classified as having complicated disease [9]. Intravaginal agents used in the treatment of VVC are 5 g of 2% butoconazole cream intravaginally for 3 days or 5 g (sustained-release) once; 5 g of 1% clotrimazole cream for 7–14 days or 100 mg tablet intravaginally for 7 days; 5 g of 2% miconazole cream intravaginally for 7 days or 100 mg suppository intravaginally for 7 days or 200 mg suppository for 3 days or 1200 mg suppository once; Nystatin 100,000 U tablet intravaginally for 14 days; 5 g of 6.5% tioconazole ointment intravaginally once; 5 g of 0.4% terconazole cream intravaginally for 7 days or 0.8% cream 5 g intravaginally for 3 days or 80 mg suppository intravaginally for 3 days. Oral agent is fluconazole 150 mg oral tablet once.

Prolonged local intravaginal therapy regimens and addition of oral fluconazole may be required to treat non-albicans VVC [7]. Fluconazole, 100–200 mg weekly for 6 months, is also the drug for prevention of recurrent VVC, whereas 600 mg boric acid gelatine capsule intravaginally daily for 2 weeks is useful in the management of non-albicans recurrent VVC [7].

2.2. Anaerobic bacterial infection and bacterial vaginosis

Vaginal flora of a normal asymptomatic reproductive-aged woman includes multiple aerobic or facultative species as well as obligate anaerobic species [9]. Of these, anaerobes are predominant and outnumber aerobic species approximately 10–1 [20]. These anaerobes include gram-negative organisms such as *Prevotella, Bacteroides, Fusobacterium* species, and *Veillonella* species and gram-positive bacilli such as *Propionibacterium* species, *Eubacterium* species and *Bifidobacterium* species [9, 20]. These anaerobic bacteria cause non-specific vaginitis [5].

Bacterial vaginosis is characterised by a shift from normal vaginal population of lactobacilli to anaerobes such as *G. vaginalis, Prevotella, Bacteroides* and *Mobiluncus* species and other bacteria such as *Mycoplasma* and *Ureaplasma* species [20]. It is one of the most frequent conditions encountered in reproductive health clinics throughout the world [20]. The condition had been previously called *Haemophilus vaginalis* vaginitis, non-specific vaginitis and *G. vaginalis* vaginitis [5, 21].

Bacterial vaginosis has been strongly associated with poor pregnancy outcomes such as preterm delivery and low birth weight infants, and several studies have now established the associations between bacterial vaginosis, human immunodeficiency virus and puerperal sepsis [20, 22].

Bacterial vaginosis appears to be particularly common in Sub-Saharan Africa where several studies have reported high prevalence rates, ranging from 20–49% among women presenting to STD clinics with vaginal discharge to 21–52% among pregnant women attending antenatal clinic [20]. These are very much higher than the rates reported from industrialised countries with 13% in the United Kingdom [23], 11% in London [20] and 15–30% in the United States [24].

Bacterial vaginosis usually occurs in sexually active patients. Some of the other risk factors include multiple sexual partners, low socioeconomic status, lesbians, presence of intrauterine device and prior STD [5]. It is still debatable whether it is sexually transmitted; however, supporting this is the recovery of *G. vaginalis* in the urethral of male partners [5].

Bacterial vaginosis is characterised by a malodorous, profuse, thin, homogenous yellow, white or grey discharge that is adherent to the anterior and lateral vaginal walls. Typically, the patient may complain of a fishy odour during or shortly after coitus and also during menses. The alkaline nature of blood or semen (pH > 7) brings about a transient increase in the vaginal pH, and this causes the release of amines, which the patient perceives as fishy odour. This typical discharge may be found on examination in some patients who in fact have not complained of a vaginal discharge [25]. The fishy smell of the discharge is the main problem and is often responsible for sexual disharmony between partners. Vulvitis and pruritus are very minimal or totally absent. Nearly half of patients with BV have no symptoms. Obstetric complications include premature rupture of foetal membranes, late miscarriage and postpartum endometritis, whereas pelvic inflammatory disease, post-hysterectomy cuff infection and postabortal sepsis are some of the gynaecological complications [25].

Diagnosis of BV can be based on the Amsel's clinical criteria or the microbiological Nugent's scoring technique [26, 27]. In Amsel's criteria, three of the following are required to diagnose BV: (1) homogenous vaginal discharge; (2) vaginal pH greater than 4.5; (3) positive Whiff test and (4) presence of clue cells on microscopy. The Nugent's method relies on the identification of categories of vaginal microflora based on quantitative assessment of a vaginal gram-stained smear. The Nugent's method has been extensively validated in industrialised countries where assessment of vaginal microflora is an important step in understanding the pattern of flora association with BV. Culture is the least accurate in making a diagnosis of BV as there is overgrowth of many vaginal organisms in this condition [5]. Though virtually, all patients with BV have *G. vaginalis* isolated on culture, it must also be noted that the organism can also be cultured in 40–50% of women with normal flora [5].

In pregnancy, BV should be treated with metronidazole 250 mg three times a day (alternatives; metronidazole 2 g single dose, clindamycin 300 mg twice a day; or metronidazole gel) [5]. The standard treatment of BV in non-pregnant women is oral metronidazole 500 mg twice daily for 7 days; clindamycin cream 2% on applicator ful (5 g) intravaginally at bedtime for 7 days or metronidazole gel one applicator ful (5 g) intravaginally once or twice a day for 5 days [5, 10, 28].

2.3. Trichomoniasis

Trichomoniasis is the commonest sexually transmitted disease worldwide [5]. It was originally thought to be innocuous but has now been found to be associated with preterm labour, premature rupture of membranes, increased perinatal loss and pelvic inflammatory disease (PID) [5, 29]. *T. vaginalis* can be identified during perinatal examination in as many as 20% of women [29].

T. vaginitis is caused by the trichomonas organism, which is a small, flagellated, motile and anaerobic protozoan. The particular trichomonad responsible for vaginitis is *T. vaginalis*, which is the type found in the vagina. Other trichomonads, which include *Trichomonas buccalis* found in the mouth and *Trichomonas hominis* found in the anal canal and rectum, are known but do not cause vaginal discharge because they cannot survive in the vagina. *T. vaginalis* has been demonstrated in the male urethra and prostate gland.

T. vaginalis is usually transmitted sexually. The organism may survive for several hours in urine, wet towels and even on toilet seats. The possibility of transmission by these routes had been suggested but not completely proven [5]. Incubation period is 4–20 days with an average of 7 days. Males are usually asymptomatic, but they can easily infect treated female.

The prevalence of trichomoniasis in pregnancy has been found to be 7.5–19% [14, 30]. A prevalence of 10.1% has been reported from the Gambia, West Africa [20].

The vaginal discharge of trichomoniasis is malodorous, frothy and profuse, thin creamy or slightly greenish and may cause itching. The classic yellow–green discharge is found in 20–50% of patients [5]; more often, the discharge is grey or white. The patient may also complain of dyspareunia, postcoital bleeding, pruritus vulvae, frequency of micturition and dysuria.

Characteristically, vulvitis is minimal or absent compared with candidiasis. On speculum exam, apart from the discharge, a cervical erosion may be seen, and in severe cases, multiple, small punctuate haemorrhages and swollen papillae may be found on the cervix ("straw berry" cervix) and vagina [17].

The vaginal pH is usually 5–5.5 in trichomonas infection [17]. Applying litmus to the unlubricated speculum after it has been withdrawn from the vagina easily tests the pH. A saline wet mount of the swab taken from the vagina or cervix will show motile flagellated protozoa and leucocytes. Wet mount alone detects 64% infection in asymptomatic women, 75% of those with clinical vaginitis and 80% of those with characteristic symptoms [5]. The use of culture (Feinberg-Whittington or Diamond culture) gives a sensitivity of 86–97% [5]. Pap smear has a detection rate of about 50–86% [5]. Monoclonal antibody staining is also used. It is sensitive and is reported to detect 77% of those missed on wet mount [5].

Metronidazole is effective in eradicating *T. vaginalis* administered orally in a single 2 g dose [5, 10]. Ootrimazole, which is both a fungicide and trichomonacide, can be used intravaginally usually in pregnancy in the same dosage regime as in candidiasis [5]. In persistent infection, it is best to treat the patient and her male sexual partner simultaneously.

2.4. Gonorrhoea and chlamydial infection

Chlamydia and gonorrhoea can both cause vaginal discharge in pregnancy and a major cause of morbidity among women in developing countries [31]. Both infections have been associated with pregnancy-related complications [32]. These two conditions are prevalent worldwide particularly in Africa [20]. They are a major cause of acute pelvic inflammatory disease, infertility and adverse pregnancy outcomes [20].

The prevalence of *Chlamydia* and gonorrhoea among pregnant women in Africa, in several studies, is between 6–13% [4, 33] and 2–8% [4, 34], respectively. According to the WHO, globally new cases of *C. trachomatis* infection have been estimated as 92 million, including 19 million in Sub-Saharan Africa [35–37]. In Maiduguri, North-eastern Nigeria, Amin et al. reported a prevalence of 9% [38].

Chlamydia is characteristically asymptomatic [39, 40]. About one-third of patients may have symptoms including mucopurulent vaginal discharge [5]. The role of *Chlamydia* in infertility is well documented [39–42]. Tubal pathology in *Chlamydia* infection is the cause of infertility in 10–30% of couples in developed countries and in up to 85% in developing countries [36, 37, 43, 44]. The main cause of tubal pathology is PID. Several different methods to diagnose chlamydial infection are available. Great studies have been performed in the areas of reliable methods of diagnosis [40, 45]. *Chlamydia* culture is considered as the gold standard because it has near 100% specificity [40, 45]. Because only viable infectious chlamydial elementary bodies are detected by culture, this is the method of choice for medico-legal issues. The disadvantages of culture include its low sensitivity and is that it depends on the laboratory inter-personal experience [46]. Non-culture methods include enzyme immunoassay (EIA), direct fluorescent staining with monoclonal antibodies (DFA), nucleic acid amplification tests (NAATs) and nucleic acid hybridisation techniques. In the management of chlamydial infection, both the patient and her infected sexual partner must be treated. It is, therefore, important to screen the sexual partners and treat those who are infected. With the advent of single-dose therapy, patients are now diagnosed and treated with the highest convenience and reliability [47]. Antimicrobial groups effective against *C. trachomatis* include the tetracyclines, macrolides, quinolones and penicillins [47].

Most women with gonorrhoea are asymptomatic [48]. When symptoms occur, they are localised to the lower genitourinary tract and include vaginal discharge, urinary frequency or dysuria and rectal discomfort. The incubation period is only 3–5 days [48]. The vulva, vagina, cervix and urethra may be inflamed and may itch or burn. Specimens of discharge from the cervix, urethra and anus should be taken for culture from the symptomatic patients. A stain of purulent urethra exudates may demonstrate gram-negative diplococci in leucocytes. Similar findings in a purulent cervical discharge are less conclusively diagnostic of *Neisseria gonorrhoea*. Gram-negative diplococci that are oxidase positive and obtained from selective media (Thayer-Martin or Transgrow) usually signify *N. gonorrhoea*. Carbohydrate fermentation tests may be performed, but in addition to being time consuming and expensive, they occasionally yield other species of Neisseria. Therefore, cultures are reported as presumptive for *N. gonorrhoea*. In addition, other techniques for detecting gonorrhoea include EIA for cervical swab or urine specimens, DNA probes for endocervical swabs and NAATs for endocervical swabs, liquid Papanicolaou specimens, vaginal swabs and urine specimens. Any patient with gonorrhoea must be suspected of having other STDs and managed accordingly. Treatment should cover *N. gonorrhoea*, *C. trachomatis* and incubating syphilis. Dual therapy has contributed greatly to the declining prevalence of *Chlamydia* infection. Therefore, if chlamydial infection is not ruled out, doxycycline (for non-pregnant women) should be added to ceftriaxone or azithromycin.

3. Outcome of study on abnormal vaginal discharge among pregnant women conducted in Maiduguri, Borno State in North-eastern Nigeria

3.1. Goal and objectives

The general objective of the study is to detect the clinical features associated with abnormal vaginal discharge and antibiotic sensitivity pattern of the causative microorganisms in pregnant women to improve the early diagnosis and prompt treatment. The specific objectives were as follows:

1. To determine the prevalence of abnormal vaginal discharge as a presenting complaint in pregnancy
2. To determine the frequency of bacterial causes of abnormal vaginal discharge in pregnancy and symptoms associated with it
3. To evaluate the sensitivity of microbial isolates from the vaginal discharge to antibiotics

3.2. Methodology

Borno State lies between latitude 10° and 14° north and longitude 14° and 45° east. It is located in the north-eastern part of Nigeria. Maiduguri is the capital city. The University of Maiduguri Teaching Hospital (UMTH) is a tertiary health institution and is the only functional teaching hospital in the north-eastern zone of Nigeria. The 2006 Nigerian provisional census puts the population of Borno State at 4,151,193 with 1,990,036 females [49].

It was a cross-sectional analytical study. The study population consisted of pregnant women presenting to the antenatal clinic with complaint of abnormal vaginal discharge while pregnant women without complaints of abnormal vaginal discharge attending the antenatal clinic of the hospital served as controls. A sample size of 800, consisting of 400 cases and 400 controls, was obtained using Taylor's and Kish's formulas [50]. Information on sexual and reproductive risk factors and symptoms was obtained. Vaginal examination was performed, and discharge was assessed. Endocervical and high vaginal swabs were collected and immediately processed in accordance with microbiological standard. Infection with *Candida* species was diagnosed by microscopy of a saline mount, which showed a highly refractile, round or oval budding yeast cells, and gram-stained smear of material from the vagina showed gram-positive pseudohyphae with budding yeast cells; *T. vaginalis* was diagnosed by microscopy of a saline mount for actively motile, spear-shaped flagellates, whereas bacterial vaginosis was diagnosed using Amsel's criteria [26]. *N. gonorrhoea* was identified by typical colonial morphology, reactions to gram stain, positive oxidase test and sugar fermentation. The antibiotic sensitivity of isolates was tested by the agar diffusion method on chocolate agar plates using oxoid multi discs with standard antibiotic concentration.

The computer program SPSS V 20.0 (2010) Inc., Illinois, United States was used to analyse the results; the association between organisms and studied variables was compared using chi-square (χ^2) and Fisher's exact tests while P value <0.05 was considered significant at 95% confidence level.

3.3. Results

During the period of study, 1280 pregnant women were seen at the antenatal booking clinic among which 800 satisfied the inclusion criteria. Four hundred of the pregnant women complained of abnormal vaginal discharge (cases), whereas 400 had no complaint of vaginal discharge, giving a prevalence of abnormal vaginal discharge in pregnancy of 31.5%.

Table 1 shows the clinical features associated with vaginal discharge in the study group. Vulval pruritus was present in 266 patients, and 200 (75%) of them complained of vaginal discharge, whereas 66 (25%) were in the control group. There was a significant association between pruritus and vaginal discharge ($\chi^2 = 1.011$, $P < 0.001$). As much as 63% of those without itching were in the control group. Dysuria showed statistically significant association with vaginal discharge ($\chi^2 = 44.008$, $P < 0.000$) with 74 (83%) of the 89 patients who complained of dysuria having vaginal discharge. There was no statistically significant association between dyspareunia and vaginal discharge ($\chi^2 = 2.082$, $P = 0.149$). The only patient that had vulval wart

http://dx.doi.org/10.5772/62599

complained of vaginal discharge, there was, however, no statistically significant association between vulval warts and abnormal vaginal discharge.

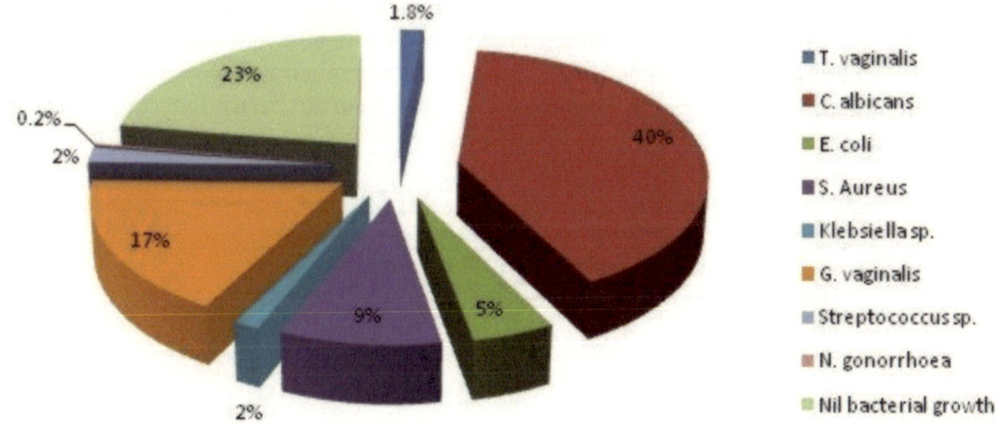

Figure 1. (Findings from culture of ECS/HVS from pregnant women with abnormal vaginal discharge (N=400)) shows outcome of culture and microscopy from vaginal discharge specimens collected from women with complaint of vaginal discharge. The prevalence of positive culture was 77% (308) among the cases and 21.3% (85) among the control group. Of the 400 patients with abnormal vaginal discharge, the commonest microorganism found was *C. albicans*, 160 (40%), whereas *N. gonorrhoea* infection was the least, 1(0.2%). *E. coli* was isolated in 20 (5%), *T. vaginalis* in 7 (1.8%), *Staphylococcus aureus* in 36 (9%), *Klebsiella* species in 8 (2%), *G. vaginalis* in 68 (17%) and *Streptococcus* species in 8 (2%) of the pregnant women. Samples from 92 (23%) patients had negative culture.

Feature		Case	Control	Total
1. Vulval itching	Yes	200 (75 %)	66 (25 %)	266
	No	200 (37 %)	334 (63 %)	534
$x^2 = 1.011$, $P < 0.001$				
2. Dysuria	Yes	74 (83 %)	15 (17 %)	89
	No	326 (46 %)	385 (54 %)	711
$x^2 = 44.008$, $P = 0.000$				
3. Dyspareunia	Yes	25 (61 %)	16 (39 %)	41
	No	375 (49 %)	384 (51 %)	759
$x^2 = 2.082$, $P = 0.149$				
4. LAT[a]	Yes	24 (60 %)	16 (40 %)	40
	No	376(49 %)	384 (51 %)	760
$x^2 = 1.684$, $P = 0.194$				
5. Vulval warts	Yes	1 (100 %)	0 (0 %)	1
	No	399 (49.9 %)	400 (50.1 %)	799
$x^2 = 1.001$, $P = 0.317$				

[a]Lower abdominal tenderness.

Table 1. Clinical features associated with vaginal discharge in the study group ($N = 800$).

Table 2 shows the association between the bacterial isolates and their antibiotic sensitivity patterns. *G. vaginalis* was sensitive to augmentin and ofloxacin in 64% of cases. *Streptococcus* sp. was most sensitive to augmentin and erythromycin in 92% (12/13) and 84% (11/13) of cases, respectively. *N. gonorrhoea* was sensitive to augmentin and ofloxacin in 100% of cases but was 100% resistant to other antibiotics. *E. coli* was sensitive to cefuroxime and gentamicin in 62% and 65% of cases, respectively. Most of the microbial isolates were resistant to ampicillin and norbactam. Only augmentin had greater than 60% sensitivity rate to all the isolated microorganisms.

Antibiotics	*S. aureus*	*Klebsiella sp.*	*E. coli*	*G. vaginalis*	*Streptococcus sp.*	*N. Gonorrhoea*
Amoxicillin	16.9	10.5	14.2	35.9	0	0
Augmentin[a]	86	61.5	75	64	92	100
Ofloxacin	75	55	12.5	64	25	100
Ciprofloxacin	64	51	25	9.2	22.5	0
Erythromycin	45	1.2	25	72	84	0
Cefuroxime	50	50	62	26	50	0
Gentamicin	61	64	65	21	30	0
Ampicillin	25	45.5	0	7.2	0	0
Norbactam	17.5	25	4.2	0	0	0

[a]Amoxicillin-clavulanic acid.

Table 2. Antibiotic sensitivity rate (%) of isolated bacteria.

4. Conclusion

Vaginal discharge in pregnancy is common, but distinguishing abnormal vaginal discharge from normal leucorrhoea of pregnancy is challenging. Since findings have showed that the trio of vaginal candidiasis, trichomoniasis and bacterial vaginosis are common causes of abnormal vaginal discharge in pregnancy; efforts must be made to exclude these conditions in pregnant patients presenting with vaginal discharge so that appropriate treatment can be instituted timely. Finally, gonococcal infection must also be excluded since though it is less prevalent than others, it is a major cause of morbidity in women in developing countries.

Author details

Sanusi Mohammed Ibrahim*, Mohammed Bukar and Bala Mohammed Audu

*Address all correspondence to: ozovehesan@yahoo.co.uk; smibrahim@unimaid.edu.ng

Department of Obstetrics and Gynaecology, University of Maiduguri Teaching Hospital, Maiduguri, Nigeria

References

[1] Witkin SS, Inglis SR, Polaneczky M. Detection of *Chlamydia trachomatis* and *Trichomonas vaginalis* by polymerase chain reaction in introital specimens from pregnant women. Am J Obstet Gynecol 1996; 175:165–167.

[2] Goldstein MS. Vaginitis. In: Chekry & Merkatz's complications of pregnancy. 5th edition. Edited by Wayne RC. Lippincott, Williams & Wilkins (Philadelphia) 2000: 47–54.

[3] Mayaud P, Mabey D. Approaches to the control of sexually transmitted infections in developing countries: old problems and modern challenges. Sex Transm Infect 2004;80:174–182.

[4] Sexton J, Garnett G, Rottingen JA. Meta analysis and meta regression in interpreting study variability in the impact of sexually transmitted disease on susceptibility to HIV infection. Sex Transm Dis 2005; 32:351–357.

[5] Agboola A. Vaginal discharge. In: Textbook of obstetrics and gynaecology for medical students. 2ndedition. Edited by Agboola A. Heinemann Educational Books Ibadan, Nigeria 2006:70–77.

[6] Kwawukume EY, Acquaah-Arhin R. Vulvovaginitis. In: Comprehensive gynaecology in the tropics. Edited by Kwawukume EY, Emuveyan EE. Graphic Packaging Ltd., Accra, Ghana 2005: 72–79.

[7] Sobel JD. Treatment of complicated *Candida vaginitis*, comparison of single and sequential dose of fluconazole. Am J Obstet Gynecol 2001; 185:363.

[8] Tricia EM, David LB. Benign disorders of the vulva and vagina. In: Current obstetrics and gynaecology diagnosis and treatment. 9thedition. Edited by Alan HD, Lauren N. Lange Medical Books, McGraw-Hill, NY 2003:651–670.

[9] Bradshaw CS, Morton AN, Garland SM, et al. Higher-risk behavioural practices associated with bacterial vaginosis compared with *Vaginal candidiasis*. Obstet Gynecol 2005; 106:105.

[10] Workowski KA, Berman SM, Centre for Disease Control and Prevention. Sexually transmitted diseases treatment guidelines. MMWR 2006; 55 (RR-11):1.

[11] Kazmierczak W, Wnek M, Kaminski K. Frequency of vaginal infections in pregnant women in the Department of Perinatology and Gynaecology in Zabrze. Ginekol Pol 2004;75: 932–936.

[12] Akende J, Abhitimen P, Okonofua F. Prevalence of asymptomatic genital infection among pregnant women in Benin City, Nigeria. Afr J Reprod Health 2002; 6: 93–97.

[13] Marai W. Lower genital tract infections among pregnant women: a review. East Afr Med J 2001; 78: 581–585.

[14] Klufio CA. Prevalence of vaginal infections with bacterial vaginosis, *Trichomonas vaginalis* and *Candida albicans* among pregnant women at the Port Moresby General Hospital Antenatal Clinic. PNG Med J 1995; 38: 163–171.

[15] Puri KJ, Mdan A, Benjal K. Evaluation of causes of vaginal discharge in relation to pregnancy status. Indian J Dermatol Venereol Leport [semal online] 2003; 69:129–130.

[16] Sobel JD. Vulvovaginal candidiasis. In: Sexually transmitted diseases. 3rd edition. Edited by Holwes KK, Mardh PA, Sparling PF, et al. Mc Graw Hill, New York 1999: 629–639.

[17] Omnia MS, Robert WH. Vulvovaginitis 2005. Retrieved from Emedicine.com. Updated 20 July 2005, accessed 11 November 2010.

[18] Sobel JD. Vulvovaginal candidosis. Lancet 2007; 369:1961.

[19] Bornstein J, Lakovsky Y, Lavi I. The classic approach to diagnosis of Vulvovaginitis: a critical analysis. Infect D Obstet Gynecol 2001; 9:105[PMID: 11495550].

[20] Edward D, Linda M, Maarten S. Bacterial vaginosis, vaginal flora patterns and vaginal discharge syndrome in the Gambia, West Africa. BMC Infectious Disease 2005; 12.DOI: 10.1186/1471-2334-5-12. Retrieved fromwww.biomedcentral.com

[21] Joharah MA. Patients with vaginal discharge: a survey in a University Primary Care Clinic in Riyadh City. Ann Saudi Med 2000; 20:3–4.

[22] Schmid G, Markowitz L, Koumans E. Bacterial vaginosis and HIV infection. Sex Transm Infect 2000; 76: 3–4.

[23] Morris MC, Rogers PA, Kinghorn GR. Is bacterial vaginosis a sexually transmitted infection? Sex Transm Infect 2001; 77: 63–68.

[24] Holzman C, Leventhal JM, Qlu H. Factors linked to bacterial vaginosis in non-pregnant women. Am J Public Health 2001; 91: 1664–1670.

[25] Edmonds DK. Benign disease of the vagina, cervix and ovary. In: Dewhurst's textbook of Obstetrics and Gynaecology. 7th edition. Edited by Edmonds DK. Blackwell Publishing, Oxford, UK 2007: 606–613.

[26] Amsel R, Totten PA, Spiegel CA, Chen KC, Eschenback D, Holmes KK. Non-specific vaginitis. Diagnostic criteria and microbial and epidemiologic associations. Am J Med 1983; 74:14–22. Retrieved from www.sfcityclinic.org

[27] Nugent RP, Krohn MA, Hillier SL. Reliability of diagnosing bacterial vaginosis is improved by a standardized method of Gram stain interpretation. J Clin Microbiol 1991; 29: 297–301. Retrieved from www.sfcityclinic.org

[28] American College of Obstetricians and Gynaecologists. Assessment of risk factors for preterm birth. Practice Bulletin 31, 2001.

[29] Wendel KA, Workowski KA. Trichomoniasis: challenges to appropriate management. Clin Infect Dis 2007; 44:S123.

[30] Fernandez LO. Prevalence of *Candida albicans* and *Trichomonas vaginalis* in pregnant women in Havana city by an immunologic latex agglutination test. Med Gen Med 2004; 6: 50.

[31] Maria R, Johanne S, Manonmany V. Chlamydia and gonorrhoea in pregnant Botswana women: time to discard the syndromic approach? BMC Infect Dis 2007; 7:27.

[32] Botswana Ministry of Health. Management of STI: reference manual for health workers. Gaborone, 2005.

[33] Wessel HF. Genital infections among ANC attendees in Cape Verde. Afr J Reprod Health 1998; 2: 32–40.

[34] Stum AW. Pregnant women as a reservoir of undetected sexually transmitted disease in rural South Africa: implications for disease control. Am J Public Health 1998; 88: 1243–1245.

[35] World Health Organization. Global prevalence and incidence of selected curable sexually transmitted infections - overview and estimates. WHO, Geneva 2001: 1–48.

[36] Family Health International. Preserving fertility. Network 2003; 23: 3–23.

[37] Okonofua FE. Female and male infertility in Nigeria. PhD Thesis. Karolinska Institute, Stockholm 2005.

[38] Amin JD, Zaria LT, El-Nafaty AU, Mai AM. Genital *Chlamydia trachomatis* infection in women in a Nigerian hospital. Genitourin Med 1997; 73: 146–147.

[39] Land JA, Evers JL. Chlamydial infection and subfertility. Best Pract Res Obstet Gynecol 2002; 16: 901–912.

[40] Manavi K. A review on infection with *Chlamydia trachomatis*. Best practice and research. Clin Obstet Gynecol 2006; 20: 941–951.

[41] Valentine A. Tubal damage in infertile women: prediction using *Chlamydia* serology. Hum Reprod 2003; 18: 1845–1847.

[42] Thomas K, Simms I. *Chlamydia trachomatis* in subfertile women undergoing uterine instrumentation. Human Reprod 2002; 17: 1431–1432.

[43] Okonofua F. Infertility and women's reproductive health in Africa (editorial). Afr J Reprod Health 1999; 3: 7–9.

[44] Omo-Aghoja LA, Okonofua FE, Onemu SO, Larsen U, Bergstrom S. Association of *Chlamydia trachomatis* serology with tubal infertility in Nigerian women. J Obstet Gynecol Res 2007; 33: 688–695.

[45] Ostergaard L. Microbiological aspects of the diagnosis of *Chlamydia trachomatis*. Best practice and research. Clin Obstet Gynecol 2002; 16: 789–799.

[46] Macmillan S, McKenzie H, Flett G, et al. Which women should be tested for *Chlamydia trachomatis*? Br J Obstet Gynecol 2000; 107: 1088–1093.

[47] Manavi K. A review on infection with *Chlamydia trachomatis*. Best practice &research. Clin Obstet Gynaecol 2006; 20(6): 941–951.

[48] Centres for Disease Control and Prevention. Sexually transmitted diseases, treatment guidelines. MMWR Rep 2002; 51(RR-6): 1.

[49] Federal Government of Nigeria. Report on 2006 census final results. Federal Government Printer Abuja 2009; 96: B39.

[50] Kish L. Survey sampling. J Royal Statist Soc 1969; 132(2): 272–274.

Section 2

Andrologic Genital Infections

Chapter 5

Genital Tract Infection as a Cause of Male Infertility

Nourhan Mesbah and Hosni Khairy Salem

Additional information is available at the end of the chapter

http://dx.doi.org/10.5772/62740

Abstract

Although infection is one of the preventable causes of human infertility, it is always missed or neglected. History of urethral discharge has been reported in about 45% of the black men attending the outpatient clinic with infertility complaint.

Implicated in this aspect is sexually transmitted disease (STD), including chlamydia, gonorrhea, and human immunodeficiency virus (HIV). Nonsymptomatic chronic prostatitis and seminal vesiculitis have been associated with poor semen quality and infertility. Infection may affect male fertility in different ways, including impairment of spermatogenesis, induction of autoimmune mechanisms, obstruction of the ejaculatory ducts, and dysfunction of the ejaculated sperms, decrease in the motility of the spermatozoa, and induction of reactive oxygen species (ROS).

In this chapter, the following points are discussed: 1. Types of genital tract infections that may cause infertility. 2. Prevalence of infection in infertile males. 3. Mechanism by which genital tract infection can cause infertility. 4. Fertility preservation by early diagnosis and treatment of STD. 5. Future perspectives.

Keywords: Infections, Urinary tract infections, Infertility in males, Sexually transmitted diseases, Chlamydia, Gonorrhea

1. Introduction

Infertility can be defined as a failure to conceive in a couple trying to reproduce for a period of 2 years of constant unprotected sex [1]. Of all sexually active couples, 12–15% is infertile [2]. Male component represents around 50% of the time either in isolation or in combination with a female factor [1, 3]. Infertility can be attributed to many causes. Infectious agents can interfere with the reproductive function in both sexes. Infections of male genital urinary tract account for about 15% of the case of male infertility. Different sites can be affected in the male reproductive system, such as the testis, epididymis, and male accessory sex glands. Spermatogenesis itself can be affected by urogenital infections at different levels of development, maturation, and transport of spermatozoa. These infections can be both sexually transmitted and nonsexually transmitted. Among the most common microorganisms involved in sexually transmitted infections, thus interfering with male fertility, are the *Chlamydia trachomatis* and *Neisseria gonorrhea*. Less frequently, male infertility may be due to nonsexually transmitted epididymo-orchitis, mostly caused by *Escherichia coli*. Infections of the lower genital tract seem to have little importance. However, such infections, as well as those involving other parts of the male genital urinary tract, may cause a microbial colonization of the semen [4].

2. Types of genital tract infections that may cause infertility

Epididymitis usually caused by gonorrhea, tuberculosis, chlamydia, urea plasmas, *Pseudomonas*, and coliform. Orchitis usually caused by mumps and tuberculosis. Tuberculosis and trichomoniasis are implicated in seminal vesiculitis. Urethritis usually caused by gonorrhea, chlamydiae, ureaplasmas, and trichomoniasis [5–10].

Many infectious organisms can affect fertility. These organisms include bacteria, viruses, yeasts, parasites, tropical infections, and other rare conditions.

2.1. Bacterial infections

Urethritis caused by *Neisseria gonorrhea* can affect fertility only if the testes were affected in rare situations. After the human immunodeficiency virus (HIV) epidemic in Western countries, more sexual precautions and hygiene were adopted, and this lead to marked decrease in the incidence of *N. gonorrhea* infection in the male genital tract [5].

Chlamydia trachomatis can affect both sexes but has a much greater impact on females than on males. Chlamydial infections may remain silent [6]. In men, *C. trachomatis* is the most common agent of nongonococcal urethritis, particularly serovars D and K and may cause epididymitis-orchitis, prostatitis, and sperm tract obstruction, in this way, impairing male fertility [7]. When *Chlamydia trachomatis* incubated with human spermatozoa in vitro, it seems to impair sperm motility, and cause premature death, perhaps as an effect of the chlamydial lipopolysaccharide [8]. There is evidence that an infection by trachomatis is related to the production of antisperm antibodies (ASA) that may affect fertility [9]. Also, an infected male partner, even if asymptomatic may transmit the infection to his female partner [10]. Also, results of human and animal inoculation studies support the notion that ureaplasmas are a cause of nonchlamydial and nongonococcal urethritis (NGU) in men [11]. According to a study, overnight incubation with *Mycoplasma* hominis can produce small but statistically significant differences in motility, morphology, and fertilization potential inhuman spermatozoa [12]. In addition, *Urea plasma urealyticum* is associated with the production of reactive oxygen species [13].

Escherichia coli are the most common cause of nonsexually transmitted epididymo-orchitis and are involved in the 65–80% of total acute or chronic prostatitis cases. *E. coli* may, therefore, be implicated in the genesis of infertility [14].

2.2. Viral infections

Adverse semen analysis parameters (poor sperm count and reduced motility) have been reported in infertile patients with positive herpes simplex virus (HSV) in semen. These adverse parameters were reversed after initiation of antiviral treatment [15].

Human papilloma virus (HPV) was found in testicular biopsies of azoospermic men, and when present inside sperm cells, they may be related to impaired sperm motility and asthenozoospermia [16]. It was found that there is an association between HPV and infertility, particularly between the presence of these agents and tubal factor infertility that cause a sort of infertility [16]. HIV may impair semen production by itself and certainly deteriorates the outcome of concomitant genital infections; in addition, the specific anti-HIV therapies can cause serious effects on the male reproductive system [17].

2.3. Fungal infections

Candida albicans commonly colonizes the urethra. It can be found in the semen and may affect in vitro fertilization. *C. albicans* has an inhibitory effect on human sperm motility and impairs the ultrastructure of human spermatozoa, which could be associated with male infertility [18].

2.4. Protozoa infections

Trichomonas vaginalis is a common parasite of the male genital tract. The organism can, in rare cases, cause a nongonococcal urethritis, prostatitis, and other genital tract disorders. Proteinases released by *T. vaginalis* can also inhibit sperm motility in vitro, even after the microorganism has been removed from the culture medium [19].

3. Prevalence of infection in infertile males.

Infections of male genital urinary tract account for about 15% of the case of male infertility. Different sites can be affected in the male reproductive system, such as the testis, epididymis, and male accessory sex glands. Spermatogenesis itself can be affected by urogenital infections at different levels of development, maturation, and transport of spermatozoa [3].

Leucocytospermia has been reported among 10–20% of infertile male patients. Twenty-five percent of patients with abnormal semen function have been proved to have antibodies to *C. trachomatis* [5–9, 20].

4. Mechanism by which genital tract infection can cause infertility

Infection may affect male fertility in different ways, including impairment of spermatogenesis, induction of autoimmune mechanisms, obstruction of the ejaculatory ducts, dysfunction of the ejaculated sperms, decrease in the motility of the spermatozoa, and induction of reactive oxygen species (ROS) [4–12].

5. Fertility preservation by early diagnosis and treatment of sexually transmitted disease

The organisms involved in sexually transmitted diseases (STDs) can be diagnosed nowadays with accuracy by the polymerase chain reaction (PCR) technique using the primer pairs that are specific for each organism. This gene amplification technology can amplify the DNA of the organism in any sample up to 1 million fold in few hours. The traditional approaches like the in vitro culture system or the DNA hybridization techniques are less accurate than the gene amplification technique [21].

6. Future perspectives

The preventative screening campaign can be effective in reducing the incidence of infection-related infertility. On the horizon, chlamydial and gonococcal vaccines may be seen in the near future [21].

7. Conclusion

Infectious agents can affect fertility in male. This can be done through different mechanisms. They can cause inflammation in different parts of male genital tract and affect sperm count, motility, and quality.

Author details

Nourhan Mesbah and Hosni Khairy Salem*

*Address all correspondence to: Dr_hosni@kasralainy.edu.eg

Faculty of Medicine, Cairo University, Cairo, Egypt

Different databases were used, including PubMed, Google Scholar, and Cochrane.

References

[1] Poongothai J, Gopenath TS, Manonayaki S. Genetics of human male infertility. Singapore Med J 2009; 50(4):336–347.

[2] Mosher WE. Reproductive impairments in the United States, 1965–1982. Demography 1985; 22:415–430.

[3] Tielemans E, Burdorf A, te Velde E, Weber R, van Kooij R, Heederik D. Sources of bias in studies among infertility clients. Am J Epidemiol 2002; 156:86–92.

[4] Wiser HJ, Sandlow J, Köhler TS. Causes of male infertility. In: Parekattil SJ, Agarwal A, editors. Male Infertility: Contemporary Clinical Approaches, Andrology, ART and Antioxidants. New York: Springer Science+Bussiness Media; 2012; 12–15.5.

[5] Hughes G, Fenton KA. Recent trends in gonorrhea an emerging public health issue? Eur Surveill 2000; 5:1–2.

[6] Wong T, Singh A, Mann J, Hansen L, McMahon S. Gender differences in bacterial STIs in Canada. BMC Womens Health 2004; 4:S26.

[7] Motrich RD, Cuffini C, Mackern Oberti JP, et al. Chlamydia trachomatis occurrence and its impact on sperm quality in chronic prostatitis patients. J Infect 2006; 53:175–183.

[8] Eley A, Passey AA, Galdiero M, Galdiero M, Galdiero F. Can Chlamydia trachomatis directly damage your sperm? Lancet Infect Dis 2005; 5:53–57.

[9] Witkin SS, Klingman I, Bongiovanni AM. Relationship between anasymptomatic exposure to Chlamydia trachomatis and an autoimmune response to spermatozoa. Hum Reprod 1995; 10:2952–2955.

[10] Eggert-Kruse W, Neuer A, Clussmann C, et al. Seminal antibodies to human 60 kDa heat shock protein (HSP60) in male partners of sub fertile couples. Hum Reprod 2002; 17:726–735.

[11] Taylor-Robinson D. Infections due to species of Mycoplasma and Ureaplasma: an update. Clin Infect Dis 1996; 23:671–684.

[12] Rose BI, Scott B. Sperm motility, morphology, hyperactivation, andionophore-induced acrosome reactions after overnight incubation with mycoplasmas. Fertil Steril, 1994; 61:341–348.

[13] Taylor-Robinson D. Mycoplasma genitalium—an update. Int J STD AIDS 2002; 13:145–151.

[14] Weidner W, Krause W, Ludwig M. Relevance of male accessory gland infection for subsequent fertility with special focus on prostatitis. Hum Reprod Update 1999; 5:421–432.

[15] Kapranos N, Petrakou E, Anastasiadou C, Kotronias D. Detection of herpes simplex virus, cytomegalovirus, and Epstein-Barr virus in the semen of men attending an infertility clinic. Fertil Steril 2003; 79:1566–1570.

[16] Martorell M, Gil-Salom M, Perez-Valles A, Garcia JA, Rausell N, Senpere A. Presence of human papillomavirus DNA in testicular biopsies from nonobstructive azoospermic men. Arch Pathol Lab Med 2005; 129:1132–1136.

[17] Gray GE, McIntyre JA. Effect of HIV on women.AIDS Read 2006; 16:365–368; 373–377.

[18] Tian Y-H, Xiong J-W, Hu L, Huang D-H, Xiong C-H. Candida albicans and filtrates interfere with human spermatozoal motility and alter the ultrastructure of spermatozoa: an in vitro study. Int J Androl 2007; 30:421–429.

[19] Schwebke JR, Burgess D, Trichomoniasis. Clin Microbiol Rev 2004 ; 17:794–803.

[20] Wolff H: The biologic significance of white blood cells in semen. Fertil Steril 1995; 63: 1143–1157.

[21] Oh MK, Richey CM, Pate MS et al: High prevalence of *Chlamydia trachomatis* infections in adolescent females not having pelvic examinations: utility of PCR-based urine screening in urban adolescent clinic setting. J Adolesc Health 1997; 21: 80.

Chapter 6

Decrease in Sperm Quality due to Infection of Human Papilloma Virus and *Chlamydia trachomatis*

María del Carmen Colín-Ferreyra, Maria Victoria Domínguez-García and Miriam V. Flores-Merino

Additional information is available at the end of the chapter

http://dx.doi.org/10.5772/63717

Abstract

Male infertility can have different causes, one of which may be the presence of etiologic agents that cause sexually transmitted infections. Among the most important sexually transmitted infections are human papillomavirus and *Chlamydia trachomatis*, which are associated with infertility in females – whether they cause infertility in men is controversial. The purpose of the chapter is to review the effect of these two pathogens on male fertility, the evidence suggests that the most important infertility effect is linked to the condition of the sperm. However, it is noteworthy that there are few studies with respect to infertility in regard to both pathogens, so it is important to further research this to elucidate the mechanisms by which these pathogens act on male infertility.

Keywords: Human papillomavirus, *Chlamydia trachomatis*, male infertility, sperm, infertility

1. Introduction

Sperm production is considered a complex process that can be affected by many factors, such as infections by viruses or bacteria. These may cause changes in motility, shape and sperm function. This chapter reviews the role of human papilloma virus (HPV), the bacterium *Chlamydia trachomatis* (*C. trachomatis*) single infections and co-infection by both pathogens in male infertility.

2. Human papilloma virus

HPV belongs to the family Papillomaviridae. Members of this family are small viruses of 45–60 nm in diameter with icosahedral capsid. This family includes more than 189 genotypes, which are distributed in 29 genera [1, 2]. The main features of human papillomavirus are listed in Table 1.

	Human Papillomavirus	*Chlamydia trachomatis*
Type of biological agent	Virus	Bacteria
Size	45-60 nm	200-400 nm
Morphology	Icosahedral capsid	Body elemental body and reticulum
Genotypes	189 genotypes	15 genotypes
Cellular position	Intracellular	Intranuclear
Clinic manifestations	Sexually transmitted infection Warts Nonspecific lesions Squamous intraepithelial lesions Cervical cancer and laryngeal Infertility	Sexually transmitted infection Trachoma Pelvic inflammatory disease Lymphogranuloma venereum Infertility

Table 1. Features Human Papillomavirus and *Chlamydia trachomatis*

The HPV genome consists of double-stranded DNA and is divided into three regions: the long control region (LCR), the early region (E), and the late region (L). Late proteins L1 and L2 code for capsid proteins [3, 4]. Region E is involved in the formation of non-structural proteins (E1–E7). E1 and E2 genes are involved in viral replication and transcription. E5, E6 and E7 genes encode proteins involved in oncogenesis related to HPV. E6 and E7 are involved in the viral transformation process, binding cellular proteins p53 and Rb, respectively, interfering with the cell cycle and inhibiting apoptosis [5].

The infection of HPV in both women and men may be asymptomatic or manifest itself in different forms: typical is the wart. However, atypical squamous intraepithelial lesions may culminate in the development of cancer. This has been studied particularly well for cervical cancer [5], leading to an increased investigation in this area. Because infection with this virus can be initially hard to detect it can allow progress to a chronic persistent infection or can cause changes in the infected cell disrupting the normal cell cycle. HPV is generally associated with cancer [6].

It has been established that genital tract infections have an effect on fertility, however, the effect of infection with HPV remains uncertain. It is recognized that HPV is one of the most common sexually transmitted infections in the world. There have been various studies that show a wide range in prevalence (from 1.4% to 44%) in the general population [7, 8]. Specifically it is reported to cause 16% infertility in men [9]. A review indicated that prevalence may be between 1.3% and 72.9% [10].

Moreover, male infertility is multi-factorial, including etiologic agents. The human papilloma virus has been identified as a possible cause of male infertility, but not all studies confirm the mechanisms by which this happens.

There have been controversial studies on the role of HPV on fertility. A study reported that in infertile couples only 7.8% were positive for DNA from HPV genotypes, however, in this study it was reported that it does not have an effect on semen quality [11]. Other studies show that HPV is reported in infertile couples.

Different studies have linked infection with HPV in men with different clinical symptoms such as: genital warts, anal or penile intraepithelial lesions and different types of cancer in different regions – penis, anus, prostate and urethra [12, 13]. It has been found that human papillomavirus could be infecting and persisting in different areas, such as the male accessory glands, penis, exfoliated cells, semen and sperm. Some research into these effects is referred to below.

In a study, it was reported that patients with accessory gland infection and HPV have been diagnosed with infertility. It was observed that there are significant changes in sperm quality. Particularly, there is a slight lower sperm motility, despite to have normal morphology, indicating that the co-infection could be an additional risk factor for infertility [14]. Moreover, infection has been observed in epithelial cells and exfoliated cells [15].

Studies in men showing persistent HPV (penis and semen samples) indicated higher levels in the penis (22.5 months) than in semen (15.3 months). This may demonstrate that men can transmit the disease to women despite being asymptomatic [16]. Different genotypes have been found in infertile men such as HPV-45, HPV-52, HPV-18, HPV-59 and HPV-16, which have been recognized as high-risk genotypes [11, 17]. It has been observed that HPV can infect both sperm and cell desquamation [18]. However, another study showed that sperm have low motility [19, 20].

Different techniques have been used in the diagnosis of HVP: *in situ* hybridization, dot blot, hybrid capture, real-time PCR, ELISA peptides, fused E6/E7 [21, 22, 23]; these methods have allowed a more accurate and timely diagnosis. The description of existing diagnostic methods is not discussed here, but it is important to mention that each has its own advantages and disadvantages – new technologies have become more accurate in diagnosis.

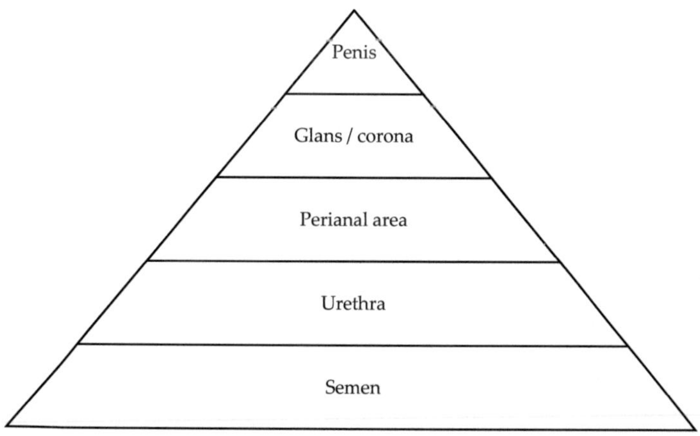

Figure 1. Pyramid showing the greatest location HPV in men, beginning with the penis at the top of the pyramid and the semen ending at the base of the pyramid.

Among the most studied area of HPV is the association with penile, larynx, head and neck cancers. It is estimated that HPV is the causative agent of 5% of human cancers [24].

In the review of Silva *et al.*, 2013 data show a prevalence in men, for different anatomical regions, in this order: penis, glans/corona, scrotum, perianal area, urethra and semen (Figure 1). This author also mentions that prevalence depends on the area, the technique used in detection and the geographical location of the patient [23].

3. *Chlamydia trachomatis*

In 1907, *Chlamydia* was first observed in the epithelium of a conjunctival scraping from an infected orangutan. This discovery is attributed to Halberstaedter and von Prowazek [25]. However, for years, trachoma was known as a blinding ocular disease in humans [26]. Although, Macchiavello reported the culture of trachoma agent in 1944, Tang and coworkers have the credit for their culture. The use of McCoy cells by Gordon and Quan was a major step to understanding chlamydial infections [27, 28]. Nowadays, it is well known that *Chlamydia trachomatis* is an intracellular pathogen and a gram-negative bacterium. In order to infect new cells, it must complete a bi-phasic developmental cycle. It contains approximately 1MB of DNA and 1000 open-reading frames (ORFs), which is considered a small genome [28]. The main features of *Chlamydia trachomatis* are listed in Table 1.

Chlamydia trachomatis can cause several clinical complications, especially in women. This bacteria not only affects the health of individuals in certain countries, it is a worldwide problem with high prevalence. For instance, it has been reported as the most common infection in the United States since 1994. The costs and the consequences of the *Chlamydia trachomatis* infection, make it a major health problem [27, 28, 29, 30]. In most cases it is asymptomatic leading to an untreated infection. It is reported that in approximately 50% of men and in 75% of women the primary infection does not show any symptoms [31]. However, it is estimated that the ratio of infected people with *Chlamydia* who develop symptoms vary depending on the study and the methodology. One major consequence in women is the pelvic inflammatory disease (PID), which is a cause of infertility. Also, there is the risk of passing the infection to the fetus in pregnant women [32, 33]. Main complications in women, which are the most affected, include: urethritis, endometritis and mucopurulent cervicitis. In men it can cause urethritis [29].

According to the World Health Organization (WHO), 101 million chlamydial infections are detected annually worldwide [34]. In adolescents and young adults between 12 and 24 years old the prevalence of *Chlamydia* is higher. For example, it was reported that in the United States the cases of *Chlamydia Trachomatis* were frequent in the young population (< 25 years old) [11]. Since young adults are in an age of sexual activity, it is a population with high-risk, therefore a higher susceptibility. In general, there are few data on the prevalence of *Chlamydia* in certain parts of the world. Most of the studies usually focus on some populations with small samples. For example, in a study carried out in Argentina (2015), 204 participants with an average age of 19 were screened for *Chlamydia trachomatis*. It was found that the prevalence was of 3.5% [31].

In Germany (2012) they studied a population of 1003 sexually active volunteers, they found a prevalence of 4.3% in women and 4.6 % in men [35].

As a mention before, *Chlamydia* can be a 'silent' infection. However, symptoms can appear after several weeks of the first exposure with the bacterium. Symptomatic infected men typically present a mucoid or watery urethral discharge and dysuria. An uncommon clinical signal is the development of epididymitis with unilateral testicular pain, tenderness and swelling. In women, some clinical signs include mucopurulent endocervical discharge, pyuria, dysuria and urinary frequency. If the infection spreads to the upper reproductive tract, the typical symptom is abdominal and/or pelvic pain, along with signs of cervical motion tenderness and uterine or adnexal tenderness on examination. It is worth mentioning that *Chlamydia* can also be found in the throats of women and men. Also, chlamydial conjunctivitis can be found in both men and women due to contact with infected genital secretions [28].

The effects of *Chlamydia trachomatis* infection in men have focused on semen parameters. However, the results of these studies have shown opposite outcomes. Some claim that there is not an association between the infection and the poorest semen quality. On the other hand, in some literature it has been reported that *Chlamydia trachomatis* affects semen quality. These contradictory results could be due to the different methodologies and techniques used, which can be difficult to compare [36, 37].

There are several methods available to detect *Chlamydia Trachomatis*. Cell culture is one of the traditional screening techniques to identify this pathogen. Briefly, this method consists of inoculate specimens (i.e., urethral swabs) in a monolayer cell culture. A stain is used to observe chlamydial inclusions. The specificity is 100%, however it can take up to 72 hours to observed sufficient viable microorganisms [38]. Recently, the molecular methods of detection have proved to be a useful tool in diagnosis. One of the first molecular methods was the *in situ* hybridization. However, this technique was not sensitive enough. Polymerase chain reaction (PCR) and ligase chain reaction (LCR) are useful to detect *Chlamydia trachomatis* infections in asymptomatic patients and populations with low prevalence [39]. Other methods include the identification of antibodies in serological samples. However, serological tests have several limitations, one example of these is that there is no specific *Chlamydia trachomatis* antibody test [40].

The most recent development is the real-time or quantitative PCR that detects *Chlamydia trachomatis* DNA copy numbers. The advantage of this method includes high sensitivity and specificity, also it is a less time-consuming method. It is very clear that there have been improvements in *Chlamydia* detection. However, there are still several challenges such as the creation of lower cost tests without sacrificing any accuracy or speed obtaining results [39].

4. Co-infection of HPV and *Chlamydia trachomatis*

It has been confirmed in different studies that HPV can be part of a co-infection with *Chlamydia trachomatis*. This is important since sexually transmitted diseases and there association with the development of cancerous and precancerous lesions has been shown in several studies. In Honduras, in women aged 18–35 years, the prevalence of *Chlamydia trachomatis* and HPV was found to be 6% and 28%, respectively; 19 genotypes were detected – proving to be the most common were HPV-5 and 11 [41]. In a previous study of our working group we found that of 77 patients with squamous intraepithelial lesions 13% had a co-infection with HPV and *Chlamydia trachomatis*; 46% only HPV infection and 13% only *Chlamydia trachomatis* infection [42].

In another study, it was found that patients with *Chlamydia trachomatis* and HPV had a prevalence of 74 %. However, only 13% of patients were negative to HVP and positive to *Chlamydia trachomatis* [43]. In the case of sexually transmitted infections *Chlamydia trachomatis* was found in 50% and HPV in 30% [44]. Other studies show that *Chlamydia trachomatis* infection is associated with multiple HPV genotypes and changes in signaling mechanisms in cancer and precancerous lesions [45, 46].

As mentioned in the above paragraphs the relationship between infection of HPV and *Chlamydia trachomatis* is confirmed, however, few studies exist regarding infertility in men with high prevalence. It has been found that men who have HPV present *Chlamydia trachomatis* 82.8% compared to a negative HPV of 17.2% [47]. In another study a prevalence of HPV in the semen of men with conjugal infertility was of 38.5 %, meanwhile the prevalence of *Chlamydia trachomatis* with HSV (types 1 and 2) was 9.6 % [48].

There are few studies showing the association of the two pathogens as co-factors with male infertility, however, there are multiple studies showing their coexistence, so it is important to know how each of these pathogens affects infertility.

5. HPV and *Chlamydia trachomatis* co-infection in the decrease of sperm quality

It has been written that the cause of infertility may be multifactorial and its etiology – viral and bacterial agents – is of particular interest because of its prevalence. HPV and *Chlamydia trachomatis* are common sexually transmitted infections that could be associated with infertility.

Infection with HPV has been identified as one of the possible causes associated with male infertility, although the mechanisms that may be using this virus are not yet clear. However, it was found that HPV can act both at conception and gestational development. Although there are different places where HPV may be infecting, as mentioned in the first section, the main concern linked to infertility is regarding the quality of sperm [18].

Other studies confirm this last statement which demonstrates a significant reduction in sperm motility while other parameters were not affected (semen volume, pH, normal morphology, viability, sperm concentration) [49] and cell desquamation. Sperm infected by HPV can go on to introduce the virus to the oocyte when being fertilized, which can have different consequences such as underdevelopment of the fetus. It has been observed that couples undergoing *in vitro* fertilization and abortion are at high risk of HPV from semen samples [18]. Therefore, diagnosis of HPV should be included in the diagnosis of infertility especially when considering cases of pregnancy loss [20] (Figure 2).

http://dx.doi.org/10.5772/63717

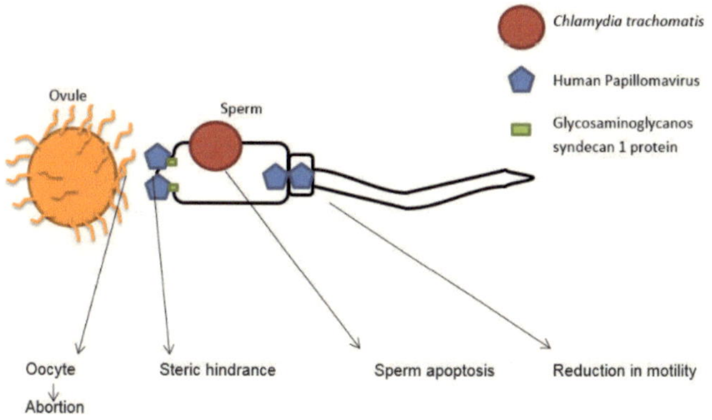

Figure 2. Effect of human papillomavirus and *Chlamydia trachomatis* in sperm

Currently, molecular techniques have detected HPV in different samples (i.e. semen, scrape of the epithelium in different parts of the masculine reproductive apparatus) in heterosexual men with a maximum prevalence of 21 % [50]. Another molecular technique, fluorescent *in situ* hybridization has allowed location of HPV on the sperm head and on the surface of sperm cells. The presence of the virus on the surface of sperm suggests that glycosaminoglycans, or soluble factors similar in chemical structure, could be involved in the binding of the sperm and HPV [49, 51]. Another study demonstrated that glycosaminoglycans syndecan-1 protein may be the unifying factor, particularly HPV L1 capsid protein because it has been unable to locate these two molecules in the sperm head [18]. We suggest that this may be a feature that explains infertility due to the fact that HPV on the head of the sperm, and on its surface, may prevent entry of the sperm to the egg because of steric hindrance since receivers can be occupied by HPV. On the other hand if fertilization is accomplished then infection of the embryo may occur. HPV in this manner could affect male fertility and that of the couple.

Despite this evidence understanding has not been achieved fully regarding the role of HPV in male infertility so the study of *Chlamydia trachomatis* as a co-factor was suggested.

With respect to *Chlamydia trachomatis* they have been reported in several studies as a major cause of female infertility [52, 53, 54]. However, male infertility has not been investigated as thoroughly.

Chlamydia trachomatis, as a sexually transmitted disease, is suggested as a factor that may be involved in the infertility of the couple. Recent studies have shown that *Chlamydia trachomatis* infection has shown an important role in chronic prostatitis [55] that could allow *Chlamydia trachomatis* to move to different areas of the male reproductive system allowing the infection to reach areas of sperm production.

It has been suggested that the cause of apoptosis of sperm is the lipopolysaccharide of the *Chlamydia* cell wall [56, 57] (Figure 2). This effect is even more serious because it would kill the sperm, preventing fertilization due to a lack of sperm, giving the bacteria a central role in male infertility.

There is little research studying the effect of these two infections as co-factors in regard to male infertility. In a study of men from Denmark it was reported that *Chlamydia trachomatis* infection may be a risk factor that allows the acquisition of an additional type of a genotype of HPV [57]. In a multivariate analysis, it was found that infection with *Chlamydia trachomatis* is significantly associated with HPV [59].

It is proposed that co-factors such as genital tract infections could have an important role in the evolution and outcome of HVP. For example, the association of HVP with *Chlamydia trachomatis* could be associated with increased risk of cervical cancer and with the reduction in cell mediated immunity [60]. This was reported in the cervix, but the same could be happening in the male reproductive system. Therefore, *Chlamydia trachomatis* infection could be a predisposing factor for the acquisition of HPV factor, which becomes more relevant if we consider that more than 50% of *Chlamydia trachomatis* infections are asymptomatic in men [61]. It has been observed that men with *Chlamydia trachomatis* infection are at increased risk of contracting an HPV infection [47].

In a study, it was found that heterosexual men, with prostatitis symptoms attributable to *Chlamydia trachomatis* and with papillomavirus had a lower motile sperm motility. Also, the morphology was lower compared with patients that were infected only with *Chlamydia trachomatis*. However, the results did not show any significant relationship depending on the HPV genotype presented [62].

Both HPV and *Chlamydia trachomatis* are sexually transmitted infections that have become important because of their prevalence, and it has been suggested that their association may be related to the development of other complications, as in the case of sperm quality.

In conclusion, the presence of *Chlamydia trachomatis* plays an important role in male infertility as well as sperm production and also facilitates entry of HPV, which contributes to a large degree the affectation of sperm. Therefore, HPV and *Chlamydia trachomatis*, and their associations, are two important pathogens that should be included in diagnostic tests for male infertility and the infertility of couples.

Author details

María del Carmen Colín-Ferreyra[1,2*], Maria Victoria Domínguez-García[2] and Miriam V. Flores-Merino[2]

*Address all correspondence to: mdcolinf@uaemex.mx

1 Centro de Investigación en Ciencias Médicas (CICMED), Universidad Autónoma del Estado de México Toluca, Estado de México, México

2 Facultad de Medicina, Universidad Autónoma del Estado de México, Toluca, Estado de México, México

References

[1] Bernard HU, Burk RD, Chen Z, *et al.* Classification of papillomaviruses (PVs) based on 189 PV types and proposal of taxonomic amendments. *Virology*. 2010; 401: 70–79. DOI: 10.1016/j.virol.2010.02.002

[2] De Villiers EM, Fauquet C, Broker TR, *et al.* Classification of papillomaviruses. *Virology*. 2004; 324: 17–27.

[3] Letian T, Tianyu Z. Cellular receptor binding and entry of human papillomavirus. *Virology Journal*. 2010; 7(2): http://www.virologyj.com/content/7/1/2.

[4] Horvath CA, Boulet GA, Renoux VM, Delvenne PO, Bogers JP. Mechanisms of cellentry by human papillomaviruses: an overview. *Virol J*. 2010; 20(7): 11. DOI: 10.1186/1743-422X-7-11

[5] Moody CA, Laimins LA. Human papillomavirus oncoproteins: pathways to transformation. *Nat Rev Cancer*. 2010; 10: 550–60.

[6] Muñoz N, Bosch FX, de Sanjosé S, Herrero R, Castellsagué X, Shah KV, Snijders PJ, Meijer CJ; International Agency for Research on Cancer Multicenter Cervical Cancer Study Group. Epidemiologic classification of human papillomavirus types associated with cervical cancer. *N Engl J Med*. 2003; 348(6): 518-27. PubMePMID: 12571259.

[7] Bosch FX, Lorincz A, Munoz N, *et al.* The causal relation between human papillomavirus and cervical cancer. *J Clin Pathol*. 2002; 55: 244–265.

[8] Dursun P, Senger SS, Arslan H, *et al.* Human papillomavirus (HPV) prevalence and types among Turkish women at a gynecology outpatient unit. *BMC Infect Dis*. 2009; 9: 191. DOI: 10.1186/1471-2334-9-191

[9] Laprise C, Trottier H, Monnier P, *et al.* (2014). Prevalence of human papillomaviruses in semen: a systematic review and meta-analysis. *Hum Reprod*. 29; 640–651. DOI: 10.1093/humrep/det453

[10] Dunne EF, Nielson CM, Stone KM, Markowitz LE, Giuliano AR. Prevalence of HPV infection among men: A systematic review of the literature. *J Infect Dis*. 2006; 194(8): 1044–57.

[11] Schillaci R, Capra G, Bellavia C, *et al.* Detection of oncogenic human papillomavirus genotypes on spermatozoa from male partners of infertile couples. *Fertil Steril*. 2013; 100(5): 1236–40. DOI: 10.1016/j.fertnstert.2013.06.042

[12] Petersen I, Klein F. HPV in non-gynecological tumors. *Der Pathologe*. 2008; 29(2): 118–22. DOI: 10.1007/s00292-008-1051-x

[13] Giuliano AR, Lazcano-Ponce E, Villa LL, Flores R, Salmeron J, Lee J-H, *et al.* The human papillomavirus infection in men study: human papillomavirus prevalence and type distribution among men residing in Brazil, Mexico, and the United States. *Can-*

cer Epidemiol Biomarkers Prev. 2008; 17(8): 2036–43. DOI: 10.1158/1055-9965.EPI-08-0151

[14] La Vignera S, Vicari E, Condorelli RA, *et al*. Prevalence of human papilloma virus infection in patients with male accessory gland infection. *Reprod Biomed Online*. 2015; 30(4): 385–91. DOI: 10.1016/j.rbmo.2014.12.016

[15] Foresta C, Pizzol D, Moretti A, Barzon L, Palù G, Garolla A. Clinical and prognostic significance of human papillomavirus DNA in the sperm or exfoliated cells of infertile patients and subjects with risk factors. *Fertil Steril*. 2010; 94(5): 1723–7. DOI: 10.1016/j.fertnstert.2009.11.012

[16] Capra G, Nyitray AG, Lu B, *et al*. Analysis of persistence of human papillomavirus infection in men evaluated by sampling multiple genital sites. *Eur Rev Med*. 2015; 19(21): 4153–63.

[17] Yang Y, Jia CW, Ma YM, Zhou LY, Wang SY. Correlation between HPV sperm infection and male infertility. *Asian J Androl*. 2013; 15: 529–32. DOI: 10.1038/aja.2013.36

[18] Garolla A, Pizzol D, Foresta C. The role of human papillomavirus on sperm function. *Curr Opin Obstet Gynecol*. 2011; 23(4): 232–7. DOI: 10.1097/GCO.0b013e328348a3a4

[19] Garolla A, Pizzol D, Bertoldo A, De Toni L, Barzon L, Foresta C. Association, prevalence, and clearance of human papillomavirus and antisperm antibodies in infected semen samples from infertile patients. *Fertil Steril*. 2013; 99(1): 125–31. DOI: 10.1016/j.fertnstert.2012.09.006

[20] Garolla A, Pizzol D, Bertoldo A, *et al*. Sperm viral infection and male infertility: focus on HBV, HCV, HIV, HPV, HSV, HCMV, and AAV. *J Reprod Immunol*. 2013; 100(1): 20–9. DOI: doi: 10.1016/j.jri.2013.03.004

[21] Cañadas MP, Lloveras B, Lorincz A, Ejarque M, Font R, Bosch FX, Silvia de Sanjosé. Evaluación de las técnicas de detección del VPH en los programas de cribado para cáncer de cuello uterino. *Salud pública de méxico*. 2006; 48(5): 373–378.

[22] Concha RM. Diagnóstico y terapia del virus papiloma humano. *Rev Chil Infect*. 2007; 24 (3): 209–214.

[23] Silva R, León D, Brebi P, Ili C, Roa JC, Sánchez, R. Diagnóstico de la infección por virus papiloma humano en el hombre. *Rev Chilena Infectol*. 2013; 30 (2): 186–192.

[24] de Martel C, Ferlay J, Franceschi S, Vignat J, Bray F, Forman D, *et al*. Global burden of cancers attributable to infections in 2008: a review and synthetic analysis. *Lancet Oncol*. 2008; 13(6): 607–15. DOI: 10.1016/S1470-2045

[25] Budai I. Chlamydia trachomatis: milestones in clinical and microbiological diagnostics in the last hundred years: a review. *Acta Microbiol Immunol Hung*. 2007, 54: 5–22. DOI: 10.1556/AMicr.54.2007.1.2

[26] Resnikoff, S, *et al*. Global data on visual impairment in the year 2002. *Bull World Health Organ*, 2004. 82: 844–51. DOI: 10.1590/S0042-96862004001100009

[27] Ripa KT. Microbiological diagnosis of Chlamydia trachomatis infection. *Infection*. 1982, 10: S19–S24. DOI: 10.1007/BF01640710

[28] Tan M and Bauvoil P. *Intracellular Pathogens I: Chlamydiales*. Washington, DC, USA: ASM Press; 2012.

[29] Torrone E, Papp J, Weinstock H. Centers for Disease Control and Prevention (CDC). Prevalence of Chlamydia trachomatis genital infection among persons aged 14-39 years--United States, 2007-2012. *MMWR Morb Mortal Wkly Rep*. 2014, 63: 834–838.

[30] Hogben M, Leichliter JS. Social determinants and sexually transmitted disease disparities. *Sex Transm Dis*. 2008, 35: S13–S8. DOI: 10.1097/OLQ.0b013e31818d3cad

[31] Occhionero M, Paniccia L, Pedersen D, *et al*. Prevalence of *Chlamydia trachomatis* infection and factors with the risk of acquiring sexually transmitted infections in college students. *Rev Argent Microbiol*. 2015, 47(1): 9–16. DOI: 10.1016/j.ram.2014.11.003

[32] Oakeshott P, Kerry S, Aghaizu A, *et al*. Randomised controlled trial of screening for Chlamydia trachomatis to prevent pelvic inflammatory disease: the POPI (prevention of pelvic infection) trial. *BMJ*. 2010, 340: c1642. DOI: 10.1136/bmj.c1642

[33] Paavonen J, Eggert-Kruse W. Chlamydia trachomatis: impact on human reproduction. *Hum Reprod Update*. 1999, 5: 433–47. DOI: 10.1093/humupd/5.5.433

[34] Geneva: World Health Organization; 2011. Global prevalence and incidence of selected curable sexually transmitted diseases: Overview and estimates. Centers for Disease Control and Prevention. Sexually transmitted disease surveillance 2011. U.S. Department of Health and Human Services, Atlanta, GA (2012)

[35] Fieser N, Simnacher U, Tausch y, *et al*. *Chlamydia trachomatis* prevalence, genotype distribution and identification of the new Swedish variant in Southern Germany. *Infection*. 2013, 41: 159–66. DOI: 10.1007/s15010-012-0301-2

[36] Samplaski MK, Domes T, Jarvi KA. Chlamydial Infection and its role in male infertility. *Advances in Andrology*. 2014, 2014:1–11. DOI: 10.1155/2014/307950

[37] Hosseinzadeh S, Eley A, Pacey A. Semen quality of men with asymptomatic chlamydial infection. *J Androl*. 2004, 25: 104-109. DOI: 10.1002/j.1939-4640.2004.tb02764.x

[38] Chernesky MA. The laboratory diagnosis of *Chlamydia trachomatis* infections. *Can J Infect Dis Med Microbiol*. 2005, 16(1): 39–44.

[39] Harkins AL, and Munson E. Molecular diagnosis of sexually transmitted *Chlamydia trachomatis* in the United States. *ISRN Obstet Gynecol*. 2011: 2011: 279149. DOI: 10.5402/2011/279149

[40] Johnson AM, Horner P. A new role for *Chlamydia trachomatis* serology?.*Sex Transm Infect*. 2008, 84: 79–80. DOI: 10.1136/sti.2007.028472

[41] Tabora N, Zelaya A, Bakkers J, *et al.* Chlamydia trachomatis and genital human papillomavirus infections in female university students in Honduras. *Am J Trop Med Hyg*. 2005; 73: 50–53.

[42] Colín-Ferreyra MC, Mendieta-Zerón H, Romero-Figueroa MS, Martínez-Madrigal M, Martínez-Pérez S, Domínguez-García MV. Expression of gamma interferon during HPV and Chlamydia trachomatis infection in cervical samples. *Enferm Infecc Microbiol Clin*. 2015; 33(2): 105–9. DOI: 10.1016/j.eimc.2014.05.014

[43] Tamim H, Finan RR, Sharida HE, *et al.* Cervicovaginal coinfections with human papillomavirus and *Chlamydia trachomatis*. *Diagn Microbiol Infect Dis*. 2002; 43: 277–281.

[44] Gopalkrishna V, Aggarwal N, Malhotra VL *et al. Chlamydia trachomatis* and human papillomavirus infection in Indian women with sexually transmitted diseases and cervical precancerous and cancerous lesions. *Clin Microbiol Infect*. 2000; 6: 88–93.

[45] Lehtinen M, Ault KA, Lyytikainen E, *et al. Chlamydia trachomatis* infection and risk of cervical intraepithelial neoplasia. *Sex Transm Infect*. 2011; 87: 372–376. DOI: 10.1136/sti.2010.044354

[46] Paba P, Bonifacio D, Di BL *et al.* Co-expression of HSV2 and *Chlamydia trachomatis* in HPV-positive cervical cancer and cervical intraepithelial neoplasia lesions is associated with aberrations in key intracellular pathways. *Intervirology*. 2008; 51: 230–234. DOI: 10.1159/000156481

[47] Alberts CJ, Schim van der Loeff MF, Papenfuss MR, da Silva RJ, Villa LL, Lazcano-Ponce E, Nyitray AG, Giuliano AR. Association of Chlamydia trachomatis infection and herpes simplex virus type 2 serostatus with genital human papillomavirus infection in men: the HPV in men study. *Sex Transm Dis*.2013; 40(6): 508–15. DOI: 10.1097/OLQ.0b013e318289c186

[48] Gimenes F, Medina FS, Abreu AL, *et al.* Sensitive simultaneous detection of seven sexually transmitted agents in semen by multiplex-PCR and of HPV by single PCR. *PLoS One*. 2014; 9(6): e98862. DOI: 10.1371/journal.pone.0098862

[49] Foresta C, Garolla A, Zuccarello D, *et al.* Human papillomavirus found in sperm head of young adult males a ▪ ects the progressive motility. *Fertil Steril*. 2010; 93: 802–6. DOI: 10.1016/j.fertnstert.2008.10.050

[50] Vardas E, Giuliano AR, Goldstone S, *et al.* External genital human papillomavirus prevalence and associated factors among heterosexual men on 5 continents. *J Infect Dis*. 2011; 203: 58–65. DOI: 10.1093/infdis/jiq015

[51] Pérez-Andino J, Buck CB, Ribbeck K. Adsorption of human papillomavirus 16 to live human sperm. *PLoS One*. 2009; 4: e5847. DOI: 10.1371/journal.pone.0005847

[52] Ghosh M, Choudhuri S, Ray RG, Bhattacharya B, Bhattacharya S. Association of genital Chlamydia trachomatis infection with female infertility, study in a tertiary care

hospital in Eastern India. *Open Microbiol J.* 2015; 9: 110–6. DOI: 10.2174/1874285801509010110

[53] Verweij SP, Kebbi-Beghdadi C, Land JA, Ouburg S, Morré SA, Greub G. Waddlia chondrophila and Chlamydia trachomatis antibodies in screening infertile women for tubal pathology. *Microbes Infect.* 2015; 17(11–12): 745–8. DOI: 10.1016/j.micinf.2015.09.019

[54] Steiner AZ, Diamond MP, Legro RS, *et al;*. Reproductive Medicine Network. Chlamydia trachomatis immunoglobulin G3 seropositivity is a predictor of reproductive outcomes in infertile women with patent fallopian tubes. *Fertil Steril.* 2015; 104(6): 1522–6. DOI: 10.1016/j.fertnstert.2015.08.022

[55] Mazzoli S, Cai T, Addonisio P, Bechi A, Mondaini N, Bartoletti R. Chlamydia trachomatis infection is related to poor semen quality in young prostatitis patients. *Eur Urol.* 2010; 57(4): 708–14. DOI: 10.1016/j.eururo.2009.05.015

[56] Eley A, Hosseinzadeh S, Hakimi H, *et al.* Apoptosis of ejaculated human sperm is induced by co-incubation with Chlamydia trachomatis lipopolysaccharide. *Hum Reprod.* 2005a; 20: 2601–2607.

[57] Sellami H, Znazen A, Sellami A, *et al.* Molecular detection of Chlamydia trachomatis and other sexually transmitted bacteria in semen of male partners of infertile couples in Tunisia: the effect on semen parameters and spermatozoa apoptosis markers. *PLoS One.* 2014; 9(7): e98903. DOI: 10.1371/journal.pone.0098903

[58] Kjaer SK, Munk C, Winther JF, Jørgensen HO, Meijer CJ, van den Brule. Acquisition and persistence of human papillomavirus infection in younger men: a prospective follow-up study among Danish soldiers. *Cancer Epidemiol Biomarkers.* 2005; 14(6): 1528–33.

[59] Shigehara K, Kawaguchi S, Sasagawa T, *et al.* Prevalence of genital mycoplasma, ureaplasma, gardnerella, and human papillomavirus in Japanese men with urethritis, and risk factors for detection of urethral human papillomavirus infection. *J Infect Chemother.* 2011; 17: 487–492. DOI: 10.1007/s10156-010-0203-0

[60] Castle PE, Giuliano AR. Chapter 4: Genital tract infections, cervical inflammation, and antioxidant nutrients-assessing their roles as human papillomavirus cofactors. *J Natl Cancer Inst Monogr.* 2003; 31: 29–34.

[61] Manavi K. A review on infection with Chlamydia trachomatis. *Best Pract Res Clin Obstet Gynaecol.* 2006; 20: 941–951.

[62] Cai T, Wagenlehner F.M.E, Mondaini N, *et al.* Effect of human papillomavirus and Chlamydia trachomatis co-infection on sperm quality in young heterosexual men with chronic prostatitis-related symptoms. *BJUI International.* 2013; 113: 281–287. DOI: 10.1111/bju.12244

Chapter 7

Microbial Infections and Male Infertility

Manonmani Samiappan and Poongothai Jayaramasamy

Additional information is available at the end of the chapter

http://dx.doi.org/10.5772/62895

Abstract

Microbial infections can happen on a daily basis. There are specific microbial infections that are associated with the reproductive health. Infertility is a devastating health problem. It is estimated that out of 15% of infertility worldwide, around 50% is due to male partner. Infections due to *Chlamydia trachomatis, Mycoplasma genitalium,* hepatitis B virus, tuberculosis, *Streptococcus faecalis,* and mumps are found to be associated with male infertility. Although most of the life-threatening microbial infections have dramatically declined since the introduction of the childhood vaccination program, there are concerns about few outbreaks and the associated risk of male infertility. This chapter deals with few microbial infections, their association with male infertility, prevention, symptoms, diagnosis, treatment, and control measures.

Keywords: Microbial infections, male infertility, genital infections, *Streptococcus faecalis, Chlamydia trachomatis, Mycoplasma genitalium*

1. Introduction

With enormous growth of population, India ranks second in world with 1.28 billion. Rather population growth is a major concern, yet infertility is a devastating health problem. According to World Health Organisation (WHO), infertility is the inability of the female partner to attain pregnancy after 1 year or more of the unprotected sex. Infertility affects about 15% of the couple of which half of the reproductive problems are associated with the male counterpart [1]. Many factors, including genetic causes, intoxication, microbial infections in genital tract, changes in lifestyle, stress, and the recent trend of late marriages, contribute to this occurrence. Table 1 highlights infertility due to male genital infections. Despite enormous progress in the understanding of human reproductive physiology, the underlying cause of male infertility remains undefined in about 50% of cases, which are referred to as idiopathic infertility [2, 3].

STD:*Chlamydia trachomatis* and ***Mycoplasma genitalium***
Urinary tract: *Streptococcus faecalis*
Orchitis: Small pox, mumps, measles, and tuberculosis
Damaging spermatozoa: Hepatitis B viral infection

Table 1. Male genital tract infections that may cause infertility

2. Rationale

Globally, 5.0–7.0% of the general male population was affected by infertility and the trend may increase in the future, considering the apparent decline of sperm count in industrialized countries [4]. Male infertility, a multifactorial complex disease, has been a source of concern in India lately. Recent statistics reports that the percentage of male infertility has elevated to 60% now against 40% in 1980s (New Indian express, 2015). The magnitude of the problem calls for urgent action, particularly when the infertility is avoidable in the majority of cases.

3. Causes of male infertility

Primary (when no pregnancy has ever occurred) and secondary (there has been a pregnancy, regardless of the outcome) infertility are the two forms of infertility. The former is found in 67–71% and latter in 29–33% of patients, respectively. Approximately 50% of the infertility is due to male of which 30% is due to male factors and 20% with both male and female factors. However, in approximately 30% of cases, the origins of reduced male infertility are unknown called as idiopathic. Male infertility has been associated with several genetic and nongenetic conditions.

3.1. Molecular genetics of male infertility

Genetic abnormalities, such as numerical and structural chromosomal abnormalities, were identified in men with unexplained oligozoospermia and azoospermia [5]. Chromosomal disorders, mitochondrial DNA (mtDNA) mutations, monogenic disorders, and multifactorial disorders are the genetic factors involved in male infertility.

3.1.1. Chromosomal disarrays

Renowned chromosomal abnormalities, such as Klinefelter syndrome (XXY) and specific translocations are well-documented causes of male infertility [6]. Point mutations in the androgen receptor and the cystic fibrosis transmembrane conductance regulator (CFTR) gene commonly associated with congenital vas deferens abnormalities are the two important gene defects conclusively associated with spermatogenic failure.[7]

3.1.1.1. *Y chromosome microdeletion*

Microdeletion of the long arm of the Y chromosome (Yq) is one of the prominent causes of male infertility. It was shown by 13% of azoospermic men, 1–7% of severely oligozoospermia men, and 5% of men with severe primary testicular failure and with a sperm density of less than 5 million/mL [6]. Recombination events between long stretches of highly repetitive DNA sequences during meiosis or early preimplantation development cause de novo deletions of Yq [8]. Intracytoplasmic sperm injection (ICSI), an artificial reproduction technique, may allow for the transmission of Y chromosome microdeletions to the next generation [9].

3.1.1.2. *Mutations in Mitochondrial DNA*

Mitochondria have their own genome, capable of producing many essential components of the respiratory chain, which in turn have a profound blow on sperm motility. Environmental and genetic factors may affect the quality and quantity of sperm production. Adenosine triphosphate (ATP) production by sperm mitochondria is essential because of the high demand of energy for these cells [10].

3.1.1.3. *Monogenic disorders*

Monogenic genetic disorders are an inherited disease controlled by a single pair of genes. Such disorders are inherited in a simple pattern according to Mendel's laws. Male infertility is associated with 50 monogenic disorders.

3.1.1.4. *Complex or multifactorial disorders*

Complex or multifactorial disorders result from mutations in multiple genes, often together with environmental causes. A mutation (C677T) in the gene, methylenetetrahydrofolate reductase (MTHFR), is known to increase susceptibility to various multifactorial disorders [11].

3.2. Nonheritable causes of male infertility

Nonheritable causes include **genital infections**, hypogonadotrophic hypogonadism, testicular maldescence, structural abnormalities of the male genital tract (obstruction of spermatic ducts, agglutination of sperm), impotency, previous scrotal or inguinal surgery, varicoceles, chronic illness, medication, exposure to chemicals, environmental factors, and immunological causes.

3.2.1. *Hormonal causes*

Fertility is questioned when endocrine system is affected on exposure to certain environmental compounds. Elevated concentrations of luteinizing hormone (LH) and follicle-stimulating hormone and low concentrations of gonadal steroids cause gonadal failure, a reason for infertility. In the male, elevated concentrations of LH can result from hypergonadotrophic hypogonadism (HH), which could be due to various reasons, such as primary testicular failure, seminiferous tubule dysgenesis (Klinefelter syndrome), Sertoli cell failure, and anorchia [12].

3.2.2. Hypogonadotrophic hypogonadism

Patients with this condition show decreased levels of gonadotrophins.

3.2.3. Erectile dysfunction

Of all males are affected by impotence or erectile dysfunction and can be emotionally and psychologically disabling for men and their partners; 80% of erectile dysfunction cases may be due to physical factors, such as drugs, blood flow abnormalities, nerve impulse abnormalities, and hormonal abnormalities. Remaining cases may be due to psychological factors and may be attributed to stress, performance anxiety, or misinformation about sexuality.

3.2.4. Previous scrotal or inguinal surgery

Gonorrhea and chlamydia cause acute inflammation of the scrotal contents (usually unilateral) in young men. Painless swellings in the scrotum are common. Most of these are small, round, epididymal cysts, or spermatoceles, and no investigation or treatment is required [13]

3.2.5. Varicocele

Varicocele, a condition of palpably distended veins of the pampiniform plexus of the spermatic cord, is the most common identifiable cause of male subfertility [14].Varicoceles feel like a bag of worms in the scrotum and can be associated with infertility [13]. "Subclinical varicocele" refers to a lesion too small to be detected by physical examination.

3.2.6. Exposure to chemicals

Various chemicals have been implicated as reproductive toxicants. Air pollutants are present in the blood, urine, and semen of exposed men and may affect sperm quality [15]. Sperm function tests have shown that high lead levels in semen samples reduce the ability of the sperm to bind to the egg and also to penetrate and fertilize the egg.

3.2.7. Environmental factors

Decreasing human sperm concentrations worldwide is alarming fact. Sperm morphology is affected by occupational heat exposure, which is a significant risk factor for male infertility, resulting in delayed conception. The male reproductive system is particularly vulnerable to the effects of the chemical and physical environment. This may be due to dramatic events or to endemic conditions of the environment, which involves industrial and agricultural pollution. Idiopathic male infertility may be due to exposure to environmental toxicants that alter the reproductive hormones, spermatogenesis, or sperm function. Semen quality has been shown to be altered on exposure to environmental ozone [16]. Environmental reproductive hazard studies report that sperm counts have declined in certain industrialized countries.

3.2.8. Immunological factors

Because immunological factors operate at almost every step in the human reproductive process, antibodies-induced damage to gametes is a major cause of immunological infertility.

Lifestyle and environmental factors [17], including smoking, can affect gamete, leading to subfertility/infertility

3.2.9. Genital infections

Acute and chronic genital tract infections are well-known causes of infertility in men. Most diseases of the reproductive system are sexually transmitted diseases (STDs), which lead to deterioration of spermatogenesis, impairment of sperm function, and/or obstruction of the seminal tract. Genital tract infections and antisperm antibody formation in men can lead to immune-mediated infertility in women [18, 19]. A strong association between inflammation of the male reproductive system and infertility has been reported [20, 21].

3.3. Sexually transmitted infection by *Chlamydia trachomatis* and *Mycoplasma genitalium*

3.3.1. Chlamydia trachomatis

It is well studied that chronic prostatitis (CP) due to *C. trachomatis* (CT) infection has a significant impact on a couple's reproductive health [22]. Tissue culture was an early method for the diagnosis of CT infection. In this method, bacterium was inoculated with specimen, such as urine, grown on cell monolayers. However, cell culture was too insensitive for noninvasive samples, such as urine and semen that were also found to be toxic to the growth and maintenance of the monolayer [23]. Molecular methods, such as in situ hybridization (ISH) and nucleic acid amplification testing (NAAT), were early methods used. NAATs were more effective in detecting asymptomatic chlamydial infection on noninvasive samples, such as urine. ISH was superseded once the NAAT become widely available. In-house, polymerase chain reaction (PCR) is the first test used to detect *C. trachomatis* in clinical samples during the development of NAAT. NAAT is more reliable because of its high sensitivity, whereas ample variation in the results was observed with in-house PCR [26]. Molecular methods, such as ligase chain reaction (LCR) and PCR, showed better sensitivities than nonmolecular methods, such as enzyme immunoassay (EIA) test or direct immunofluorescence (DIF), for detection of *C. trachomatis* antigen [25].

Alternatively, sperm can also be used as a sample for all molecular methods. In case of NAAT, an important issue to be considered in selecting semen as a test specimen is there are more NAAT inhibitors [25]. Another difficulty in using sperm as a sample is that during ejaculation, semen may become contaminated with elementary bodies in the urethra, and also the organism has the ability to adhere to sperm and is not always removed from sperm by density centrifugation prior to intrauterine insemination (IUI) or in vitro fertilization (IVF)/ICSI [25].

3.3.2. CT and male infertility

C. trachomatis can cause urethritis, epididymitis, and orchitis in men, and it is also found to affect sperm by decreasing sperm motility, deteriorating sperm morphology and viability and increasing proportion of sperm abnormalities. Nongonococcal urethritis (NGU) is the most common clinical genital syndrome seen in the male. Both acute and chronic infection can cause partial or complete obstruction of sperm transport (oligozoospermia or azoospermia). Chronic inflammatory changes in the seminiferous tubules in orchitis expected to disrupt the normal process of spermatogenesis and cause alterations in sperm number and quality [24].

Inflammation may act as a co-factor of infertility. Pressure-induced rupture of the epididymal duct will disrupt the blood–testis barrier, activate an immunological defense reaction, and induce the production of antisperm antibodies (ASA) [26]. Kokab et al. found that men infected with *C. trachomatis* had lower percent progressive sperm motility, a higher leukocyte count, and a raised concentration of interleukin (IL)-8 in semen compared with men without infection [26]. Mazzoli et al., 2010 [26] demonstrated that there is a correlation between *C. trachomatis* infection and some important sperm parameters, such as sperm concentration and motility. The attachment of *C. trachomatis* to human spermatozoa was first observed immunofluorescence tests and transmission electron microscopy. Sperm penetration tests revealed that spermatozoa, while progressing forward, can carry chlamydiae attached to them [26]. Chlamydial pathology may alter male fertility since male genital organs are potential targets for CT [28].

Numerous different causes have been observed to affect the sperm, including reactive oxygen species (ROS) generation and the induction of sperm apoptosis. Other causes include cigarette smoking, malignancies, elevated body mass index, insulin-dependent diabetes, drugs, and increasing male age [26].

3.3.3. Mycoplasma genitalium

MG is a member of Mollicutes class, which is of 0.3 μm in diameter and it lacks a cell wall. MG is one of the smallest self-replicating organisms usually present in the human genital tract [25]. In 1981, MG was first isolated from the urethra of two men with NGU. MG is considered as sexually transmitted infection (STI). Even though there is no STI symptoms associated with MG, there is a strong association found between risky sexual behavior and MG infection. It is also found to be strongly associated with area-level deprivation and ethnicity having high range of sexual risk behaviors. Sonnenberg et al [29] in 2015 reported high prevalence of MG infection in the United Kingdom at 2.1% in men aged 25–34 years, whereas in women, prevalence peaked at 2.4% in 16–19 years old and decreased with age.

3.3.4. MG and male infertility

It is suggested that 15% of male infertility is related to genital tract infection. The prevalence of MG in male of infertile couples found to be higher than normal. The impact of MG infection on male infertility remains unclear.

3.4. Urinary tract infection by *Streptococcus faecalis*

The incidence of oligozoospermia and teratozoospermia was significantly ($P<0.05$) higher in men whose semen samples contained *S. faecalis* [30]. *Enterococcus faecalis* are associated with poorer semen quality and may warrant treatment [31].

3.5. Hepatitis B viral infection leading to infertility

Hepatitis B virus (HBV) belongs to the class of Hepadnaviridae has a partially double-stranded DNA. HBV is 42 nm in size, and it contains a surface antigen called hepatitis B surface antigen (HBsAg) and the lipoprotein coat [49]. HBV found to be in the blood either in free form, which is predominate, or a viral particle bound protein form [32].

HBV infection is one of the threatening viral infections causing liver diseases in patients. According to Ocama *et al* (2005), approximately 2 billion people worldwide have been infected with HBV, and around 400 million live with chronic infection [33]. China, with a prevalence of 9%, has the highest rate of HBV infection in the world. The prevalence of HBV infections in the Netherlands is 2.2% in 184 men [34]. More than 300 million people in the world are affected with chronic HBV [35].

Hepatitis is an inflammation of the liver, initially recognized as an illness causing jaundice. There were two types of hepatitis: infectious/epidemic hepatitis and serum hepatitis. The HBsAg is responsible for serum hepatitis, which is an envelope protein present in HBV. Epidemic hepatitis is caused by hepatitis A virus (HAV). There are other viruses, namely hepatitis C virus (HCV), hepatitis delta virus (HDV), and hepatitis E virus (HDV) [36].

3.5.1. HBV and male infertility

Hepatitis viruses may cause diseases, which can be acute or chronic [37]. HBV antigens were detected in human semen [38], and it is well established that this biological fluid is a vector for the spread of HBV [39, 40]. There is an evidence that HBV can be transmitted via germ line [41]. The genital tract may act as a reservoir and this infection may get transmitted sexually.

HBV infection was found to be associated with reduced sperm function [42], instability of sperm chromosome, and impaired sperm viability and normal morphology. Recently, HBV DNA and RNA was detected in oocytes and embryos from HBV discordant couples, confirming the possibility of vertical transmission of HBV via germ line during IVF. However, the impact of HBV infection on pregnancy rate and live birth rate is still controversial.

3.6. Small pox, mumps, measles, and tuberculosis infections leading to infertility

Mumps is a condition caused by an RNA virus of the paramyxovirus group. In men, orchitis is the most common complication. Orchitis develops in 5–37% of all adult patients infected with mumps [43]. This causes testicular atrophy in 40–70% of patients with orchitis [44]. Orchitis can be unilateral or bilateral. Bilateral orchitis leads to oligospermia and testicular atrophy in 13% of those patients [45].

4. Symptoms, diagnosis and treatment of the infection

CP due to CT infection is found to have a significant impact on young male fertility. The main challenge in the chlamydial infection is up to 50% men have asymptomatic infection [46]. Many young people at risk for of CT infection may not seek sexual health care due to the asymptomatic nature of the bacterial infection [47]. HBV infection symptoms include nausea, anorexia, vomiting, flu-like complaints, fatigue, vasculitis, immune complex nephritis, and polyarteritis nodosa. There are approximately 5 % of adults (especially men) develop chronic HBV infection, which is often asymptomatic [32].

4.1. Diagnosis

MG can be found using real-time PCR technique or cell culture. MG culture is time consuming and slow process, and it requires cocultivation in Vero or equivalent cells [26]. Acute HBV infection has an incubation period of 6 weeks to several months. Most of the infected adults will show elevations in Alanine aminotransferase (ALT). Patients with acute HBV infection are mostly seropositive for anti-HBc-IgM antibody, and hepatitis B e antigen (HBeAg) marker correlates with high infectivity. The presence of antibody to HBeAg (anti HBe) shows a less infectious state and also HBV-DNA in serum or plasma indicates active HBV infection [50].

4.2. Treatment

Antibiotic therapy in the eradication of *C. trachomatis* infection does not always result in recovery of semen quality. Prulifloxacin is a drug used to treat patients with CP. Combination of antibiotic drugs and phytotherapeutic agents, such as FERTIMEV, can improve the clinical efficacy of prulifloxacin. l-arginine, l-carnitine, and acetyl-l-carnitine are found to be effective in increasing semen quality, can stimulate the activity of endothelial nitric oxide (NO) synthase, and can enhance sperm motility and function. NO synthase appears to be involved in sperm motility, metabolism, and capacitation. l-arginine in spermatozoa is a source of NO [29].

Based on Centers for Disease Control and Prevention and the Australasian Sexual Health Alliance, 1 g of azithromycin is generally recommended as standard treatment for MG due to its superior cell penetration efficiency. There is an association between MG organism load and azithromycin treatment failure [50]. However there is also an evidence of azithromycin, treatment failure is found due to macrolide resistance mutations. Single nucleotide polymorphisms (SNPs) in region V of the 23S rRNA gene of MG were found to be strongly associated with increased MICs to azithromycin in clinical isolates and treatment failure [28]. Moxifloxacin, doxycycline, gatifloxacin, and sitafloxacin are used as second-line treatment for MG [48]. However, its considerable expense and risk of serious adverse events, including hepatotoxicity, make this agent unsuitable for initial treatment. Recent study shows that single-dose azithromycin therapy is better than doxycycline therapy in the treatment of MG [51].

Lamivudine, one of the novel antiviral agents, is a deoxycytosine analog, which inhibits HBV DNA synthesis and suppresses serum HBV DNA levels in chronic hepatitis B (CH-B) patients. A significant enhancement in CD4-mediated T cell response to HBV nucleocapsid antigen was detectable after lamivudine treatment. One of the most effective treatments for CH-B is interferon (IFN) therapy [35].

Active vaccination is highly effective in preventing HBV infection. *Active prophylaxis* is a recombinant vaccine. Recombivax HB and Engerix-B are the commercial products available

[32]. Successful vaccination strategies have led to significant decrease in HBV prevalence [36]. In case of adult patients, 90% of them recover from HBV infection. However, 90% HBV-affected children ≤4 years of age develop chronic infection [32].

5. Conclusion

Microbiota refers to the microorganisms present in a particular site. Microbiota when is disrupted can cause infection on that site. Male genital tract infections are one of the reasons for male infertility, which can be prevented by proper sanitation. Proper precaution and awareness should be exercised among population.

Author details

Manonmani Samiappan and Poongothai Jayaramasamy*

*Address all correspondence to: poongothai_jp@yahoo.co.in

PSG College of Technology, Coimbatore, India

References

[1] Kim MJ, Choi HW, Park SY, Song IO, Seo JT, Lee HS. Molecular and cytogenetic studies of 101 infertile men with microdeletions of Y chromosome in 1,306 infertile Korean men. J Assisted Reprod Genet. 2012; 29 (6): 539–546.

[2] Ferlin A, Arredi B, Foresta C. Genetic causes of male infertility. Reprod Toxicol. 2006; 22(2): 133–141.

[3] Naito M, Terayama H, Hirai S, Qu N, Lustig L, Itoh M. Experimental autoimmune orchitis as a model of immunological male infertility. Med Mol Morphol. 2012; 45(4): 185–189.

[4] Plaseska-Karanfilska D, Noveski P, Plaseski T, Maleva I, Madjunkova S, et al. Genetic causes of male infertility. Balkan J Med Genet. 2012; 15: 31–34.

[5] handley AC. Chromosome anomalies and Y chromosome microdeletions as causal factors in male infertility. Hum Reprod 1998; 13: 45–50.

[6] McLachlan RI, Mallidis C, Ma K, Bhasin S, de Kretser DM. Genetic disorders and spermatogenesis. Reprod Fertil Dev. 1998; 10: 97–104.

[7] Dohle GR, Veeze HJ, Overbeek SE, et al. The complex relationships between cystic fibrosis and congenital bilateral absence of the vas deferens: clinical, electrophysiological and genetic data. Hum Reprod. 1999; 14: 371–374.

[8] Edwards RG, Bishop CE. On the origin and frequency of Y chromosome deletions responsible for male infertility. Mol Hum Reprod. 1997; 3: 549–554.

[9] Gazvani R, Lewis-Jones DI. Cystic fibrosis mutation screening before assisted reproduction. Int J Androl. 2004; 27: 1–4.

[10] Díez-Sánchez C, Ruiz-Pesini E, Lapeña AC, et al. Mitochondrial DNA content of human spermatozoa. Biol Reprod. 2003; 68: 180–185.

[11] Singh K, Singh SK, Sah R, Singh I, Raman R. Mutation C677T in the methylenetetrahydrofolate reductase gene is associated with male infertility in an Indian population. Int J Androl. 2005; 28: 115–119.

[12] Franchimont P, Heynen G, Reginster M, Denis F. [Calcitonin: nature, secretion, mechanism, therapeutic possibilities]. Brux Med. 1973; 53:719–727 (French).

[13] Richens J. Main presentations of sexually transmitted infections in men. BMJ. 2004; 328:1251–1253.

[14] World Health Organization. The influence of varicocele on parameters of fertility in a large group of men presenting to infertility clinics. Fertil Steril. 1992; 57: 1289–1293.

[15] Selevan SG, Borkovec L, Slott VL, et al. Semen quality and reproductive health of young Czech men exposed to seasonal air pollution. Environ Health Perspect. 2000; 108: 887–894.

[16] Sokol RZ, Kraft P, Fowler IM, et al. Exposure to environmental ozone alters semen quality. Environ Health Perspect. 2006; 114: 360–365.

[17] Benoff S, Jacob A, Hurley IR. Male infertility and environmental exposure to lead and calcium. Hum Reprod Update. 2000; 6: 107–121.

[18] Witkin SS. Production of interferon gamma by lymphocytes exposed to antibody-coated spermatozoa: A mechanism for sperm antibody production in females. Fertil Steril. 1988; 50: 498–502.

[19] Witkin SS, Chaudhry A. Circulating interferon-γ in women sensitized to sperm: new mechanisms of infertility. Fertil Steril. 1989; 52: 867–869.

[20] Comhaire F, Verschraegen G, Vermeulen L. Diagnosis of accessory gland infection and its possible role in male infertility. Int J Androl.1980; 3: 32–45.

[21] La Vignera S, Vicari E, Condorelli RA, D'Agata R, Calogero AE. Male accessory gland infection and sperm parameters (review). Int J Androl. 2011; 34: e330–e347.

[22] Cai T, Wagenlehner FME, Mazzoli S, Meacci F, Mondaini N, Nesi G, Tiscione D, Malossini G, Bartoletti R. Semen quality in patients with *Chlamydia trachomatis* genital in-

fection treated concurrently with prulifloxacin and a phytotherapeutic agent. J Androl. 2012; 33(4): 615- 623.

[23] Eley A. How to detect *Chlamydia trachomatis* in males? J Androl. 2011; 32(1): 391- 401.

[24] Rangel GJ, Avila GG, Gonzalez BR, Cuevas SA, Garcia AMM, Sanchez JJ, Maldonado ICM Garcia AN, Rodriguez JA, Martinez MO. The role of *Chlamydia trachomatis* in male infertility. 2012. Chlamydia, Mihai Mares (Ed.), InTech. ISBN: 978-953-51-0470-4. http://www.intechopen.com/books/chlamydia/the-role-of-chlamydia-trachomatis-in-male-infertility

[25] Eley A, Pacey AA. The value of testing semen for *Chlamydia trachomatis* in men of infertile couples. Int J Androl. 2011; 34: 391–401.

[26] Mazzoli S, Cai T, Addonisio P, Bechi A, Mondaini N, Bartoletti R. *Chlamydia trachomatis* infection is related to poor semen quality in young prostatitis patients. Eur Urol. 2010; 57: 708–714.

[27] Oberti JPM, Motrich RD, Breser ML, Cejas C, Cuffini C, Maccioni M, Rivero VE. Male rodent genital tract infection with Chlamydia Muridarum: persistence in the prostate gland that triggers self-immune reactions in genetically susceptible hosts. J Urol. 2011; 186: 1100-1106.

[28] Tagg K, Jeoffreys NJ, Couldwell DL, Donald JA, Gilbertb GL. Fluoroquinolone and macrolide resistance-associated mutations in *Mycoplasma genitalium*. J Clin Microbiol. 2013; 51(7): 2245–2249.

[29] Sonnenberg P, Ison CA, Clifton S, Field N, Tanton S,Soldan K, Beddows S, Alexander S,Khanom R, Saunders P, Copas AJ, Wellings K, Mercer CH, Johnson AM. Epidemiology of Mycoplasma genitalium in British men and women aged 16–44 years: evidence from the third National Survey of Sexual Attitudes and Lifestyles. Int J Epidemiol, 2015, 1982–1994. doi: 10.1093/ije/dyv194.

[30] Mehta RH, Sridhar H, Vijay Kumar BR, Anand Kumar TC. High incidence of oligozoospermia and teratozoospermia in human semen infected with the aerobic bacterium Streptococcus faecalis. Reprod Biomed Online. 2002; 5(1):17–21.

[31] Rodin DM, Larone D, Goldstein M. Relationship between semen cultures, leukospermia, and semen analysis in men undergoing fertility evaluation. Fertil Steril. 2003; 79(3):1555–1558.

[32] Gitlin N. Hepatitis B: diagnosis, prevention, and treatment. Clin Chem. 1997; 43:8(B): 1500–1506.

[33] Ocama P, Opio CK, Lee WM. Hepatitis B virus infection: current status. Am J Med. 2005; 118: 1413.

[34] Trum JW, Ben W, Pannekoek Y, Spanjaard L, Wertheim P, Bleker P, Veen F. Value of detecting leukocytospermia in the diagnosis of genital tract infection in subfertile men. Fertil Steril.1998; 70(2): 315–319.

[35] Boni C, Bertoletti A, Penna A, Cavalli A, Pilli M, Urbani S, Scognamiglio P, Boehme R, Panebianco R, Fiaccadori F, Ferrari C. Lamivudine treatment can restore T cell responsiveness in chronic hepatitis B. J Clin Invest. 1998; 102(5): 968–975.

[36] Lavanchy D, Kane M. Global epidemiology of hepatitis B virus infection. Hepatitis B virus in human diseases. Mol Transl Med. 2016; 187–203.

[37] Dejucq N, Je Gou B. Viruses in the mammalian male genital tract and their effects on the reproductive system. Microbiol Mol Biol Rev. 2001; 65(2): 208–231.

[38] Judson FN. Epidemiology of sexually transmitted hepatitis B infections in heterosexuals: a review. Sex Transm. Dis. 1981; 8: 336–343.

[39] Davidson AJ, Freeman SA, Crosier KE, Wood CR, Crosier PS. Expression of murine interleukin 11 and its receptor alphachan in adult and embryonic tissues. Stem Cells. 1997; 15: 119–124.

[40] Fagan EA, Alexander GJ, Davison F, Williams R. Persistence of free HBV DNA in body secretions and liver despite loss of serum HBV DNA after interferon-induced seroconversion. J Med Virol. 1986; 20: 183–188.

[41] Hadchouel M, Scotto J, Huret JL, Molinie C, Villa E, Degos F, Brechot C. Presence of HBV DNA in spermatozoa: a possible vertical transmission of HBV via the germ line. J Med Virol. 1985; 16: 61–66.

[42] Zhou XL, Sun PN, Huang TH, Xie QD, Kang XJ, Liu LM. Effects of hepatitis B virus S protein on human sperm function. Hum Reprod. 2009; 24: 1575–1583.

[43] Freeman R, Hambling MH. Serological studies on 40 cases of mumps virus infection. J Clin Pathol. 1980; 33: 28–32.

[44] Beard CM, Benson RC, Jr., Kelalis PP, Elveback LR, Kurland LT. The incidence and outcome of mumps orchitis in Rochester, Minnesota, 1935 to 1974. Mayo Clin Proc. 1977; 52: 3–7.

[45] Casella R, Leibundgut B, Lehmann K, Gasser TC. Mumps orchitis: report of a mini-epidemic. J Urol. 1997; 158: 2158–2161.

[46] Malhotra M, Sood S, Mukherjee A, Muralidhar S, Bala M. Genital *Chlamydia trachomatis*: an update. Indian J Med Res. 2013; 138(3): 303–316.

[47] Theunissen K, Hoebe C, Kok G, Crutzen R, Kara-Zaïtri C, Vries N, Bergen J, Hamilton R, Sande M, Dukers-Muijrers N. A web—based respondent driven sampling pilot targeting young people at risk for *Chlamydia trachomatis* in social and sexual networks with testing: a use evaluation. Int J Environ Res Public Health. 2015; 12: 9889–9906.

[48] Manhart LE, Jensen JS, Bradshaw C, Golden MR, Martin D. Efficacy of antimicrobial therapy for *Mycoplasma genitalium* infections. Clin Infect Dis. 2015: 61(8):802-817.

[49] Krajden M, McNabb G, Petric M. The laboratory diagnosis of hepatitis B virus. Can J Infect Dis Med Microbiol. 2005:16(2):65–72.

[50] Jensen JS, Bradshaw CS, Tabrizi SN, Fairley CK, Hamasuna R. Azithromycin treatment failure in *Mycoplasma genitalium*–positive patients with nongonococcal urethritis is associated with induced macrolide resistance. Clin Infect Dis. 2008; 47: 1546–1553.

[51] Walker J, Fairley CK, Bradshaw CS, et al. Mycoplasma genitalium incidence, organism load, and treatment failure in a cohort of young Australian women. Clin Infect Dis 2013; 56:1094–1100.

Section 3

Individual Genital Tract Microorganisms

Chapter 8

Microbiome, Infection and Inflammation in Infertility

Reza Peymani and Alan DeCherney

Additional information is available at the end of the chapter

http://dx.doi.org/10.5772/63090

Abstract

The implantation mechanism and process are very complex and require a precise interaction between the embryo and endometrium. The failure to implant is thought to be due to implantation environment factors or embryonic factors.

A suitable condition of the uterine cavity is essential for successful reproduction. Inflammation can be a part of the normal physiologic process during implantation; however, there are also pathologic sources of inflammation that can adversely affect the uterine cavity and endometrial receptivity.

Chronic Endometritis is usually asymptomatic and is defined histologically by the presence of plasma cells in an endometrial biopsy. It is mostly associated with the gonorrheal or chlamydial also non-sexually transmitted infections including E-coli, streptococcus, staphylococcus, enterococcus faecalis, mycoplasma, urea plasma and yeast. However, often a causal organism can not be identified.

Available evidence suggests that chronic subclinical endometritis is relatively common in women with symptomatic lower genital tract infections, including cervicitis and recurrent bacterial vaginosis and may not be altogether rare even in asymptomatic infertile women.

Mucopurulent cervicitis is highly associated with chlamydial and mycoplasma infections and both organisms, in turn, are associated with chronic endometritis, which likely plays a role in the pathogenesis of tubal factor infertility.

There is also a growing interest in the Microbiome of the reproductive tract. The Vaginal and Uterine Microbiome have been partially characterized and shown to be related to obstetric outcomes. Given the large number of unexplained IVF failures, it is reasonable to consider the uterine Microbiome and its impact on female fertility.

Although routine serologic testing, cervical cultures and endometrial biopsies may be difficult to justify, further evaluation and treatment are appropriate and prudent in infertile women with clinical cervicitis, chronic or recurrent bacterial vaginosis or other symptoms that suggest pelvic infection as well as in women with unexplained IVF failures.

Compared to culture-dependent methods, culture-independent methods are estimated to have increased bacterial detection in the uterine cavity by about 50% and increased number of detected species by up to fivefold. The detection of bacteria in the intrauterine cavity by PCR, in the absence of signs of infection, confirms the proposition of a non-sterile uterus.

This chapter will focus on chronic endometritis, uterine microbiome and hydrosalpinges and will review the diagnosis, pathophysiology and the recommended treatments of these specific inflammatory processes that contribute to implantation failure.

Keywords: Uterine Microbiome, Chronic Endometritis, Hydrosalpinges, Implantation Failure, Infertility

1. Introduction

1.1. Inflammation and implantation

Implantation has a complex and multistep process and mechanism, resulting in the blastocyst being embedded in the uterine endometrium, which is often viewed as the rate-limiting step for the in vitro fertilization (IVF) success. Implantation failure is related to either maternal factors or embryonic causes. Maternal factors include uterine anatomic abnormalities, thrombophilia, non-receptive endometrium and immunological factors.

Although uterine abnormalities are considered to have a relevant impact on the chances to conceive through IVF, conventional infertility investigations, based on ultrasound and hysterosalpingography (HSG), may miss subtle intrauterine lesions. Fatemi et al. demonstrated that the prevalence of unsuspected intrauterine abnormalities in hysteroscopy before IVF ranges from 11 to 45% accordingly, recent reports suggest that hysteroscopy in the cycle preceding ovarian stimulation, could be useful for patients with recurrent implantation failure (RIF). It is well established that the success of embryo implantation depends on embryo quality and uterine integrity, including endometrial receptivity.

Although embryo quality is the most consistent factor for predicting implantation and pregnancy rates in IVF patients, this cannot be evaluated independently from uterine integrity or endometrial receptivity [1, 2].

The definition of RIF remains controversial, generally being defined as failure to conceive following two or three embryo transfer (ET) cycles, or cumulative transfer of >10 good-quality embryos [3].

Patients with RIF comprise a heterogeneous group that presents with diverse clinical problems, and need a thorough evaluation.

Evaluation of a couple with RIF includes assessment of maternal and paternal karyotypes, testing for antiphospholipid antibodies, and thorough assessment of the uterine cavity, including sampling of the endometrial lining.

Endometrial biopsy is one inexpensive and minimally invasive method to assess and study the physical and hormonal endometrial environment. If abnormalities are identified and corrected, implantation rates can be improved.

Chronic endometritis (CE) is a persistent inflammation of the endometrial lining. Histologically, the diagnosis of CE is generally based on finding plasma cells, which infiltrates in endometrial biopsies [4]. CE is thought to be related to infertility and spontaneous abortion, and is mostly asymptomatic and rarely suspected clinically [2, 5, 6].

Implantation is believed to be a process with physiologic inflammation, involved with inflammatory mediators, such as leukocytes, chemokines and other pro inflammatory mediators [7].

The great effect of inflammation on implantation was shown in mice by the localized implantation defect after the blockade of the pre-implantation cellular influx into one of the two uterine horns [8]. There is also notable histologic [9] and biochemical [10] supports on the role of physiologic inflammation in labor at term.

The decidua in human uterus has a great number of immune cells such as macrophages [11], natural killer (NK) cells [12, 13], T cells [14] and stromal cells [15] capable to produce soluble factors (e.g., prostaglandins, chemokines and cytokines) involved in regulating the immune response [16].

Wegmann et al. [17], through the classification of T cells into two subgroups by their cytokine profile (Th-1 producing INF, interleukin (IL)-2, and Th-2 producing IL-4, IL-5), suggested that pregnancy takes place in the content of a predominant Th-2 response, and that increase toward Th-1 levels would decrease the chance of successful pregnancy [11].

Although the discovery of newer cytokines and complexity of the inflammatory response at the feto-maternal interface has increased the understanding of the role of specific cellular subtypes (e.g., dendritic cells, natural killer cells, and regulatory T cells) [16] on implantation and pregnancy, the evidence that a Th-1 response in the human decidua may lead to spontaneous abortion remains substantial.

Regardless of how the micro organisms and inflammation effect the implantation, one thing is clear: the cause, prevalence and results of subclinical infection and inflammation in the endometrium and their effect on pregnancy failure (infertility, implantation failure, spontaneous abortion, preterm birth) deserve great attention as a mechanism of pathology [12].

The presence of high concentrations of endotoxins (components of gram negative Bacteria) induces a reaction of TH1 inflammatory cells. TH1 cells may predispose a hostile endometrial environment and thereby cause implantation failure, spontaneous abortion or even premature labor. Endometritis is also considered to be an inflammatory reaction. In contrast to acute endometritis, in CE, usually no causal pathogen can be identified.

2. Chronic endometritis

CE is the continuous inflammation of the uterine endometrium. The prevalence of CE ranges from 0.8 to 19% in the general population and 0.2 to 46% in patients with infertility, based on the population type and the diagnostic criteria of the studies [18]. The pregnancy rate following one cycle of IVF/ET can be as high as 60%. However, even in the very successful units, some couples fail repeatedly. Failure could be due to many different factors, such as inappropriate ovarian stimulation, suboptimal embryo culture conditions and faults in ET techniques. CE is one of the pathologies, which can not be evaluated and diagnosed by HSG and ultrasound, since it is a subtle abnormality, which is usually asymptomatic or with only mild symptoms.

Kasius et al. demonstrated the histological detection of plasma cells (Figure 1) in the endometrial stroma as the gold standard for the diagnosis of CE. It is good to note that even histology can miss the diagnosis due to the normal presence of leukocytes in the endometrium, mostly prior to menstruation.

Matteo et al. [18] showed that CE may reduce endometrial receptivity and may cause infertility because the endometrium is characterized by an abnormal pattern of lymphocyte subsets and, consequently, an aberrant endometrial microenvironment.

In a recent study by Cicinelli et al in 2014 [29], it was demonstrated that in women with repeated abortions, CE is a frequent finding and that women who received adequate antibiotic treatment had a significantly higher rate of successful pregnancies compared with women who were not treated or with persistent disease.

Moreover, in a research study by Quaas and Dokras [109], CE was identified in 30.3% of patients with repeated implantation failure at IVF, and women diagnosed with CE had lower implantation rates (11.5%) after an IVF cycle.

2.1. Chronic endometritis and IVF

Although CE has been related to infertility and recurrent abortion, it is usually asymptomatic, and the diagnosis is rarely clinically suspected [13]. It has also been demonstrated that a present or a recent inflammation of the upper genital tract can affect uterine receptivity and be implicated in worse results in IVF and ET (IVF-ET) [19].

The uterine cavity and its receptivity, despite the constant progress in the assisted reproductive technologies, seem somewhat left behind [20]. ET and implantation are the stages of IVF procedures that have the highest failure rate, and it seems that endometrial abnormality is an important causative factor in this failure. Consequently, any endometrial abnormality should be detected and treated before an IVF-ET cycle to improve pregnancy rates [21].

Approximately, 8% of all couples seek for infertility treatment during their reproductive life. Although the frequency of infertility etiologically depends on the population studied, pelvic infections and their sequelae have been considered important causative factors. CE has been related to infertility and recurrent abortion, particularly because it could affect uterine receptivity and embryo implantation [22].

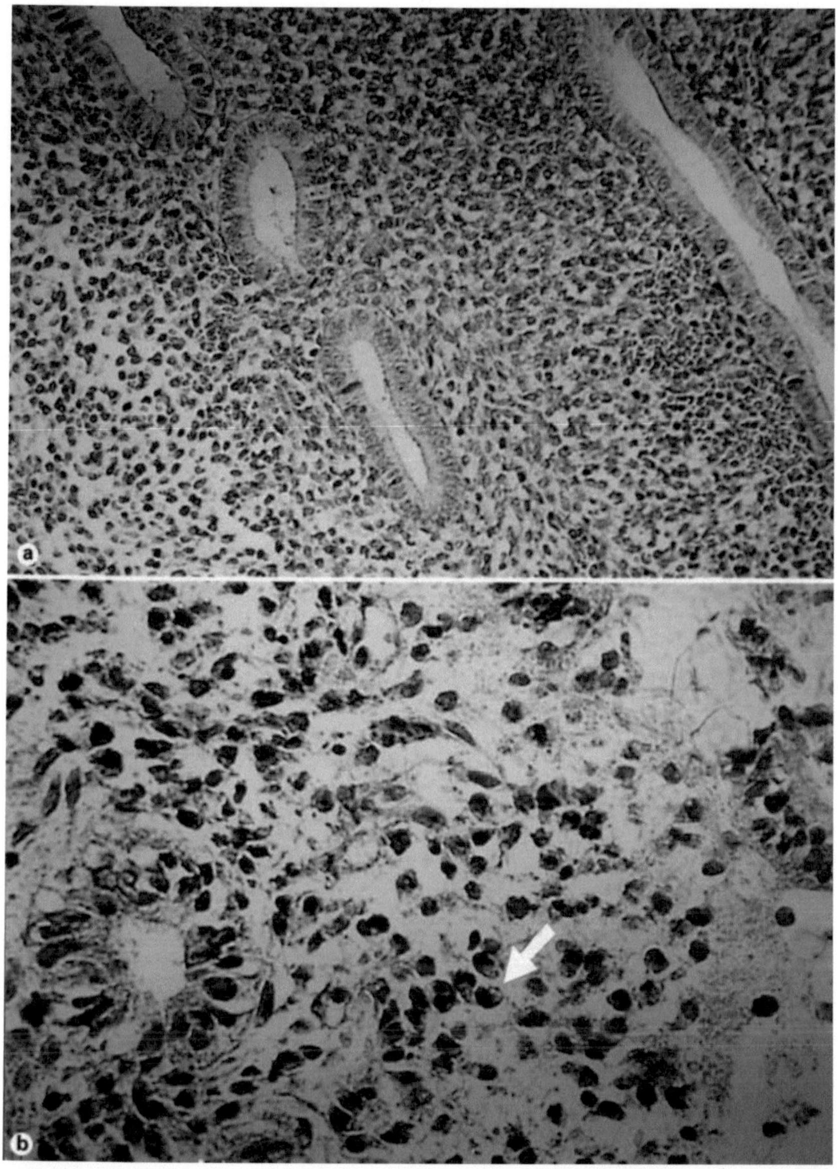

Figure 1. A. Photomicrograph of an endometrial biopsy specimen showing a proliferative endometrium. B. Photomicrograph of an endometrial biopsy specimen showing plasma cell endometritis (arrow).

A specific therapy is required in these cases; so it is important to have a reliable diagnostic test to detect the pathology. Endometritis causes specific stromal, vascular, and glandular modifications that can be detected by hysteroscopy.

Very few studies have investigated the value of diagnostic hysteroscopy in the detection of CE in infertile patients, and they failed in analyzing the real value of this method in these cases.

In evaluating the role of diagnostic hysteroscopy (Figure 2) in the detection of asymptomatic endometritis in infertile patients, a high negative predictive value (89.1%) is identified. This means that when the hysteroscopy shows a negative result for endometritis, it is highly probable that the result is correct and that the patient does not really have an endometrial inflammation.

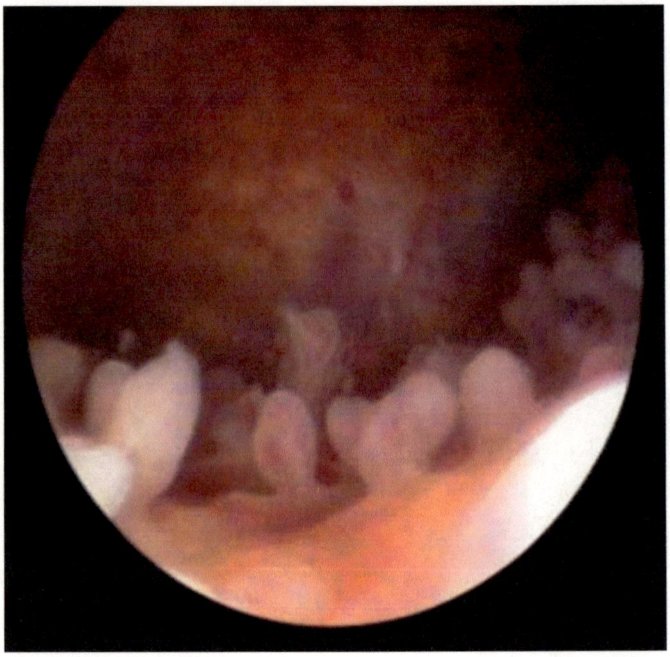

Reproduced with the permission from Cicinelli. Microorganisms and chronic endometritis. Fertil Steril 2008;89 (3).

Figure 2. Chronic endometritis at fluid hysteroscopy. Endometrial mucosa appears thick, edematous, hyperemic and covered by micropolyps (less than 1 mm size), which float into the uterine cavity.

If a diagnostic hysteroscopy shows the absence of endometritis, it is possible to assert, with a good margin of safety, that the patient does not exhibit an endometrial inflammation, which could hinder embryo implantation.

Hysteroscopy is also found to have a low positive predictive value in the detection of endometritis. This means that when the hysteroscopy shows a positive result for endometritis, it is better to consider that this could be an incorrect result and that the patient could have a normal endometrium.

Gump et al. [23] studied 204 infertile patients attending an infertility clinic, and all but 1 had negative cultures for *Chlamydia trachomatis* in cervical and endometrial specimens. These authors have found a significant correlation between prevalence of chlamydial antibodies and prior pelvic inflammatory disease (PID), as documented by HSG and/or laparoscopy. From these data, Gump et al. [23] concluded that antecedent infection caused by *C. trachomatis*, as measured by antibody prevalence, is an important factor in infertility of tubal origin, but they could not find infections in the cervical or in the endometrial specimens.

In conclusion, data suggest that hysteroscopy is not useful in the screening for CE in asymptomatic infertile women.

2.2. Chronic endometritis and recurrent miscarriage

Recurrent miscarriage (RM) is defined as three or more miscarriages before 20 weeks of gestation and it affects 3% of couples.

Genetic abnormalities, anti-phospholipid syndrome, endocrine disorders, and uterine abnormalities have been diagnosed in 50% of these couples. The other 50% are diagnosed as with unexplained RM. The competence of the uterine environment is an issue of big interest these days. The regular infertility investigations, such as HSG and ultrasounds, are unable to detect small intrauterine pathologies, and the prevalence of unsuspected intrauterine abnormalities in hysteroscopy has been shown to range between 11% and 45%.

In recent years, the focus on CE, a slight and mostly asymptomatic inflammation of the endometrial lining, is growing [24, 25].

A retrospective pilot study [26] showed a relationship between RM and chronic endometrial inflammation, which could have several clinical implications.

First, they showed that CE is a common finding in women with RM. Second, this study showed that mycoplasmas and the bacteria are the most frequently involved micro organisms in CE.

Third, the study demonstrated hysteroscopy as a reliable diagnostic technique for CE and that the previously noted endometrial pathologies [26, 27] such as micropolyps, stromal edema, and diffuse or focal hyperemia are clearly related to the inflammatory state of the endometrium. Moreover, results indicated an improved reproductive outcome and a normal hysteroscopic exam after an appropriate antibiotic treatment in patients with CE.

Fourth, the results showed a restored fertility status in women with CE after appropriate antibiotic treatment, suggesting the appropriateness of performing a hysteroscopy in women with RM.

Fifth, the sustained signs of CE in hysteroscopy after treatment, even with negative endometrial cultures, were related to a worse reproductive outcome.

Their results are in concordance with those from the PID Evaluation and Clinical Health (PEACH) study, which showed non-gonococcal, and non-chlamydial infection in approximately 60% of women with PID [28].

Considering the high prevalence of bacterial vaginosis and the fact that ascending bacteria can colonize the uterine cavity, those data are not surprising [29]. In fact, bacterial vaginosis has been associated with PID and, in ART, may decrease implantation rates, increase early miscarriages, and may also increase the risk of preterm labor [30]. This study suggested Mycoplasma and *Ureaplasma urealyticum* to be responsible for CE in about 24% of the cases.

This data do not disagree with the recent opinion that the uterine cavity is normally not sterile and that the presence of microorganisms does not mean inflammation [31–33]. Therefore, the main issue that causes the pathology is rather the interactions between the infectious agents and the endometrial environment than just the presence of infectious agents within the uterine cavity [30].

Fluid mini-hysteroscopy is a minimally invasive procedure that can be performed in an office without anesthesia [34], so the benefit in terms of evaluation, diagnosis and treatment sufficiently overcome the cost of hysteroscopy. The improvement of the reproductive outcome after both antibiogram-guided antibiotic therapy and the CDC guideline-based treatment supported the value of the hysteroscopic evaluation in women with RM.

Another important finding in the mentioned study data was that in the subjects with a negative endometrial culture, the ones with persistent CE diagnosed by hysteroscopy had a worse reproductive outcome compared to patients without CE in hysteroscopic evaluations after treatment. This shows that the hysteroscopic evaluation in patients with endometrial inflammation has a higher sensitivity than cultures and that a normal hysteroscopic evaluation could be more accurate in predicting of a successful pregnancy after treatment.

In conclusion, although some limitations are related to retrospective studies, in this study, Cicinelli et al, evaluating a large number of patients, demonstrated that CE is a condition commonly associated with RM. Mycoplasma and common bacteria were most prevalent microorganism for CE.

In women with RM, hysteroscopy reliably detects the existence of CE. The normalization of the hysteroscopic endometrial pattern seems to be associated with a significant improvement in the reproductive outcome [25].

In one study by Kitaya et al [36] using immuno-histochemical analysis of the stromal plasmacyte marker syndecan-1, CE was identified in approximate 10% of the women with RMs. In patients with RMs of unknown etiology, its prevalence was approximately 12-13%. It was lower compared with the reported prevalence (approximately 30%) in repeated embryo implantation failure after IVF-ET [35] and unexplained infertility [36]. All patients with CE had a history of RMs in the first trimester of pregnancy. Amassment of stromal B cells was observed in all the endometrium exhibiting CE. A flow cytometric study demonstrated that the proportion of B cells in endometrial mononuclear cells was threefold higher in the patients with RMs than in fertile women during the mid-secretory phase [37].

In addition, another morphometric study found that 2 of 22 patients with unexplained RMs had more endometrial B cells than any other patient or fertile woman in the mid-secretory phase [38].

2.3. Diagnosis

Most of the patients with CE are asymptomatic, which causes some diagnostic challenge.

http://dx.doi.org/10.5772/63090

The gold standard for diagnosis of CE remains the histopathologic evaluation of the endometrial biopsy specimen, which is through the identification of plasma cells in the stroma of the endometrium by immunohistochemistry [4].

This method of diagnosis is limited by

1. Inadequate sampling of the endometrium
2. Inadequate staining of the specimen
3. Dependency on the existence of plasma cells, that can be hard to localize
4. Confounding factors like fibrotic stromal cells that can mimic plasma cells
5. Unknown clinical significance of the presence of few plasma cells

Considering these limitations, physicians have studied the role of hysteroscopic evaluation of the endometrium to diagnose CE with mixed results. The suggested hysteroscopic findings for the diagnosis for CE have been mucosal edema, areas of hyperemia, and micropolyps [39].

A study by Yang et al in patients with RIF showed a sensitivity and specificity of 35% and 68%, respectively, for diagnosis of CE by hysteroscopy. In addition, hysteroscopic and histological evaluations resulted in identification of 66% and 44% of CE cases, respectively [39].

Proponents of hysteroscopy as a diagnostic tool for CE argue that hysteroscopy allows a complete evaluation of the uterine cavity, whereas the endometrial biopsy is a random biopsy of the uterine cavity and therefore may miss focal points of inflammation.

The isolation of infectious agents (common bacteria, *Neisseria gonorrhea, Chlamydia trachomatis, Mycoplasma* species, *Ureaplasma urealyticum* and yeast) from the endometrial cavity is the last method of diagnosis for CE. A study completed by Cicinelli et al showed that among 483 women with hysteroscopic-diagnosed CE, 73% had at least a single microorganism isolated from endometrial cultures vs. 5% in the control group [18].

Syndecan-1 (Figure 3) is a plasma cell, cell membrane marker. It has been broadly used to detect plasma cells in flow cytometry and is a useful marker to detect both malignant and benign plasma cells in paraffin-embedded bone marrow biopsies [40]. Syndecan-1 is a cell surface proteoglycan that facilitates cell to cell adhesion, cell to extracellular matrix adhesion, cell proliferation and migration [41].

Syndecan-1 expression was evaluated in CE and dysfunctional uterine bleeding. In all subjects with CE, plasma cells were noted by light microscopic study of both hematoxylin and eosin (H&E) and syndecan-1 dyed slides. Immunohistochemical staining with syndecan-1 increased the plasma cell detection. Plasma cells have characteristic "clock-face chromatin in an eccentrically placed nucleus with a perinuclear halo" appearance. This characteristic can be easily visible by syndecan-1 staining. This staining also showed that some plasma cells lacking some of the classic features, were actually plasma cells.

Identifying plasma cells in the endometrial stroma of CE can be very challenging.

Some conditions can present with the histologic findings of CE or affect the search for plasma cells. These conditions are early proliferative endometrium or late menstrual, monocytic

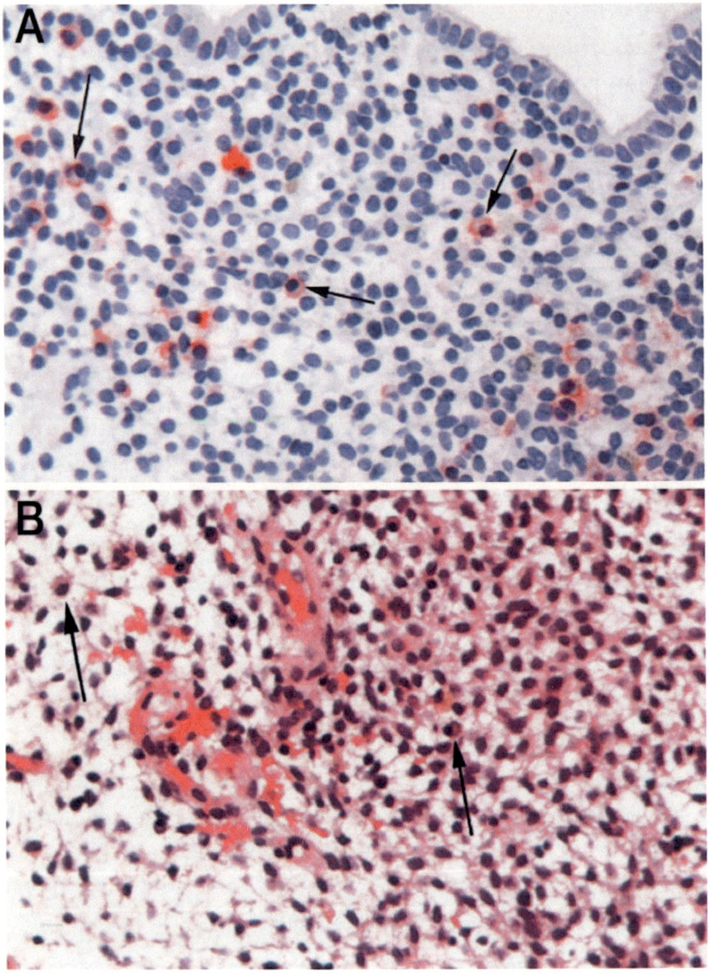

Figure 3. A. Plasma cells membrane staining with syndecan-1 in endometrial tissue showing a prominent spindle cell stromal component in chronic endometritis. B. H&E staining of the same field showing plasma cells.

inflammatory infiltrates, ample stromal mitoses, the plasmacytoid appearance of stromal cells, stromal cell proliferation or a marked pre-decidual reaction in a late secretory endometrium [4, 42].

This is notable that plasmacytoid stromal cells and macrophages do not stain with syndecan-1 and plasma cells can be recognized by immunohistochemical staining with syndecan-1 even in conditions that may interfere with their identification on H&E.

The search to localize plasma cells, in order to establish CE, does not always involve a quick examination of the specimen. It is usually a time-consuming task. Many times there are suspicious for CE, when plasma cells cannot be detected in H&E slides, and syndecan-1 immunohistochemistry staining helps in identifying the plasma cells and then the diagnosis of CE can be documented. Immunohistochemical syndecan-1 staining decreases the time consumption looking for plasma cells in patients suspicious for having CE, and will help the diagnosis in cases with other histological findings that can interfere with the detection of plasma cells.

It is of importance to mention that CE should not be the diagnosis when only mere number of plasma cells are detected, since endometrial stroma can contain limited number of plasma cells without an inflammatory process [43]. Only in the presence of a characteristic setting of CE, the diagnosis can be considered and the detection of plasma cells will be confirmatory.

In conclusion, syndecan-1 staining can be a great assistance and tool identifying the plasma cells and aid in the diagnosis of CE in patient with suspected CE when plasma cells can not be localized in H&E stained also when there are other histologic findings interfering the detection of plasma cells [44].

2.4. Pathophysiology

Studies characterizing the distribution of leukocytes in CE have noted an abnormal pattern of leukocytes. Not only the overall number of leukocytes rise, but also the accumulation of the leukocytes is superficial under the endometrial surface as well as around the superficial blood vessels and glands [4].

Plasma cells have been also identified in unusual locations, such as within the lumen of the glands or the intraepithelial [36]. It is believed that these plasma cells provide an abnormal local micro-environment, that decreases the endometrial receptivity.

Since plasma cells are in a minimal number in a healthy endometrial cavity, their presence in larger numbers in CE is considered pathologic. Immature B cells only normally express IgM immunoglobulins. Yet, when naïve B cell meets a particular antigen, a class-switch DNA recombination occurs, causing its differentiation into a plasma cell [45].

Based on the type of inflammatory response, plasmacells are able to produce a variety of immunoglobulins. The majority of the immunoglobulins in the endometrial cavity are IgM and IgA in the epithelial cells and IgG in the stromal cells.

The density of the Ig-bearing stromal cells, including IgM, IgA and IgG, is higher in patient with CE compared to people with normal healthy endometrium. Specially, IgG2 cells are noted to have an extremely higher density than other immunoglobulin subclasses in the endometrial stroma cells of the patients with CE [46]. This special Ig subclass expression is suggested to be a possible mechanism contributing to CE and implantation failure.

The role of matrix metalloproteinases (MMPs) is another interesting hypothesis contributing to inflammation, CE and implantation failure. Lately, a difference in the expression profile of several inflammatory cytokines has been demonstrated through endometrial gene expression studies in women with CE and infertility [47]. Endometrial stromal and epithelial cells by down-regulating the IL-11,could cause a dysregulation of trophoblast invasion. The noted significant decline in CCL4 in CE, may also increase the employment of NK cells and macrophages into the endometrial environment [48].

2.5. Treatment

Mostly due to non-standardized treatment protocols and conflicting results about pregnancy outcomes, so far the management of CE to increase in the implantation rate has been controversial.

Some authors recommend treating CE first with of doxycycline for 2 weeks, then with persistent inflammation in a second biopsy, and ciprofloxacin and metronidazole for another 2 weeks [49]. Some others base the treatment on the identified infectious agent and the antibiotic sensitivity profile, giving ciprofloxacin for gram-negative bacteria, amoxicillin/clavulanate for gram-positive bacteria, and wide spectrum antibiotics (metronidazole ceftriaxone, doxycycline) for even negative cultures [18].

In one study, a treatment of antibiotics plus steroid was used to treat women with increased MMP activity in uterine fluid lavage [48].

The efficacy of treatment of CE to increase endometrial implantation and pregnancy rate is unclear. In a cohort study, clinical pregnancy per embryo transferred and live birth rates showed no change between the treated and non-treated patients with CE undergoing their first IVF/ICSI cycles. Both groups underwent endometrial biopsy and hysteroscopy as part of a larger RCT [18].

Another study on RIF compared treated women with a positive biopsy for CE (10) to women with a negative biopsy (23). Even after antibiotic therapy, the implantation rates stayed lower in women with CE (11.5 vs. 32.7%) [49]. Cicinelli et al, in a recently published retrospective study of women with RIF, showed an improvement in pregnancy rates and live birth rates with antibiotic treatment in patient with CE compared with the patient with persistent CE, 65 versus 33% and 60.8 versus 13.3%, respectively [18]. To date, this is the only study showing a significant higher live birth rates after antibiotic therapy of CE. Although, it is good to note before generalizing these results as subjects in this research had hysteroscopic evaluation as a first diagnostic module for diagnosis of CE, which can be subjective. Also, instead of blastocyst-stage embryos, cleavage-stage embryos, were transferred, which may not be applicable to all practices.

2.6. Summary

Physicians mostly look for the diagnosis of CE, in cases of RIF; however, because the lack of a universally accepted definition for RIF indirectly biases the pool of patients who are worked up for CE. The diagnosis of CE becomes even more complex and difficult by limitations in microbiology and immunohistopatholog, and the subjective nature of hysteroscopy. Management of CE is also non-standardized. Taken all together, the absence of definitive evidence to establish improved pregnancy outcomes after the treatment of CE precludes establishing a standard of care [48].

3. Hydrosalpinges

Hydrosalpinx is defined as a chronic inflammatory condition in which a fallopian tube is filled with fluid as the result of distal obstruction.

PID caused by chlamydia or gonorrhea is considered as the primary cause of hydrosalpinx; however, other conditions that may cause tubal obstruction include adhesions from previous surgery, endometriosis, non-tubal infections (i.e., appendicitis, inflammatory bowel disease), salpingitis isthmica nodosa and pelvic tuberculosis.

The diagnosis rate of hydrosalpinges ranges from 10 to 13% by ultrasound, and up to 30% by laparoscopy or HSG [50]. Hydrosalpinges are documented in ultrasound as cystic elongated masses in the adnexa that can sometimes wrap around the ovaries [51].

There is some controversy for the definition of a "clinically significant hydrosalpinx," with some studies proposing that the diagnosis should be only made when hydrosalpinges are visible in ultrasound [52]. Findings of distal tubal occlusion on hysterosalpingogram would not qualify. Studies have shown low intra-observer reliability in detecting hydrosalpinges on HSG (kappa -0.28), when the intra-observer reliability for distal tubal obstruction was higher (kappa -0.71) [53]. This demonstrates the fact that hydrosalpinx and distal tubal occlusion are not synonymous conclusions.

A recent survey performed from members of the Society for Reproductive Surgeons and the Society for Reproductive Endocrinology and Infertility has highlighted the variation in clinical practice. The results showed that 60% of the members would make the diagnosis based on transvaginal ultrasound and 70% would make the diagnosis upon visualization of a dilated tube that is distally occluded on laparoscopy. However, commonly 80% of members would diagnose a hydrosalpinx based on a dilated tube that is distally occluded on hysterosalpingogram [54].

The presence of unilateral or bilateral hydrosalpinges has been shown to adversely affect implantation or pregnancy rates for IVF in different clinical studies. There were two main meta-analyses performed. The first meta-analysis included over 6,700 treatment cycles from 11 studies, which identified that the implantation rate and the clinical pregnancy rate were 50% lower in patients with hydrosalpinges compared to patients without hydrosalpinges. Miscarriage in patients with hydrosalpinges had also a twofold higher rate [55].

3.1. Pathophysiology

There are multiple hypothesis as to how hydrosalpinges can affect and predispose to implantation failure. These include a direct embryotoxic effect, [56] decrease in subendometrial and endometrial blood flow [57] decrease in endometrial receptivity, [50] possible developmental abnormalities of the endometrium [58] and tubal fluid, which can compromise the contact between the embryo and the endometrial surface as mechanical effect [59].

In a retrospective case-control study, inflammation and inflammatory markers in hydrosalpinges were investigated. This study evaluated 21 cases of hydrosalpinges and 9 cases of chronic salpingitis, and it was shown that the cases with hydrosalpinx were found to have an increase in inflammatory cells in the endometrium, including neutrophils and basophils. This correlation was statistically significant [60]. This case-control study showed that 65% of cases had high-intensity staining of IL-2, a marker for generalized inflammation, compared with only 7.4% in control group.

Inflammatory markers, especially Th-1 inflammatory cytokines, have been implicated in recurrent pregnancy loss, which is in favor of these markers playing a critical role in implantation failure [61]. In the presence of hydrosalpinx, similar to LIF, the expression of $\alpha v\beta 3$ integrins has been reported to be decreased [62] with an increase and return to normal levels following salpingectomy [63]. Integrins mainly play a role in cell-cell and cell-matrix adhesion and interaction in a variety of physiological processes, which include immune defense mechanisms and wound healing and should not be specifically considered inflammatory markers. Interestingly, $\beta 3$ integrins are cell-cycle-specific and are mainly expressed between cycle days 20-24, proposing the hypothesis that they might play a role during the window of implantation [64].

Poor outcomes have been seen with hydrosalpinx and the reasons are not clearly understood. The unfavorable effect seems to be directly related to the presence of a hydrosalpinx, rather than an embryo or oocyte factor.

Some investigators have researched the affect of the fluid from hydrosalpinx on the embryo and whether it has an embryotoxic effect or not and have determined that there might be an embryotoxic affect. On the contrary, recent studies have raised doubt about this toxin-induced effect. To further investigate this hypothesis, Strandell et al. [65] cultured human embryos in 50% hydrosalpinx fluid and realized that these embryos developed to blastocysts at the same degree as human embryos grew in a standard culture media.

The poor IVF outcomes seen in patients with a hydrosalpinx have been hypothesized to be related to tubal inflammation. A chronic inflammatory process can be present for multiple reasons. It could be observed with recurrent bacterial infections, including chlamydia, as a more common cause, or other bacteria. Acute inflammation can happen during an IVF procedure because of bacterial seeding of the hydrosalpinx during either ET or oocyte retrieval. As there is open communication between the tubes and the endometrium, the inflammatory process could directly spread from the fallopian tubes to the endometrium. The outcome of this process could then impact the development of the pre-implantation embryo and causes a change in the endometrial environment [66].

3.2. Treatment

The American Society of Reproductive Medicine has proposed that based on the clinical studies there is evidence that for every six women with hydrosalpinges, one more ongoing pregnancy will be successful if salpingectomy is performed prior to initiating IVF treatment [67].

A known approved alternative to salpingectomy for hydrosalpinges is laparoscopic proximal tubal occlusion.

A randomized control trial was performed to evaluate the efficacy of laparoscopic salpingectomy and laparoscopic proximal tubal occlusion in 115 patients with bilateral or unilateral hydrosalpinges undergoing IVF treatment. These women were randomized to three groups: two treatment and one control. The outcome in group with laparoscopic proximal tubal occlusion was better than control (no surgery) group and compared to the laparoscopic salpingectomy group [68].

In a recent meta-analysis of eight RCTs evaluating the efficacy of salpingectomy versus proximal tubal occlusion in hydrosalpinges, same results as above was achieved in which the implantation and clinical pregnancy rates were not significantly different between the treatments, odds ratio (OR), 0.86 (95% CI: 0.53–1.4) and OR, 1.56 (95% CI: 0.81–3.0), respectively [69].

The use of hysteroscopic Essure microinsert placements to occlude hydrosalpinges has been studied, mainly in women who have contraindications to laparoscopic procedure. The Essure system is a spring device composed of nickel–titanium and Dacron fibers. The Food and drug Administration (FDA) has approved the Essure system as a sterilization method. The device is space occupying, and can induce an inflammatory response that can cause fibrosis in the tubal lumen. To this date, the studies and literature on the use of Essure for occluding hydrosalpinges is limited to small case series with unclear outcomes and mixed results.

The first live birth from IVF using Essure, following proximal occlusion of a hydrosalpinx, was reported by Rosenfield et al in 2005. This was performed in a 31-year-old nulligravid woman with a history of significant pelvic adhesions and a body mass index of 50 [70]. This unfavorable surgical candidate delivered a dichorionic-diamniotic twins at 34 weeks of gestation after the transfer of three cleavage-stage embryos.

In a case series of 15 patients who underwent Essure placement, 6 were reported to have successful pregnancies. On the other hand, there are also reports of complications using the Essure device, such as unsuccessful placement of the device, subsequent expansion of the hydrosalpinx and PID, which could potentially require an emergency laparotomy and bilateral adnexectomy. There also seems to be a hypothetical concern for having the Essure coils in the uterine cavity [48]. Larger scale studies and prospective multicenter clinical trials should be performed before recommendations regarding hysteroscopic tubal occlusion can become part of standard of care in patients with hydrosalpinx.

Retrospective studies have shown that the larger the hydrosalpinx, the worse the outcome after IVF, which raises the question of embryo toxic effect of the fluid.

Whatever the exact mechanism, an interruption of the communicating hydrosalpinx appears appropriate to improve the implantation in the endometrial environment [71].

In a study performed by Hurst et al, patients with an increased quantitative serum *Chlamydia trachomatis* IgG antibody titer were considered for treatment with doxycycline 100 mg twice daily for a total of 10 days before the first IVF cycle was initiated. This group also included 75% of the patients who had hydrosalpinx. The outcome of the study, which was implantation and pregnancy rates, was slightly lower in the group with hydrosalpinx than in the control group; however, this difference was not statistically significant. In summary, patients treated with doxycycline for extended periods whom had hydrosalpinx did not have lower IVF success rates. On the contrary, the highest implantation rate was present in the group with hydrosalpinx [66].

An unfavorable effect of a hydrosalpinx could be caused by a chronic or acute tubal bacterial infection that could potentially affect the endometrium. This detrimental effect could be suppressed and become ineffective by using extended antibiotic therapy. In addition, healthcare cost can be prevented and minimized if initiating treatment with a 2-week course of an inexpensive antibiotic provides the same outcome comparable to surgical treatment of a hydrosalpinx prior to IVF treatment.

4. Salpingectomy

Studies have shown that patients with hydrosalpinx visible by ultrasound, are generally the ones that benefit from salpingectomy. As a result, this group of patients are the ones who are recommended to perform prophylactic salpingectomy prior to IVF treatment.

The psychological impact of this surgery and the removal of the tubes in an infertile patient are significantly important and should be emphasized. Even if a patient has a clear candidate for salpingectomy, it is essential that she is psychologically prepared for the procedure. At times, it has been necessary for the patient to undergo a few failed cycles before one can bring up the discussion of surgery and salpingectomy. Obviously, the final decision to perform salpingectomy should be based on appropriate evaluation of the tubal mucosa at laparoscopy and therefore avoid unnecessary surgery for the patient. It is crucial that surgeons identify carefully that whether a hydrosalpinx should be excised or is acceptable enough for a surgical repair [71].

4.1. Tubal ligation vs. salpingectomy

There are no results from randomized trials to answer this question. The data from two retrospective studies by Surrey/Schoolcraft [77], did not show any significant differences in pregnancy outcome, but the number of patients has been too low to allow for any conclusion. Today, there is no evidence that transvaginal aspiration is as effective as salpingectomy, but it is an option for patients who will not undergo salpingectomy, and for those who develop tubal fluid during stimulation.

Hydrosalpinges with destroyed mucosa are not suitable for reconstructive surgery. However, patients with these also have an impaired success rate after IVF, possibly due to the leakage of fluid into the uterus. Salpingectomy is the only method that has been properly evaluated as a surgical approach to overcome the negative influence of the hydrosalpingeal fluid.

From the Scandinavian study, a clear conclusion was drawn: patients with hydrosalpinges large enough to be visible on ultrasound examination can be recommended laparoscopic salpingectomy prior to IVF in order to enhance their chance of a full-term pregnancy. Patients

http://dx.doi.org/10.5772/63090

with large hydrosalpinges and without prospect of spontaneous conception should be recommended a salpingectomy, which truly increases their chances of a successful IVF treatment [71].

4.2. Surgical vs. medical management

Different hypothesis on medical management for hydrosalpinx have been considered. This is not just prophylactic antibiotics to patients after the puncture of hydrosalpinx. Sharara et al. in 1996 suggested giving prophylactic antibiotics to selected groups of patients with elevated serum Chlamydia trachomatis IgG antibody titers or considered as a routine before oocyte retrieval for all patients.

Nevertheless, this hypothesis of antibiotic treatment specifically in hydrosalpinx patients has not been studied or evaluated prospectively.

Hurst et al. in 2001 in a retrospective study worked on hydrosalpinx and antibiotic treatment. In this study, patients with hydrosalpinx who received prolonged doxycycline treatment during an IVF cycle were compared to those who did not receive antibiotics and had other conditions, such as (endometriosis/unexplained infertility or tubal occlusion without hydrosalpinx/adhesions). Implantation and pregnancy rates were similar in all groups. This concludes that antibiotic treatment could also minimize the detrimental effect of hydrosalpinx. Even though this method is simple and safe, its benefits should be evaluated in a prospective trial before it becomes a standard of care [71].

4.3. Salpingectomy vs. proximal tubal occlusion

One of the secondary benefits salpingectomy provides, is the removal of a mass that may possibly be infected and could also be a source of torsion. Hydrosalpinx left in situ, can potentially have a negative impact because it can cause an increase in the risk of infection and decrease in access to the ovary during oocyte aspiration.

On the contrary, there are potential disadvantages to the performance of salpingectomy. Salpingectomy is a procedure that would need expertise because it would be difficult to perform in patients with extensive pelvic adhesions, also considered an invasive procedure and could potentially increase the possibility of injury to the surrounding tissues and structures. In addition, transection of the tube too close to the cornua may also increase the risk of an interstitial pregnancy after ET, a devastating complication [72].

Salpingectomy could also hypothetically result in a decrease in ovarian perfusion, as part of the blood supply to the ovaries is provided by branches of the uterine artery and the mesosalpingeal vascular arcade [73]. Acute reduction in ovarian blood flow may have a direct impact on ovulatory function in the rat model [74]. In a study by Lass et al. [75], it was shown that fewer follicles were developed and fewer oocytes were retrieved from the ipsilateral ovary in women who had undergone unilateral salpingectomy.

On the contrary, Dar et al. [76] reported that ovarian response in assisted reproductive technology cycles that was performed before and after laparoscopic salpingectomy for ectopic pregnancy was not affected by surgery [76].

Of note, proximal tubal occlusion constitutes a significantly less invasive approach that includes minimal surgical intervention and less time allocated for the surgery, while at the same time eliminating retrograde flow of hydrosalpingeal fluid into the endometrial cavity. The current study demonstrated that laparoscopic proximal occlusion of the affected fallopian tube with bipolar cautery had similar ovarian response and IVF-ET cycle outcome as that of controls or as of those who have undergone laparoscopic salpingectomy [77].

In conclusion, prophylactic surgical management of hydrosalpinges by either proximal tubal occlusion or laparoscopic salpingectomy demonstrated statistically similar responses to controlled ovarian hyperstimulation and IVF-ET cycle outcomes. There is no evidence of any compromise in ovarian response induced by either surgical procedure [77].

4.4. Spontaneous or surgical drainage of the hydrosalpinx

Studies have shown that draining hydrosalpinges surgically or with the help of ultrasound guidance have improved pregnancy and implantation rates [78].

Even though this technique would potentially decrease the overall volume of hydrosalpingeal fluid, drainage cannot eliminate its source or its ability to flow into the endometrial cavity even in decreased amounts. Sowter et al. [79] have shown that surgical drainage of distended hydrosalpinges offered no benefits in enhancing implantation or pregnancy rates over untreated controls. In addition, Bloechle et al. [59] have demonstrated re-accumulation of hydrosalpingeal fluid within 3 days of aspiration performed at oocyte retrieval, which would precede the time of embryo implantation. As a result, this would hypothetically eliminate the benefit of drainage alone.

It appears that the drainage of a hydrosalpinx might not have much benefit to implantation. Generally, re-accumulation of fluid in the tubes can cause subsequent drainage into the uterus, resulting in the distention of the uterine cavity, which has been reported by Mansour et al. in 1991 [110] and many others.

Failure to benefit from drainage of hydrosalpinges might not necessarily be a result of incomplete drainage leaving some fluid to spill into the uterine cavity or from fluid re-accumulation. There could potentially be a functional destruction to the tube which would enhance retrograde passage of transferred embryos, both increasing the risk of ectopic pregnancy, and also contributing by wastage of embryos to the observed decrease of intrauterine implantation. If, indeed, this was a notable mechanism causing decreased intrauterine implantation, there would also be no advantage from undertaking distal salpingostomy simply to maintain tubal drainage.

The study results highly recommend that transvaginal drainage of hydrosalpinges provides no benefit at the time of oocyte retrieval for IVF treatment [80].

http://dx.doi.org/10.5772/63090

4.5. Summary

Hydrosalpinges is a chronic inflammatory condition that could unfavorably affect the chance of endometrial receptivity.

Several studies have shown changes in the inflammatory and immunological markers in the endometrium of patients exposed to hydrosalpingeal fluid. Markers identified were IL-2, NK-κB, and LIF.

Today, prior to IVF treatment, the routine approach is a surgical intervention performing laparoscopic salpingectomy or proximal tubal occlusion.

Some studies have demonstrated the most surgical benefit in the subset of patients with bilateral hydrosalpinges or ultrasound visible hydrosalpinges.

5. Microbiome of the reproductive tract

As more is learned about the human microbiome, it is becoming evident that it meaningfully affects the physiologic function of virtually every organ where bacteria are present.

The human body is colonized with an order of magnitude more bacteria than human cells in the body [81]. The majority of published medical literature focuses on the subset of the microbiome involved in pathogenesis, and only a subset focuses on the physiologic role that the microbiome plays.

The importance of this was recognized in 2001 at the time of the human genome published [82], when scientists called for a "second human genome project" that would investigate the normal microbiome colonies at various sites to understand the synergistic interactions between the microbiome and its host [83]. Several initiatives commenced worldwide, and in the United States the Human Microbiome Project led by the National Institutes of Health was launched in 2007, using high throughput sequencing technologies to characterize the human microbiome in 250 normal healthy volunteers at multiple body sites [81].

The female reproductive tract has long been known to have an active microbiome (Figure 4). Although the greatest focus has been on the vaginal milieu, data have been accumulating for decades demonstrating that the remainder of the female reproductive axis is not sterile. In fact, with more than 20 studies completed, virtually all of them have found that there is a small but active microbiome in the uterine cavity.

Importantly, many of these studies obtained their samples at the time of surgery with the use of transfundal collection techniques where there was no potential for contamination from transiting the vagina or endocervical canal. The majority of these studies were done with the use of traditional culture techniques to identify any bacteria that were present.

More recently, metagenomic techniques are confirming earlier findings and providing a more comprehensive definition of the endometrial microbiome.

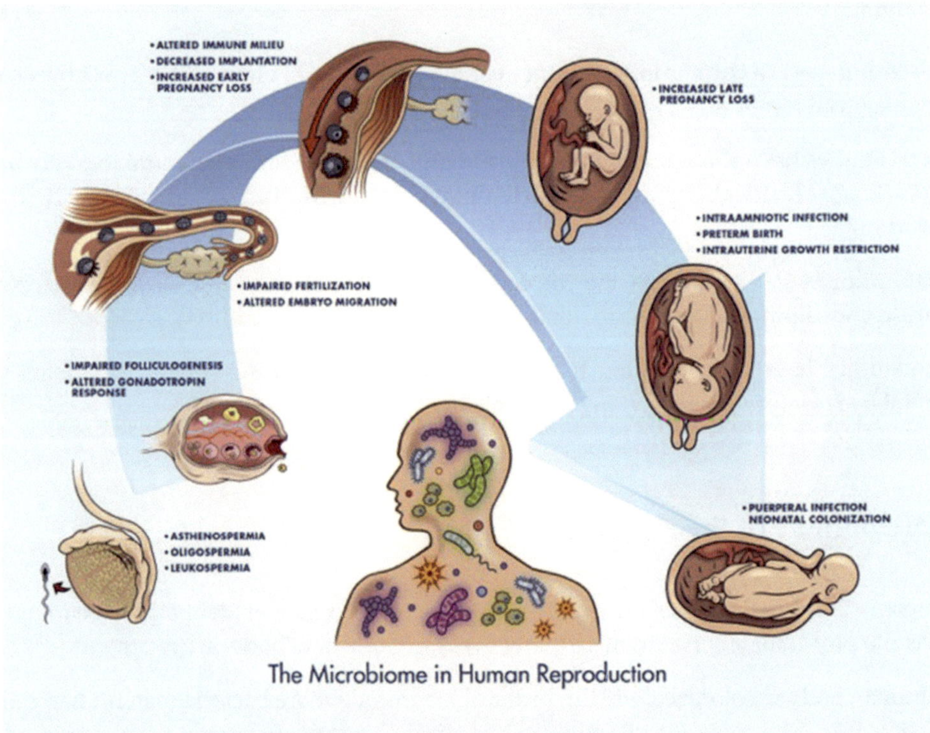

Figure 4. The human microbiome affects all facets of reproduction from gametogenesis, to fertilization and embryo migration, to implantation with implications in early pregnancy failure, to involvement in late pregnancy loss, and poor obstetric outcomes during gestation and parturition in terms of intrauterine infection and preterm birth, among other things. A more complete characterization of this complex symbiosis is imperative as we understand its implications in human health and disease.

Interestingly, the microbiome extends above the endometrial cavity. Some studies have demonstrated bacteria in the fallopian tubes of women without obvious tubal pathology. Additional studies have demonstrated that the intra-follicular milieu may have an active microbiome in some patients.

Finally, there are now studies showing that the microbiome of the male reproductive axis is more complex than previously appreciated. The addition of metagenomic tools allowed descriptions of much broader and more complex microbiome, even in men without evidence of acute or chronic inflammation of their reproductive tract.

As the microbiome of the female and male reproductive axis has become more clearly defined, studies evaluating the clinical impact on ART treatment have followed. Given the influence which the microbiome has in virtually every organ systems, it is not surprising that subtle changes in the microbiome are associated with meaningful changes in gamete quality and ultimate clinical outcomes. In some cases, changes in the microbiome may provide insight into previously unexplained treatment failure [82].

http://dx.doi.org/10.5772/63090

5.1. Diagnosis

It is important to briefly recognize that microbiome data are procured in one of two ways: culture-based or sequencing-based technology.

The various techniques available in metagenomics (fingerprinting, DNA microarrays, targeted sequencing, and whole genome sequencing) supply both strengths and weaknesses depending upon the primary purpose of the analysis.

Much of the early work describing the human microbiome comes from culture-based approaches using the 16S rRNA analysis of highly conserved genes as a way to characterize the diversity of the microbiome in a given environment [84]. However, data from the vaginal microbiome suggest that many organisms can not be identified with the use of culture-based techniques, which results in underestimating the diversity of the ecosystem as well as failing to identify potentially important organisms when describing their relationship to health and disease [85]. Thus, culture-based data, though still informative, must be interpreted within the limits of the technology.

Data presented more recently have relied on 16S rRNA gene sequencing, specifically the hypervariable regions within the gene, which serves as a molecular fingerprint down to the genus and species level [86]. Although to date, data that describe the microbiome of the reproductive tract have not widely used this technique, metagenomics is becoming an increasingly widespread approach to describing the microbiome [87]. Using this method, also termed community genomics, analysis of microorganisms occurs by means of direct extraction and cloning of DNA from a grouping of organisms. It allows analysis that extends beyond phylogenetic descriptions and attempts to study the physiology and ecology of the microbiome [82].

The study of the microbiome and its relationship to the efficiency of conception and early pregnancy maintenance is just beginning. Although there have been efforts to distinguish between normal or favorable microbiomes and those that impair or limit clinical outcomes, early investigations are also identifying alterations in several physiologic processes. These alterations provide insight into reproductive failure in some patients. They may also provide the foundational information to guide the development of new therapeutic interventions that could improve outcomes and previously recalcitrant clinical circumstances.

The association between clinically evident infection, inflammation, and altered reproductive function is well established. Much of this inflammation involves secretion of a number of pro-inflammatory cytokines and growth factors secreted by immune cells, which are activated in response to the presence of apparent pathogens. In the case of small shifts in the microbiome, the resulting subtle changes in the local milieu are typically not clinically evident but may remain clinically meaningful; however, the exact molecular mechanisms are not well characterized.

Accumulations of a particular interleukin or some other cytokine are described, but detailed mechanisms are still lacking. It is possible that the influence of some components of the microbiome is not via direct interaction with the local organ system.

The microbiome of the vagina is typically dominated by Lactobacilli [88]. In fact, a normal milieu is defined by the presence of specific subspecies of Lactobacilli that are capable of acting as probiotics and inhibiting the overgrowth of other bacterial species. For example, Lactobacilli species capable of producing high levels of H_2O_2 are generally considered to be most favorable. This demonstrates an important concept that some components of the microbiome's principal function may be to alter or limit some other component of the microbiome. A direct interaction with the actual tissue may occur but is not essential.

It is becoming increasingly evident that the aggregate microbiome is not a simple accumulation of free-floating bacteria on the surface of a human tissue. In many cases, complex three-dimensional lattices are formed, which may have one layer or may have an inner and an outer layer.

A protective outer coating composed of polysaccharide, nucleic acid, and protein may develop. At times, these biofilms may inhibit immune detection and reduce the effectiveness of antimicrobial treatment [89]. These three-dimensional structures spread across the surfaces of the tissues where they are located and are termed biofilms.

Biofilms are the subject of intensive investigation and may have important physiologic and pathophysiologic roles. Biofilms are routinely present in the vagina but commonly extend into the endometrial cavity [90] and even up into the fallopian tubes (Figure 5). Although no definitive conclusions regarding the role of biofilms of the reproductive axis have been established, it is important to understand that the relationship between the microbiome and the mullerian system may be more complex than the simple presence or absence of various species or bacteria or even their relative concentration. The interactions that lead to different biofilms and their subsequent impact on reproduction will provide important topics for future investigation.

The influence of the microbiome, most prevalent in the mullerian system, may extend to the remainder of the reproductive axis and may even affect gametogenesis. Indeed, ovarian follicles may have an active microbiome. Some investigators have found that some bacteria may adversely influence follicular development and may even inhibit gonadotropin responsiveness. Similarly, the male reproductive axis may be adversely affected, with subtle changes in the microbiome being associated with altered semen parameters [82].

Most studies characterizing the influence of the microbiome on ART and clinical outcomes are largely association studies. Detailed mechanistic studies that could lead to new therapeutic approaches are possible but remain to be done.

5.2. Vaginal microbiome

In contrast to the Human Microbiome Project, which investigated normal healthy volunteers, several investigators have looked at the link between the vaginal microbiome and infertility in patients undergoing various forms of ART [82].

One such study prospectively analyzed 152 patients undergoing IVF. Of the 152 patients, 133 (87.5%) tested positive for one or more microorganisms and 19 (12.5%) tested completely

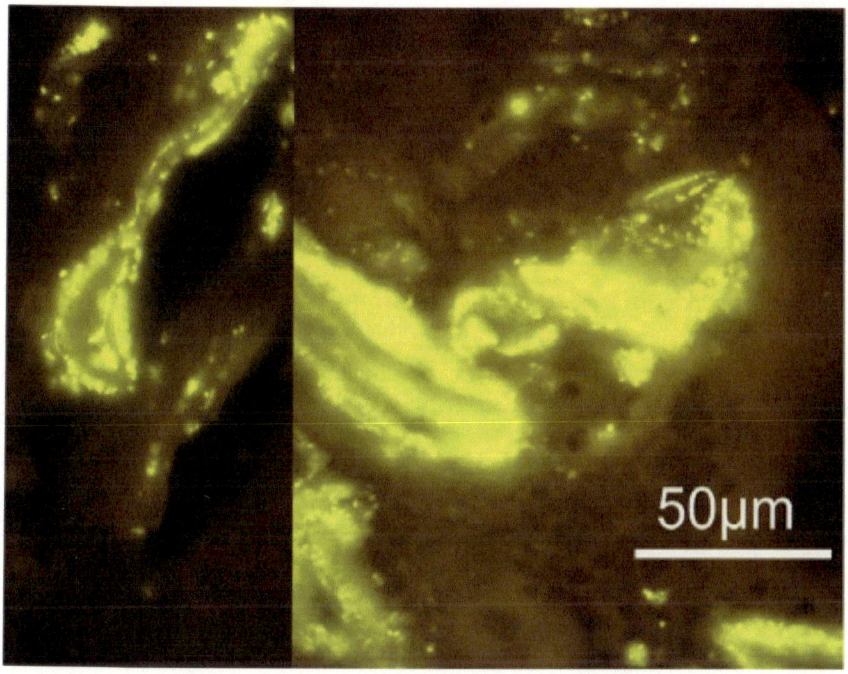

Reproduced with the permission from Swidsinski et al.Reproductive tract microbiome in ART. Fertil Steril. Copyright© 2015.

Figure 5. Polymicrobial biofilm dominated by Gardnerella attached to the endometrium. The left panel shows follicular and the right panel shows luteal endometrium.

negative for bacterial contamination. The most common microorganisms identified were *Lactobacillus* species, *Staphylococcus* species, and Enterobacteriaceae, including *Escherichia coli*, Klebsiella, and Proteus. Outcomes data showed that implantation rates were 12.4% in those with one or more bacteria present versus 14% in those completely negative (P<0.001).

Additionally, patients testing positive for Enterobacteriaceae and *Staphylococcus* had lower pregnancy rates than the negative culture group. Although this study provided some insight into the microbiome during IVF treatment, it highlighted the limitations associated with culture-based technology for evaluation of the microbiome. The fact that 12.5% of patients were completely negative for bacterial contamination suggests that the culture-based technique significantly underrepresents both the presence and the diversity of the microbiome at the time of ET.

A subsequent study with the use of 16S sequencing technology took a more robust look at the vaginal microbiome in the infertile patient undergoing IVF [90]. The investigators approached the study design with the hypothesis that, given that the vaginal microbiome has changes during the normal menstrual cycle with varied estrogen levels in the physiologic range [91], controlled ovarian hyperstimulation required to achieve success in IVF would also affect the vaginal microbiome [82].

5.3. Uterine microbiome

Just as alterations in the microbial environment affect vaginal health, these fluctuations may also predispose to upper genital tract infection, such as PID.

Direct culture or sequencing of samples from upper genital tract structures has been performed less frequently than the evaluation of vaginal samples, but available data confirm that BV-associated bacteria can be isolated from the upper genital tract [92].

In a study of 45 women with laparoscopically confirmed acute salpingitis (cases) and 44 women seeking bilateral tubal ligation (controls), 16S rDNA PCR detected bacteria in the fallopian tubes of 24% of cases and none of the controls [93]. Several of the specimens contained bacteria associated with BV, such as *Atopobium vaginae*, as well as *Leptotrichia* species and *N. gonorrhoea*.

The identification of causal microorganisms in upper genital infection is important for understanding disease pathogenesis and provides insight into why some cases are resistant to conventional treatment. The presence of certain organisms in the vagina is physiologic, and bacteria may also exist in the upper cervix and uterus during states of health.

In a study, by performing quantitative PCR on endometrial and upper cervical swabs from 58 women undergoing hysterectomy for benign conditions, at least one bacterial species was found in the upper genital tract of 95% of the subjects. The most frequently detected species were *Lactobacillus iners* (45%), *Prevotella* species (33%), and *Lactobacillus crispatus* (33%) [94].

An important consideration is that the upper cervix and uterus were grouped together as the "upper genital tract";however, these sites may contain different bacterial species or proportions of bacteria. For instance, there was a statistically significant difference in the proportion of upper genital tract bacteria based on race. African American and Hispanic women were more likely to harbor an upper genital tract microbiome dominated by a non-*Lactobacilli* species (83% and 75%, respectively) compared with Caucasian women (54%). These results mirror those of vaginal microbiome in that non-*Lactobacilli* species were more common in African American and Hispanic women, but the clinical implications of these findings are unclear.

Furthermore, there was no evidence of significant inflammation in the endometrial samples that contained bacteria typically found in the vaginal tract. Possible explanations for the lack of inflammation include vaginal contamination of the uterine samples or that molecular methods detected RNA of non-living organisms that did not affect clinical status.

Alternatively, it remains a possibility that certain bacteria in the upper cervix and uterus may serve important roles in maintaining homeostasis and may not necessarily represent pathology [92].

5.4. Ovarian follicle microbiome

Human follicular fluids have been extensively cultured and found to have an active microbiome in many patients.

Although some specimens were collected from follicular aspirate attained at the time of transvaginal oocyte retrieval, others were collected laparoscopically [95]. It is not clearly established whether the bacteria that were cultured represent true colonization or merely contamination of the ovarian follicular fluid at the time of puncture for transvaginal oocyte aspiration [96].

Studies simultaneously evaluating the vagina, endocervix, endometrium, fallopian tube, follicular fluid, and peritoneal cavity are lacking.

Current studies looking at the microbiome of the follicle have used culture techniques. Early culture studies have suggested that an active follicular microbiome does affect ART outcomes. Interestingly, the impact of the microbiome is influenced by the clinical diagnosis of the female partner.

Diminished fertilization and development rates as well as reduced transfer and implantation rates have been noted in women with endometriosis, but not in women with ovulatory dysfunction or male-factor infertility [97, 98]. This may suggest that a more complex mechanism with an altered immune response present in women with endometriosis may produce a different reaction to the presence of an active microbiome and then also influence the developing oocyte.

It may also be important to note that an active microbiome is not always a negative finding. Pelzer et al. [99] noted that outcomes improved when Lactobacilli were present. This is in sharp contrast to the presence of other species, such as *Propionibacterium* and *Actinomyces*, among others, where impaired clinical outcomes were documented. They also observed differences in the microbiome between the left and right ovaries, which were attributed to differences in hematogenous spread. The clinical relevance of this finding remains to be fully characterized [82].

At the present time, data are still accumulating regarding the significance of the follicular microbiome and the need for screening. Additional studies, particularly those using metagenomic approaches, are needed.

5.5. ART and microbiome

Data have been gathered on the microbiome at every stage and level of human reproduction from the ovary, follicle and oocyte to testes and semen/spermatozoa and to the fallopian tube, uterus, cervix, and vagina. Both the male and female reproductive tracts exhibit complexity and diversity only realized within the last decade.

Furthermore, it is not enough to simply qualitatively or even quantitatively explore the reproductive tract microbiome using metagenomics. Understanding that these bacteria are not simply free-floating on the surface of tissue, but form their own three-dimensional biofilms with inner and outer layers, adds an additional complexity and could be of great importance if they were further explored. The fact these biofilms exist from the vagina to the fallopian tubes, allows complex and dynamic interactions between the gametes and embryo, as well as the maternal tissue interface.

To date, the assisted reproductive technology literature describing attempts to alter the microbiome in the reproductive tract in order to impact outcomes has been operating on a rudimentary understanding of this complex environment at best. However, this approach, although perhaps to blunt a tool at present, may indeed be an important key to altering both the microbiome and subsequently the immune system as we further explore enhancement of reproductive competence in assisted reproductive technology.

5.6. Conclusion

Knowledge regarding the interactions between the microbiome and the human reproductive axis is growing rapidly. A deeper understanding of normal physiology, identification of different dysbioses, and characterizing the microbiome's impact on reproductive outcomes promise meaningful enhancements in clinical care. While much has been learned since the early contributions of Semmelweis, the most insightful and powerful findings may lie just ahead [100].

6. Antimicrobials and ART

Although the reproductive tract microbiome remains relatively poorly understood in terms of its relationship to reproductive outcomes, there is a long history of attempting to influence it with the use of prophylactic antibiotics at the time of procedures during ART. This has been a practice ingrained since 1978, when it was suggested that contamination during ART procedures could negatively affect outcomes [101]. Because antiseptics, such as povidone iodine, can have a negative impact on embryos, antibiotics were turned to as a way of manipulating the microbiome [102].

A common time for antimicrobial prophylaxis is at the time of ET. Given the concern for colonization of the transfer catheter tip with microbiota from the upper genital tract, antibiotics have been proposed as a way to decrease inoculation of the uterine cavity and thereby increase pregnancy rates. Despite this widespread practice, relatively little data exist to support or refute antibiotic use.

A recent Cochrane review analyzed randomized controlled trials in the literature that investigated antibiotics at ET [103]. Only four potential studies were identified, of which three were excluded. The remaining study reported on clinical pregnancy rates as the primary outcome. Although administration of antibiotics reduced microbial contamination as defined by culture of ET catheter tips, the clinical pregnancy rate was 36% in those receiving antibiotics and 35.5% in those not receiving antibiotics (odds ratio 1.02, 95% confidence interval 0.66–1.58) [104]. The reviewers concluded that more evidence is needed with live birth as the primary outcome.

http://dx.doi.org/10.5772/63090

Author details

Reza Peymani* and Alan DeCherney

*Address all correspondence to: rpeymani@hotmail.com

National Institutes of Health (NIH), Eunice Kennedy Shriver National Institute of Child Health and Human Development, Fertility and Infertility Branch, Bethesda, USA

References

[1] LaSala GB, Montanari R, Dessanti L, Cigarini C, Santori F. The role of diagnostic hysteroscopy and endometrial biopsy in assisted reproductive technologies. Fertil Steril 1998;70:378–380.

[2] Oliveira FG, Abdelmassih VG, Diamond MP, Dozortsev D, Nagy ZP, Abdelmassih R. Uterine cavity findings and hysteroscopic interventions in patients undergoing in vitro fertilization embryo transfer who repeatedly cannot conceive. Fertil Steril 2003;80:1371–1375.

[3] El-Toukhy T, Taranissi M. Towards better quality research in recurrent implantation failure: standardizing its definition is the first step. Reprod Biomed Online 2006;12:383–385.

[4] Greenwood SM, Moran JJ. Chronic endometritis: morphologic and clinical observations. Obstet Gynecol 1981;58:176–184.

[5] Polisseni F, Bambirra EA, Camargos AF. Detection of chronic endometritis by diagnostic hysteroscopy in asymptomatic infertile patients. Gynecol Obstet Invest 2003;55:205–210.

[6] Romero R, Espinoza J, Mazor M. Can endometrial infection/inflammation explain implantation failure, spontaneous abortion and preterm birth after in vitro fertilization? Fertil Steril 2004;82:799–804.

[7] Romero R, Parvizi ST, Oyarzun E, Mazor M, Wu YK, Avila C, et al. Amniotic fluid interleukin-1 in spontaneous labor at term. J Reprod Med 1990;35:235–238.

[8] Kachkache M, Acker GM, Chaouat G, Noun A, Garabedian M. Hormonal and local factors control the immunohistochemical distribution of immunocytes in the rat uterus before conceptus implantation: effects of ovariectomy, fallopian tube section, and injection. Biol Reprod 1991;45:860–868.

[9] Halgunset J, Johnsen H, Kjollesdal AM, Qvigstad E, Espevik T, Austgulen R. Cytokine levels in amniotic fluid and inflammatory changes in the placenta from normal deliveries at term. Eur J Obstet Gynecol Reprod Biol 1994;56:153–160.

[10] Saito S, Kasahara T, Kato Y, Ishihara Y, Ichijo M. Elevation of amniotic fluid interleukin 6 (IL-6), IL-8 and granulocyte colony stimulating factor (G-CSF) in term and preterm parturition. Cytokine 1993;5:81–88.

[11] Hill JA. T-helper 1-type immunity to trophoblast: evidence for a new immunological mechanism for recurrent abortion in women. Hum Reprod 1995;10 Suppl;2:114–120.

[12] Roberto et al. Can endometrial infection/inflammation explain implantation failure, spontaneous abortion, and preterm birth after in vitro fertilization? Fertil Steril 2004;82:799–804.

[13] Paavonen J, Aine R, Teisala K, Heinonen PK, Punnonen R. Comparison of endometrial biopsy and peritoneal fluid cytologic testing with laparoscopy in the diagnosis of acute pelvic inflammatory disease. Am J Obstet Gynecol 1985;151:645–650.

[14] Trundley A, Moffett A. Human uterine leukocytes and pregnancy. Tissue Antigens 2004;63:1–12.

[15] Saito S, Fukunaga R, Ichijo M, Nagata S. Expression of granulocyte colony-stimulating factor and its receptor at the fetomaternal interface in murine and human pregnancy. Growth Factors 1994;10:135–143.

[16] Saito S. Cytokine network at the feto-maternal interface. J Reprod Immunol 2000;47:87–103.

[17] Wegmann TG, Lin H, Guilbert L, Mosmann TR. Bidirectional cytokine interactions in the maternal-fetal relationship: is successful pregnancy a TH2 phenomenon? Immunol Today 1993;14:353–356.

[18] Cicinelli E, Matteo M, Tinelli R, et al. Prevalence of chronic endometritis in repeated unexplained implantation failure and the IVF success rate after antibiotic therapy. Hum Reprod 2015;30(2):323–330.

[19] Hamou JE. Hysteroscopy and Microcolpohysteroscopy: Text and Atlas, 1 ed. Paris: Appleton & Lange, 1985.

[20] Golan A, Eilat E, Ron-El R, Herman A, Soffer Y, Bukovsky I. Hysteroscopy is superior to hysterosalpingography in infertility investigation. Acta Obstet Gynecol Scand 1996;75:654–656.

[21] Dicker D, Ashkenazi J, Feldberg D, Farhi J, Shalev J, Ben-Rafael Z. The value of repeat hysteroscopic evaluation in patients with failed in vitro fertilization transfer cycles. Fertil Steril 1992;58:833–835.

[22] Kluytmans JA, Goessens WH, Mouton JW, van Rijsoort-Vos JH, Niesters HG, Quint WG, Habbema L, Stolz E, Wagenvoort JH. Evaluation of Clearview and Magic Lite tests, polymerase chain reaction, and cell culture for detection of *Chlamydia trachomatis* in urogenital specimens. J Clin Microbiol 1993;31:3204–3210.

[23] Gump DW, Gibson M, Ashikaga T: Evidence of prior pelvic inflammatory disease and its relationship to *Chlamydia trachomatis* antibody and intrauterine contraceptive device use in infertile women. Am J Obstet Gynecol 1983; 146:153–159.

[24] Fernanda et al. Detection of chronic endometritis by diagnostic hysteroscopy in asymptomatic infertile patients. Gynecol Obstet Invest 2003;55:205–210.

[25] Ettore et al. Chronic endometritis due to common bacteria is prevalent in women with recurrent miscarriage as confirmed by improved pregnancy outcome after antibiotic treatment. Reprod Sci 2014;21(5): 640-–647.

[26] Resta L, Palumbo M, Rossi R, Piscitelli D, Grazia Fiore M, Cicinelli E. Histology of micro polyps in chronic endometritis. Histopathology 2012;60(4):670–674.

[27] Cicinelli E, Resta L,Nicoletti R, Zappimbulso V, TartagniM, Saliani N. Endometrial micropolyps at fluid hysteroscopy suggest the existence of chronic endometritis. Hum Reprod 2005;20(5):1386–1389.

[28] Ness RB, Soper DE, Holley RL, et al. Effectiveness of inpatient and outpatient treatment strategies for women with pelvic inflammatory disease: results from the Pelvic Inflammatory Disease Evaluation and Clinical Health (PEACH) randomized trial. Am J Obstet Gynecol 2002;186(5):929–937.

[29] Cicinelli E, Ballini A, Marinaccio M, et al. Microbiological findings in endometrial specimen: our experience. Arch Gynecol Obstet 2012;285(5):1325–1329.

[30] Eckert LO, Moore DE, Patton DL, Agnew KJ, Eschenbach DA. Relationship of vaginal bacteria and inflammation with conception and early pregnancy loss following in-vitro fertilization. Infect Dis Obstet Gynecol 2003;11(1):11–17.

[31] Cowling P, McCoy DR, Marshall RJ, Padfield CJ, Reeves DS. Bacterial colonization of the non-pregnant uterus: a study of pre-menopausal abdominal hysterectomy specimens. Eur J Clin Microbiol Infect Dis 1992;11(2):204–205.

[32] Valli E, Zupi E, Marconi D, et al. Hysteroscopic findings in 344 women with recurrent spontaneous abortion. J Am Assoc Gynecol Laparosc 2001;8(3):398–401.

[33] Bohlmann MK, von Wolff M, Luedders DW, et al. Hysteroscopic findings in women with two and with more than two first trimester miscarriages are not significantly different. Reprod Biomed Online 2010;21(2):230–236.

[34] Cicinelli E, Parisi C, Galantino P, Pinto V, Barba B, Schonauer S. Reliability, feasibility, and safety of minihysteroscopy with a vaginoscopic approach: experience with 6,000 cases. Fertil Steril. 2003;80(1):199–202.

[35] Johnston-MacAnanny EB, Hartnett J, Engmann LL, Nulsen JC, Sanders MM, Benadiva CA. Chronic endometritis is a frequent finding in women with recurrent implantation failure after in vitro fertilization. Fertil Steril 2010;93:43741.

[36] Kitaya K, Yasuo T. Aberrant expression of selectin E, CXCL1, and CXCL13 in chronic endometritis. Mod Pathol 2010;23:1136–1146.

[37] Lachapelle MH, Miron P, Hemmings R, Roy DC. Endometrial T, B, and NK cells in patients with recurrent spontaneous abortion. Altered profile and pregnancy outcome. J Immunol 1996;156: 4027–4034.

[38] Quenby S, Bates M, Doig T, Brewster J, Lewis- Jones DI, Johnson PM, et al. Pre-implantation endometrial leukocytes in women with recurrent miscarriage. Hum Reprod 1999;14:2386–2391.

[39] Yang R, Du X, Wang Y, Song X, Yang Y, Qiao J. The hysteroscopy and histological diagnosis and treatment value of chronic endometritis in recurrent implantation failure patients. Arch Gynecol Obstet 2014;289(6):1363–1369.

[40] Wijdenes J, Voous WC, Clement C, Post J, Morard F, Vita N, et al. A plasmocyte selective monoclonal antibody (B-B4) recognizes syndecan-1. Br J Haematol 1996;94:318–323.

[41] Carey DJ. Syndecans: multifunctional cell-surface coreceptors. Biochem J 1997;327:1–16.

[42] Crum CP, Egawa K, Fenoglio CM, Richart RM. Chronic endometritis: the role of immunohistochemistry in the detection of plasma cells. Am J Obstet Gynecol 1983;147:812–815.

[43] Brudenell JM. Chronic endometritis and plasma cell infiltration of the endometrium. J Obstet Gynaecol Br Emp 1955;62:269–274.

[44] Ilene B, et al. Plasma cells in chronic endometritis are easily identified when stained with syndecan-1. Mod Pathol 2001;14(9):877–879.

[45] Xu Z, Zan H, Pone EJ, Mai T, Casali P. Immunoglobulin class-switch DNA recombination: induction, targeting and beyond. Nat Rev Immunol 2012;12(7):517–531.

[46] Kitaya K, Tada Y, Hayashi T, Taguchi S, Funabiki M, Nakamura Y. Comprehensive endometrial immunoglobulin subclass analysis in infertile women suffering from repeated implantation failure with or without chronic endometritis. Am J Reprod Immunol 2014;72(4):386–391.

[47] Di Pietro C, Cicinelli E, Guglielmino MR, et al. Altered transcriptional regulation of cytokines, growth factors, and apoptotic proteins in the endometrium of infertile women with chronic endometritis. Am J Reprod Immunol 2013;69(5):509–517.

[48] Alin L, et al. The role of inflammatory pathways in implantation failure: chronic endometritis and hydrosalpinges. Semin Reprod Med 2015;33:298–304.

[49] Johnston-MacAnanny EB, Hartnett J, Engmann LL, Nulsen JC, Sanders MM, Benadiva CA. Chronic endometritis is a frequent finding in women with recurrent implantation failure after in vitro fertilization. Fertil Steril 2010;93(2):437–441.

[50] Savaris RF, Giudice LC. The influence of hydrosalpinx onmarkers of endometrial receptivity. Semin Reprod Med 2007;25(6):476–482.

[51] Bloechle M.What is a hydrosalpinx? A plea for the use of a proper terminology in scientific discussion. Hum Reprod 1999;14(3):578

[52] de Wit W, Gowrising CJ, Kuik DJ, Lens JW, Schats R. Only hydrosalpinges visible on ultrasound are associated with reduced implantation and pregnancy rates after in-vitro fertilization. Hum Reprod 1998;13(6):1696–1701.

[53] Renbaum L, Ufberg D, Sammel M, Zhou L, Jabara S, Barnhart K. Reliability of clinicians versus radiologists for detecting abnormalities on hysterosalpingogram films. Fertil Steril 2002;78(3):614–618.

[54] Omurtag K, Grindler NM, Roehl KA, et al. How members of the Society for Reproductive Endocrinology and Infertility and Society of Reproductive Surgeons evaluate, define, and manage hydrosalpinges. Fertil Steril 2012;97(5):1095–1100.

[55] Zeyneloglu HB, Arici A, Olive DL. Adverse effects of hydrosalpinx on pregnancy rates after in vitro fertilization-embryo transfer. Fertil Steril 1998;70(3):492–499.

[56] Mukherjee T, Copperman AB, McCaffrey C, Cook CA, Bustillo M, ObasajuMF. Hydrosalpinx fluid has embryotoxic effects on murine embryogenesis: a case for prophylactic salpingectomy. Fertil Steril 1996;66(5):851–853.

[57] Ng EH, Chan CC, Tang OS, Ho PC. Comparison of endometrial and subendometrial blood flows among patients with and without hydrosalpinx shown on scanning during in vitro fertilization treatment. Fertil Steril 2006;85(2):333–338.

[58] Nackley AC, Muasher SJ. The significance of hydrosalpinx in in vitro fertilization. Fertil Steril 1998;69:373–384.

[59] Bloechle M, Schreiner T, Lisse K. Recurrence of hydrosalpinges after transvaginal aspiration of tubal fluid in an IVF cycle with development of a serometra. Hum Reprod 1997;12(4):703–705.

[60] Copperman AB, Wells V, Luna M, Kalir T, Sandler B, Mukherjee T. Presence of hydrosalpinx correlated to endometrial inflammatory response in vivo. Fertil Steril 2006;86(4):972–976.

[61] Hill JA, Polgar K, Anderson DJ. T-helper 1-type immunity to trophoblast in women with recurrent spontaneous abortion. JAMA 1995;273(24):1933–1936.

[62] Meyer WR, Castelbaum AJ, Somkuti S, et al. Hydrosalpinges adversely affect markers of endometrial receptivity. Hum Reprod 1997;12(7):1393–1398.

[63] Bildirici I, Bukulmez O, Ensari A, Yarali H, Gurgan T. A prospective evaluation of the effect of salpingectomy on endometrial receptivity in cases of women with communicating hydrosalpinges. Hum Reprod 2001;16(11):2422–2426.

[64] Lessey BA, Damjanovich L, Coutifaris C, Castelbaum A, Albelda SM, Buck CA. Integrin adhesion molecules in the human endometrium. Correlation with the normal and abnormal menstrual cycle. J Clin Invest 1992;90(1):188–195.

[65] Strandell A, Sjogren A, Bentin-Ley U, Thorburn J, Hamberger L, Brannstrom M. Hydrosalpinx fluid does not adversely affect the normal development of human embryos and implantation in vitro. Hum Reprod 1998;13:2921–2925.

[66] Bradley S, et al. Hydrosalpinx treated with extended doxycycline does not compromise the success of in vitro fertilization. Fertil Steril 2001;75: 1017–1019.

[67] Practice Committee of American Society for Reproductive Medicine in collaboration with Society of Reproductive Surgeons. Salpingectomy for hydrosalpinx prior to in vitro fertilization. Fertil Steril 2008;90(5 Suppl):S66–S68.

[68] Kontoravdis A, Makrakis E, Pantos K, Botsis D, Deligeoroglou E, Creatsas G. Proximal tubal occlusion and salpingectomy result in similar improvement in in vitro fertilization outcome in patients with hydrosalpinx. Fertil Steril 2006;86(6):1642–1649.

[69] Zhang Y, Sun Y, Guo Y, Li TC, Duan H. Salpingectomy and proximal tubal occlusion for hydrosalpinx prior to in vitro fertilization: a meta-analysis of randomized controlled trials. Obstet Gynecol Surv 2015;70(1):33–38.

[70] Rosenfield RB, Stones RE, Coates A, Matteri RK, Hesla JS. Proximal occlusion of hydrosalpinx by hysteroscopic placement of microinsert before in vitro fertilization-embryo transfer. Fertil Steril 2005;83(5):1547–1550.

[71] Strandell A. How to treat hydrosalpinges: IVF as the treatment of choice. Reprod Biomed Online; Article/180 2001;4 (Suppl. 3):37–39.

[72] Sharif K, Kaufmann M, Sharma V. Heterotopic pregnancy obtained after in-vitro fertilization and embryo transfer following bilateral total salpingectomy: case report. Hum Reprod 1994;9:1966–1967.

[73] San Filippo JS, Lincoln SR. Surgical treatment of diseases of the ovary. In: Keye WR, Chang RJ, Rebar RW, Soules MR, eds. Infertility: Evaluation and Treatment. Philadelphia: WB Saunders, pp. 539–551.

[74] Zackrisson U, Mikuni M, Peterson MC, Nilsson B, Janson P, Brannstrom M. Evidence for the involvement of blood flow-related mechanisms in the ovulatory process of the rat. Hum Reprod 2000;15: 264–272.

[75] Lass A, Ellenbogen A, Croucher C, Trew G, Margara R, Becaltini C, et al. Effect of salpingectomy on ovarian response to superovulation in an in vitro fertilization-embryo transfer program. Fertil Steril 1998;70:1035–1038.

[76] Dar P, Sachs AS, Strassburger D, Bukovsky I, Arieli S. Ovarian function before and after salpingectomy in artificial reproductive technology patients. Hum Reprod 2000;15:142–144.

[77] Surrey et al. Laparoscopic management of hydrosalpinges before in vitro fertilization–embryo transfer: salpingectomy versus proximal tubal occlusion Fertil Steril 2001; 75: 612-617.

[78] Sharara FJ, Scott RT Jr, Marut EL, Queenan JT Jr. In-vitro fertilization outcome in women with hydrosalpinx. Hum Reprod 1996;11:526–530.

[79] Sowter MC, Akande VA, Williams JAG, Hull MG. Is the outcome of in-vitro fertilization and embryo transfer treatment improved by spontaneous or surgical drainage of a hydrosalpinx? Hum Reprod 1997;10:2147–2150.

[80] Sowter MC, et al. Is the outcome of in-vitro fertilization and embryo transfer treatment improved by spontaneous or surgical drainage of a hydrosalpinx? Hum Reprod 1997;12(10):2147–2150.

[81] Peterson J, Garges S, Giovanni M, McInnes P, Wang L, Schloss JA, et al. The NIH Human Microbiome Project. Genome Res 2009;19:2317–2323.

[82] Venter JC, Adams MD, Myers EW, Li PW, Mural RJ, Sutton GG, et al. The sequence of the human genome. Science 2001;291:1304–1351.

[83] Davies J. In a map for human life, count the microbes, too. Science 2001;291:2316.

[84] Giovannoni SJ, Britschgi TB, Moyer CL, Field KG. Genetic diversity in Sargasso Sea bacterioplankton. Nature 1990;345:60–63.

[85] Verhelst R, Verstraelen H, Claeys G, Verschraegen G, Delanghe J, Van Simaey L, et al. Cloning of 16S rRNA genes amplified from normal and disturbed vaginal microflora suggests a strong association between Atopobium vaginae, Gardnerella vaginalis and bacterial vaginosis. BMC Microbiol 2004;4:16.

[86] Eckburg PB, Bik EM, Bernstein CN, Purdom E, Dethlefsen L, Sargent M, et al. Diversity of the human intestinal microbial flora. Science 2005;308:1635–1638.

[87] Handelsman J. Metagenomics: application of genomics to uncultured microorganisms. Microbiol Mol Biol Rev MMBR 2004;68:669–685.

[88] Structure, function and diversity of the healthy human microbiome. Nature 2012;486:207–214.

[89] Trinidad, A., Ibanez, A., Gomez, D., Garcia-Berrocal, J., Ramirez-Cmacho, R. Application of the environmental scanning electron microscopy for study of biofilms in medical devices. in: A. Mendez-Vilas, J Diaz (Eds.) Microscopy: science, technology, applications and education. Formatex Research Center, Spain; 2010:204–210.

[90] Swidsinski A, Verstraelen H, Loening-Baucke V, Swidsinski S, Mendling W, Halwani Z. Presence of a polymicrobial endometrial biofilm in patients with bacterial vaginosis. PLoS One 2013;8:e53997.

[91] Hyman RW, Fukushima M, Diamond L, Kumm J, Giudice LC, Davis RW. Microbes on the human vaginal epithelium. Proc Natl Acad Sci USA 2005;102:7952–7957.

[92] Green K, et al. Gynecologic health and disease in relation to the microbiome of the female reproductive tract. Fertil Steril 2015;104:1351–1357.

[93] Hebb JK, Cohen CR, Astete SG, Bukusi EA, Totten PA. Detection of novel organisms associated with salpingitis, by use of 16S rDNA polymerase chain reaction. J Infect Dis 2004;190:2109–2120.

[94] Mitchell CM, Haick A, Nkwopara E, Garcia R, Rendi M, Agnew K, et al. Colonization of the upper genital tract by vaginal bacterial species in nonpregnant women. Am J Obstet Gynecol 2015;212:611.e1–9.

[95] Artley JK, Braude PR, Cooper P. Vaginal squamous cells in follicular aspirates following transvaginal puncture. Hum Reprod 1993;8:1272–1273.

[96] Cottell E, McMorrow J, Lennon B, Fawsy M, Cafferkey M, Harrison RF. Microbial contamination in an in vitro fertilization–embryo transfer system. Fertil Steril 1996;66:776–780.

[97] Saltes B, Molo MW, Binor Z, Radwanska E. Bacterial contamination after transvaginal aspiration (TVA) of oocytes. J Assist Reprod Genet 1995;12:657–658.

[98] Weiss G, Goldsmith LT, Taylor RN, Bellet D, Taylor HS. Inflammation in reproductive disorders. Reprod Sci 2009;16:216–229.

[99] Pelzer ES, Allan JA, Cunningham K, Mengersen K, Allan JM, Launchbury T, et al. Microbial colonization of follicular fluid: alterations in cytokine expression and adverse assisted reproduction technology outcomes. Hum Reprod 2011;26:1799–1812.

[100] Franasiak et al. Introduction: microbiome in human reproduction. Fertil Steril 2015;104:1341–1343.

[101] Czernobilsky B. Endometritis and infertility. Fertil Steril 1978;30:119–130.

[102] van Os HC, Roozenburg BJ, Janssen-Caspers HA, Leerentveld RA, Scholtes MC, Zeilmaker GH, et al. Vaginal disinfection with povidone iodine and the outcome of in-vitro fertilization. Hum Reprod 1992;7:349–350.

[103] Kroon B, Hart RJ, Wong BM, Ford E, Yazdani A. Antibiotics prior to embryo transfer in ART. Cochrane Database Syst Rev 2012:CD008995.

[104] Brook N, Khalaf Y, Coomarasamy A, Edgeworth J, Braude P. A randomized controlled trial of prophylactic antibiotics (co-amoxiclav) prior to embryo transfer. Hum Reprod. (2006) 21 (11): 2911-2915.

[105] Van Voorhis BJ, Sparks AET, Syrop CH, Stovall DW. Ultrasound guided aspiration of hydrosalpinges is associated with improved pregnancy and implantation rates after in-vitro fertilization cycles. Hum Reprod 1998;13:736–739.

[106] Selman H, Mariani M, Barnocchi N, Mencacci A, Bistoni F, Arena S, et al. Examination of bacterial contamination at the time of embryo transfer, and its impact on the IVF/pregnancy outcome. J Assist Reprod Genet 2007;24:395–399.

[107] Hyman RW, Herndon CN, Jiang H, Palm C, Fukushima M, Bernstein D, et al. The dynamics of the vaginal microbiome during infertility therapy with in vitro fertilization–embryo transfer. J Assist Reprod Genet 2012;29:105–115.

[108] Hou D, Zhou X, Zhong X, Settles ML, Herring J, Wang L, et al. Microbiota of the seminal fluid from healthy and infertile men. Fertil Steril 2013;100:1261–1269.

[109] Alexander Quaas, and Anuja Dokras, Diagnosis and Treatment of Unexplained Infertility Obstet Gynecol. 2008 Spring; 1(2): 69–76.

[110] Mansour RT, Aboulghar MA, Serour GI, Riad R. Fluid accumulation of the uterine cavity before embryo transfer: a possible hindrance for implantation. J In Vitro Fert Embryo Transf. 1991 Jun;8(3):157-9.

Chapter 9

Female Infertility Associated to *Chlamydia trachomatis* Infection

Agustín Luján, Silvina Fili and María Teresa Damiani

Additional information is available at the end of the chapter

http://dx.doi.org/10.5772/62462

Abstract

Chlamydia trachomatis (CT) is the most common agent of bacterial sexually transmitted infections, both in developed and developing countries. It clearly constitutes a major burden on public health. Screening programs and current research are mainly focused on decreasing the high incidence of chlamydial infections as well as their associated morbidity.

The greater clinical impact of CT infections occurs in women of reproductive age. Acute CT infections are often associated to urethritis, mucopurulent cervicitis, endometritis, salpingitis, and pelvic inflammatory disease (PID). A vast proportion of CT infections are likely underestimated because of their asymptomatic clinical course. This leads to repeat and chronic infections, which have deleterious impact on the female reproductive health. Among the complications of the CT chronic infections are PID, ectopic pregnancy, preterm birth, tubal obstruction and female infertility, which are of great interest in the reproduction field.

Keywords: *Chlamydia trachomatis*, intracellular pathogens, bacterial sexually transmitted infections, tubal obstruction, female infertility

1. Introduction

Chlamydia trachomatis (CT) is the most frequent bacterial agent causing sexually transmitted infections (STIs) worldwide. According to the latest World Health Organization (WHO) report, approximately 100 million new infections occur annually [1]. According to the Centre for Disease Control (CDC), around 1.4 million new CT cases were reported in 2013, only in the United States [2].

In this chapter, we briefly present the current knowledge about the cell biology of the bacteria, reviewing the mechanisms of establishment of CT intracellular niche, the inducers of persistent infections, and the pathogen factors that may be involved in the damage of female reproductive tract. Then, we analyze the host factors that may contribute to the development of infertility, mainly immune response and genetic predisposition, hormonal status, and sexual behavior. Undiagnosed and untreated infections, repeat and persistent infections, and coinfections are likely responsible for the detrimental sequelae on woman fertility of CT pathogenesis.

This chapter specially focuses on the consequences of chronic diseases after CT infections, mainly pelvic inflammatory disease, tubal infertility, and adverse pregnancy outcome, which are of therapeutic interest in the reproduction field.

2. The bacteria: Intracellular life cycle, *Chlamydia trachomatis* serovars and virulence factors

2.1. Chlamydial developmental cycle and intracellular niche

CT is a highly evolved pathogen that has a reduced genome, first sequenced by Stephens and collaborators in 1998. Its chromosome consists of approximately one million base pairs and encodes for up to 600 proteins [3]. Analysis of chlamydial genes reveals that this bacterium heavily depends on host cell for nutrition and replication, indicating a complex evolution for adaptation to an obligate intracellular lifestyle.

CT has tropism for genital mucosal epithelium, which promotes its own uptake into non-phagocytic cells. Chlamydial infection and propagation rely upon a unique biphasic life cycle that begins by contact of infectious, environmentally resistant, elementary bodies (EBs) with the apical surface of the epithelial cell. Several mechanisms are involved in the invasion of host cell, likely parasite-specified phagocytosis and receptor-mediated endocytosis [4]. Multiple receptors have been proposed to mediate the interaction between the EB and the host cell, among them, the mannose receptor, the mannose 6-phosphate receptor, and the estrogen receptor [5]. Other host molecules such as heparan sulfate proteoglycans [6,7], and protein disulfide isomerase also participate in EB binding to the eukaryotic cells [8]. Concomitantly, multiple bacterial adhesins and ligands such as glycosaminoglycan [9], the major outer membrane protein (MOMP) [10], OmcB [11], and PmpD [12] facilitate EB attachment to host cells. Translocated actin-recruiting phosphoprotein (TARP) is a bacterial protein that nucleates actin and promotes host cell cytoskeleton remodeling to force bacterium uptake [13–15].

The infectious EBs enter the host cell in membrane-bound vesicles that travel toward the perinucleus and fuse to form a single vacuole termed the inclusion. Once inside this modified phagosome, EBs differentiate into metabolically active but non-infectious reticulate bodies (RBs) that are the replicative bacterial forms. RBs asynchronously multiply by binary fission within the confines of the growing inclusion. After numerous rounds of replication, RBs re-differentiate back into infectious EBs to be ready for spreading to adjacent cells [16,17]. The ability of CT to cycle between resting and replicating organisms accounts for a drawback in the eradication of this intracellular pathogen. Finally, the infectious bacteria are released by two independent mechanisms, the host cell lysis, or the extrusion of the inclusion [18]. A scheme of chlamydial developmental life cycle is shown in Figure 1.

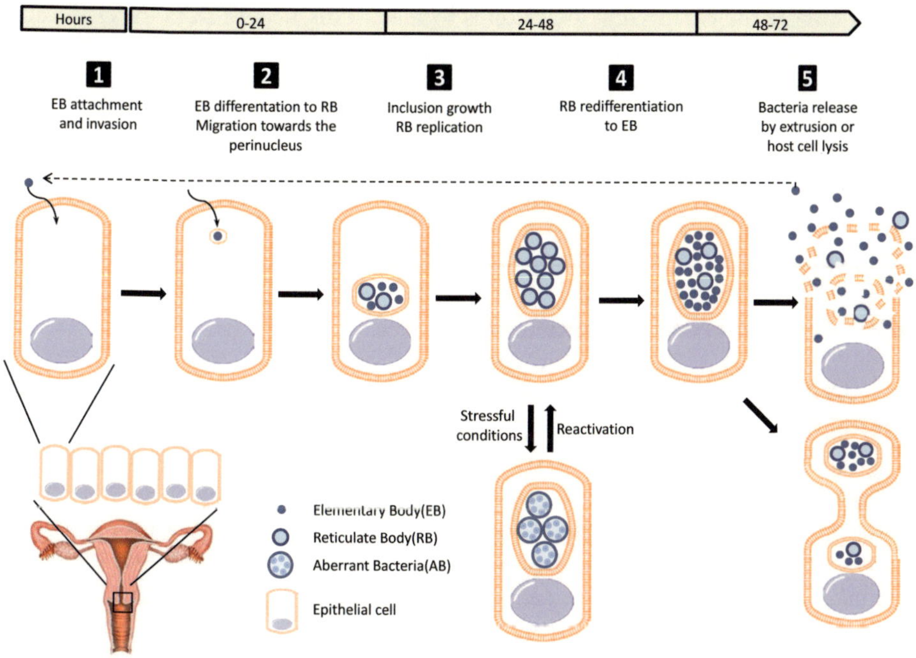

Figure 1. *Chlamydia trachomatis* developmental cycle. Chlamydial infection begins with attachment of the infectious bacterial form, the elementary body (EB) to uncharacterized host cell receptors. Signal transduction events are triggered, and EBs entry into the host cell in small vesicles. These CT-containing vesicles are actively modified by the bacteria; they travel toward the perinucleus and fuse to form a single vacuole named "the inclusion". Once internalized, EB differentiates into the replicative bacterial form, the reticulate body (RB), which multiplies by binary fission. At the end, RBs re-differentiate to EBs that are released by host cell lysis or extrusion of the inclusion. The whole cycle is completed in 40–72 hours. In a stressful environment, RBs enter a latent stage where it persists until more favorable growing conditions. These aberrant bacteria (AB) are present in persistent and chronic infections.

In response to stress, CT enters into a low replicative viable state that is termed "persistent or aberrant bacterial form", which is able to resume normal replication as soon as conditions are again favorable. Among the inducers of the persistent bacterial state stand the sphingolipid deprivation and tryptophan lack, the presence of interferon gamma (IFN-γ), or certain antibiotics such as penicillin. The evasion strategy has been linked to the capacity of these bacteria to cause latent and chronic infections. Thus, the onset of the infection is generally not detected and re-infection may occur, especially when infected couples are involved. Furthermore, the fact that CT clearance is rarely followed up, combined with the ability of this pathogen to persist, contributes to the occurrence of long-term infections [19].

Undoubtedly, an essential issue to chlamydial growth and development is the establishment of its intracellular niche. Early chlamydial gene expression is required to inclusion generation, to avoid immune system surveillance, and to hijack host cell functions [20]. These bacteria actively modify the inclusion membrane by exclusion or recruitment of selected host proteins, mainly Rab proteins, the master controllers of intracellular traffic [16,21]. Increasing evidence points out that the invading bacteria subvert trafficking not only to circumvent the lysosomal degradative route but also to facilitate the delivery of host nutrients to the growing inclusion [17,22]. As soon as the chlamydial inclusion is formed, it dissociates from the classical phagocytic pathway and barely interacts with endocytic vesicles [23]. Instead, chlamydial inclusion intersects Golgi-derived vesicles [24–27], multivesicular bodies [28], and lipid droplets [29,30]. By this strategy, these bacteria take over the infected cell for sphingomyelin, cholesterol, and neutral lipid acquisition like pirates [31–34]. In addition, CTs possess other mechanisms, such as transporter molecules, finely adapted to acquire amino acids, nucleotides, and energy from the host cell [22,35–38]. At present, the strategies developed by CTs to re-route intracellular trafficking and to co-opt host cell functions for their benefit are being actively studied.

2.2. Bacterial genotypes and virulence factors

Different strains of CT have been described based on genome sequencing and the antigenic properties of the major outer membrane protein (MOMP) [39]. There are more than 20 distinct serovars (serologically variant strains) of CT currently identified, on the basis of monoclonal antibody-based typing assays [40–42]. In general, CTs have been grouped into three main pathobiotypes: ocular infections (serovars A to C), sexually transmitted diseases (D to K), and lymphogranuloma venereum (L_1 to L_3). Serovars A, B, and C have tropism for the ocular epithelium, causing from acute conjunctivitis to trachoma, a serious eye disease endemic in Africa and Asia that is characterized by chronic conjunctivitis and can lead to infectious blindness. Serovars D through K have emerged as the major causing agents of sexually transmitted diseases. They preferentially infect squamocolumnar epithelial cells of female reproductive system and the male genitourinary tract. E and D serovars are isolated from genital tract infections with the most frequency worldwide. Occasionally, they cause conjunctivitis or pneumonia in newborns infected during labor. Serovars L1 to L3 are responsible for a systemic illness, the lymphogranuloma venereum that is associated with genital ulcer disease in tropical countries [43,44] (Table 1).

Chlamydia genotyping is useful to determine tissue tropism [45–47]. Several studies attempted to directly link disease severity with CT serovars; however, they often failed because of small number of samples and high variability in results [48]. Intensive research is conducted to confidently associate CT serotypes to higher pathogenic potential, clinical course, or disease outcome. Nevertheless, at present, bacterial ability to ascend and colonize female upper reproductive tract is not clearly associated to a particular CT serovar.

On the other hand, CT gene polymorphisms determine distinct antigenic challenge to the immune system [49]. Certain bacterial polymorphisms may induce an altered immune response [50]. In consequence, they are able to cause immunological disorders, especially in susceptible individuals. Chlamydial infections often precede the initiation of autoimmune diseases, and frequently, these bacteria are found within autoimmune lesions. Bacterial proteins similar to host self-proteins might be the underlying cause of diverse autoimmune diseases [51,52]. This molecular mimicry may elicit an immune response to both self and microbial proteins. Chlamydial heat shock protein 60, DNA primase, and OmcB proteins represent the strongest cases for molecular mimicry [53]. The most frequent autoimmune diseases connected to chlamydial infections are intestinal inflammatory pathologies and rheumatic or connective-tissue diseases [54,55]. Further research is required to unravel the molecular machinery involved in the complex pathogen-host cell interaction.

Chlamydial strains and clinical diseases			
Serovars	Host	Acute	Chronic
A–C	Newborns Both sexes	Conjunctivitis	Trachoma
D–K	Newborn	Ophthalmia neonatorum	Neonatal pneumonia
	Men	Urethritis	Proctitis Epididymitis
	Women	Urethritis Cervicitis	Mucopurulent cervicitis Pelvic inflammatory disease Tubal infertility Ectopic pregnancy Premature rupture of membranes Chorioamnionitis Premature delivery Puerperal infection Cervical neoplasia
$L_{1\text{-}3}$	Both sexes		Lymphogranuloma venereum
Different serovars and bacterial polymorphism	Both sexes		Autoimmune diseases Reactive arthritis Collagenopathies Reiter´s syndrome Inflammatory bowel disease Crohn´s disease

Table 1. Chlamydial serovars, tissue tropism and clinical diseases. Acute and chronic pathologies occur in men, women and newborns following CT infections. Serovars A to C have tropism for ocular epithelium, causing from acute conjunctivitis to infectious blindness or trachoma. Serovars D to K infect epithelial cells of the genitourinary system, generating a broad range of acute and chronic pathologies that damage reproductive tissue and may infect newborns during labor. Serovars $L_{1\text{-}3}$ cause lymphogranuloma venereum. Several autoimmune diseases are associated to diverse CT strains.

Several putative virulence factors have been postulated, including the polymorphic outer membrane autotransporter family of proteins (pmp), type III secretion system (TTSS) effectors, a large cytotoxin, and stress response proteins may contribute to increase the CT-associated pathogenicity. Pmp proteins are strongly immunogenic and trigger pro-inflammatory cytokine responses [56]. Chlamydial TTSS effectors mediate the interaction with the host as they are injected to the cytoplasm and alter host cell functioning [57–59]. Important TTSS effectors are the inclusion (Inc) proteins that are bacterial proteins present at the inclusion membrane. For instance, IncA promotes the fusion of individual CT-containing vesicles to form a single inclusion [60,61]. Natural IncA bacterial mutants are associated with reduced virulence [62]. Another TTSS effector is TARP, mentioned in the previous section, as a bacterial protein that favors CT internalization via an actin recruiting mechanism [34,63]. Additionally, a chlamydial cytotoxin glycosylates the eukaryotic protein Rac1, and thereby induces actin reorganization and promotes the invasion of host cell [64,65]. Chlamydial glycolipid exoantigens [66] and the lipopolysaccharide [67] may constitute additional virulence factors. Other proteins encoded by the cryptic plasmid or related to the ability of the bacteria to survive under stressful metabolic conditions such as iron or tryptophan deprivation are thought to increase virulence and pathogenicity [68,69]. Chlamydial stress proteins, GroEL and GroES, may activate toll-like receptors and trigger a potent inflammatory response, injuring host reproductive tissues [70–73].

In addition to CT serovars and virulence molecules, other bacterial factors may be involved in the pathogenicity and chlamydial infection outcome, such as the pathogen load, route of infection, bacterial ability to enter persistent state, ascension capacity and strength to colonize genital upper tract, resistance to antibiotic treatment, and so on. Further studies are needed to determine the contribution of each bacterial factor to the development of severe damage on the female reproductive system.

3. The host: Immunological and genetic factors, age and hormonal status, and sexual behavior

3.1. Immunological and genetic factors

An important issue that contributes to CT pathogenesis is its remarkable ability to avoid the host immune system. Several strategies are displayed by these bacteria to prevent immune degradation, such as its intracellular lifestyle, its ability to escape from phagolysosomal pathway, its resistance to interferon gamma (IFN-γ), among others lesser known bacterial molecules. Actually, host immune response has opposite results on chlamydial infection outcome. A low immune response generates a suitable environment for pathogen colonization, while a strong immune response could lead to excessive inflammation and tissue damage. Pathogens own characteristics in conjunction with host genetic susceptibility are important in determining the severity of the illness.

At the site of invasion, an intense inflammation occurs, attracting different types of cells, such as macrophages, neutrophils, T and B lymphocytes, natural killers, and dendritic cells. Locally, there is an increased production of reactive oxygen species (ROS) that produces oxidative DNA damage, lipid peroxidation, energy depletion, modulation of gene expression, and proteins synthesis. Oxidative stress provokes pathologic changes that harm reproductive tissues. In addition, a broad collection of pro- and anti-inflammatory cytokines are released including IFN-γ, tumor necrosis factor (TNF-α), interleukin (IL) IL-1β, IL-2, IL-3, IL-4, IL-5, IL-6, IL-8, IL-10, IL-12, IL-13, IL-17, IL-22, vascular endothelial growth factor (VEGF), granulocyte-macrophage colony-stimulating factor (GM-CSF), and lactoferrin. These mediators trigger cellular inflammatory responses that mediate direct damage to the tissues [74,75]. Most of them are involved in the pathophysiology of tubal infertility, birth defects, and miscarriage [76].

In addition to the inflammatory response, CT infection evokes vigorous local and systemic humoral and cell-mediated immune responses. Several CT-specific antibodies, IgG isotype rather than secretory IgA, are found in circulation and in the cervicovaginal fluid of the female genital tract. These antibodies can neutralize chlamydial antigens; nevertheless, they do not assure resolution of the infection. Antibodies toward the bacterial MOMP protein are prevalent in primary chlamydial infections, whereas antibodies against CT-hsp10 and hsp60 are present in recurrent or persistent infections and correlate with severe sequelae such as tubal infertility, ectopic pregnancy, and PID [77–79]. Regarding the cell-mediated immune response, the T-helper lymphocytes type 1 (Th1) secrete IFN-γ, IL-2, and IL-12 and play a role in the resolution of infection [80,81]. On the other hand, the T-helper lymphocytes type 2 (Th2), which support the humoral immune response, produces IL-4, IL-5, IL-6, and IL-10 and participates in the developing tubal scarring [82]. The inflammatory response occurs, at the same extent, in both initial and repeat infections, whereas T-cell responses are predominant in the latter ones [80,83].

Actually, host immune response is considered as one of the most important determinants in chlamydial infection outcome. A delicate balance between pro- and anti-inflammatory cytokines is needed to clear infection, avoiding tissue injuring. At this point, host genetic predisposition is a major player of pathology and CT-related infertility development [84].

Host genetic polymorphisms may encode aberrant or dysfunctional toll-like receptors (TLR) and nucleotide-binding oligomerization domain proteins (NOD) that do not appropriately recognize CT. These individuals have an impaired bacterial clearance and a high risk to develop an aberrant immune response, favoring CT persistence [85–88]. Identifying host genetic factors and bacterial virulence factors involved in immunoevasion and immunopathology remains a major priority in research for preventing chlamydial infection and its sequelae. Furthermore, the understanding of local innate and adaptive immune responses and their actors along the genital tract will be crucial for designing new therapeutic approaches and for developing a protective vaccine.

3.2. Age and hormonal status

CT preferentially targets young women at reproductive age. It has been reported that the highest incidence occurs in women between 16 to 24 years [89]. Therefore, the impact on female reproductive health is very important. Notwithstanding younger women are at higher risk of contracting a chlamydial infection, the rates of developing PID increase with age, being more frequent in the 30 to 40 decade [90]. After menopause, the frequency of chlamydial infections decreases substantially [91].

Accordingly, estrogen and progesterone are important for the establishment of chlamydial infection. Furthermore, estrogen receptors have been involved in the internalization of CT [92,93]. Sex hormones affect the clinical outcome of chlamydial infections; thus, follicle stimulating hormone (FSH), luteinizing hormone (LH), estradiol (E2), progesterone (P4), and prolactin (PRL) are involved not only in the establishment of chlamydial infection but also in the development of sequelae on reproductive tissue [94,95]. Additionally, oral contraceptive use was found to be a risk factor for CT infection. Several studies have attempted to elucidate the relation between the hormonal status at the time of infection and its contribution to tubal occlusion in genital chlamydial infection. Unfortunately, the role of sex steroids in infection outcome is far from being fully understood. Sex hormones have been shown to modulate immune responses and to have antioxidant effects in the female genital tract [96–98]. However, the mechanisms by which sex hormones may benefit or impair the colonization of genital tissues by pathogenic microorganisms should be further investigated.

3.3. Sexual behavior and other host factors

Sexual initiation at young age and a higher number of sexual partners are associated with increased risk of CT infection [99]. In a similar manner, having sex without protection favors CT contagion. This sexual behavior is also associated with higher incidence of sexually transmitted pathogens such as *Neisseria gonorrhoeae, Candida albicans, Human Immunodeficiency Virus*, among others [100–103]. Taken together, unsafe and high-risk sexual conduct is linked to impairment of women reproductive health, and particularly to tubal infertility. As it has been previously mentioned, some women have a genotypic predisposition to develop an abnormal immune response and severe inflammation following CT infection. In these women, there is a high rate of tubal obstruction and CT-related infertility, independent of sexual behavior [84].

In general, multiple sexual partners and unsafe intercourse increase the risk of CT recurrent infections and coinfection with other sexually transmitted pathogens. Thereby, the high chance to suffer repeat and chronic infections that target women reproductive tissue raises the infertility-associated pathologies.

4. Pathogen-host interplay: Establishment of latent, repeat, and persistent infections and coinfections

CT survival and replication heavily hinge on host cells. In fact, CT has evolved in relationship with human cells. However, little is known about the molecular basis of CT interaction with host epithelia and immune system. An increasing number of bacterial and host factors interplay for the establishment of chlamydial infection and determine the pathologic profile and clinical disease outcome. A simple scheme is shown in Figure 2 summarizing the main CT and host factors that jointly with environmental factors and the failure in diagnosis and treatment, lead to unsolved, latent, and long-term chlamydial infections.

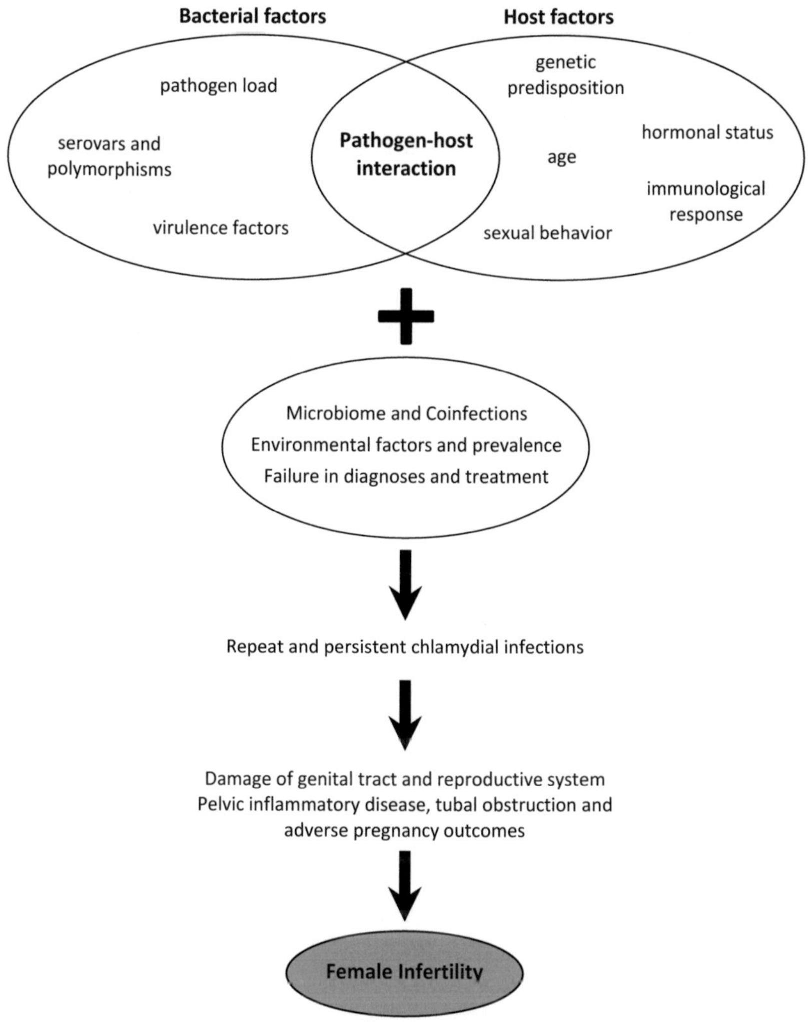

Figure 2. Bacterial and host factors involved in the development of female infertility. Bacterial factors such as CT genotypes and serovars, virulence factors, and pathogen burden, in conjunction with, host factors such as genetic predisposition and immune response, age and hormonal status, and sexual behavior participate in the establishment of the infection and pathology. Other elements that take part in the development of CT-related diseases are microbiome and coinfections with other sexually transmitted pathogens, environmental factors, and local prevalence, and most importantly, the failure in diagnosis and treatment of chlamydial infections. Taken together, these factors sustain repeat and persistent chlamydial infections that damage female reproductive health.

Microbiome (microbial flora present at the genital tract) and the presence of other sexually transmitted pathogens may be important for the colonization of reproductive tissue and the establishment of chlamydial infection. The presence of lactobacilli in the vagina confers protection against the acquisition of chlamydial infection [104]. In contrast, indole-generating bacteria present in the microbiome or bacterial vaginosis allow CT to synthesize tryptophan, and consequently, to avoid the anti-chlamydial activity of IFN-γ [45,65]. Coinfections are more frequent in vaginosis and women with high-risk sexual behavior [100]. Clearly, coinfections exacerbate host immune response and inflammation; therefore, they favor scarring and sequelae on female reproductive system and increase the likelihood of tubal infertility.

The worst scenarios involve silent and latent infections that underline chronic persistent chlamydial infection and frequent re-infections [1]. Chlamydial infections may persist in the female upper genital tract for months in the absence of treatment. They are often asymptomatic or alternate quiescent stages with periods of clinical manifestations [105]. Actually, chronic chlamydial infections may be because of the reactivation of asymptomatic latently infected deep-seated cells. The presence of aberrant bacterial forms responsible for chlamydial persistence constitutes a long-time challenge to the immune system. Host immunopathological response can damage the fallopian tube and generate female infertility [65,92].

Reinfections, persistent infections, and treatment failure account for repeat infections that represent a substantial proportion of the chlamydial infections detected annually [106]. Repeat infection is not the sole determinant of severe genital tract pathology and sequelae. However, repeat infection increases the risk of developing tubal obstruction and female infertility [76].

Increasing evidence indicates that long-term persistence of viable aberrant chlamydial organisms within host cells is associated with inflammatory and autoimmune diseases in extragenital tissues.

In definitive, the pathogen-host interplay and the concurrency of exogenous factors appear to be related to CT-induced immunopathology. In spite of the substantial worldwide impact of chlamydial disease, the bacterial and host factors that result in infertility are still not clear. Current efforts are focused on discovering what CT is doing to the host cells to prevent sequelae and undesired consequences of infection.

5. Mechanisms of pathogenicity and clinical course

CT infects both sexes; however, chlamydial infections constitute primarily a female health issue since the consequences are more damaging to the reproductive tissue in women than in men. In males, CT can infect urethra, epididymis, prostate, seminal vesicles, and testis. Usually, chlamydial infections are symptomatic, less frequent, and more easily eradicated in men than in women. Nevertheless, chlamydial infection in the male genitourinary tract might induce severe damage to seminiferous tubules, spermatogenesis, and sperm cells morphology that can result in impaired male fertility [107].

Here, we focus on chlamydial infections occurring in women. In first world countries, 3 to 5% of women younger than 30 years old will be infected by CT at any point in time [90,108]. And, in over 70% of the cases, CT infection of the female genitourinary tract is asymptomatic, spoiling the prevalence or incidence rates. Consequently, it is difficult to assess the incidence of sequelae, mainly PID, tubal obstruction, and female infertility, attributable to genital CT infection.

In women, CT is the major cause of mucopurulent cervicitis (MPC) and PID. Other manifestations of chlamydial infections are vaginitis, urethritis, salpingitis, endometritis, tubo-ovarian abscess, pelvic peritonitis, periappendicitis, and perihepatitis. The symptoms more frequently reported consist of abdominal pain, dysuria, vaginal itching, and abnormal vaginal discharge. However, the most important feature of chlamydial infection in the female genital tract is the occurrence of asymptomatic infection that remains subclinical for long periods in a high rate [109,110]. Asymptomatic ascending bacteria from the cervix may produce two groups of pathologies: (i) PID-associated complications such as chronic pelvic pain, tubal obstruction, and female infertility [111,112] and (ii) adverse pregnancy outcomes such as ectopic pregnancy, miscarriage, premature rupture of membranes, chrioamnionitis, preterm birth, stillbirths, and puerperal and neonatal infections [113–115].

General consensus in the medical community agrees that chlamydial PID is the most common preventable cause of tubal infertility and adverse pregnancy outcome [1]. However, the lack of systematic detection of the bacteria weakens these estimations, usually performed by analysis of a reduced number of cases. Approximately 20% of women with chlamydial lower genital tract infection will develop PID, 4% chronic pelvic pain, 3% tubal infertility, and 2% adverse pregnancy outcome [107]. In developing countries, the incidence and prevalence of CT infections and their harmful consequences on female reproductive tissue are not accurately known since CT infection is not routinely screened.

There is conclusive evidence that women who have suffered PID have higher risk to develop tubal infertility. A study demonstrated that 16.5% of women with abnormal laparoscopic findings likely resulting of acute PID failed to conceive, in comparison to 2.7% in control women; 10.8% developed tubal infertility, and 9.1% went through ectopic pregnancy. Therefore, PID increases the probability of permanent damage on female reproductive system. CT is the most common causing agent of PID; however, a drawback of this analysis is the lack of the identification of the infectious agent underlying the PID. Several randomized controlled trials to assess the value of CT screening found it helpful to reduce the incidence of PID among infected women [116–118]. The chance to develop tubal infertility after a single episode of PID is around 10% [112]. Furthermore, each episode of PID doubled the risk of tubal damage [119] independent of whether the infection was asymptomatic or not.

One of the most serious sequelae of PID and persistent chlamydial infections is the fibrosis and scarring obstruction of the fallopian tubes that leads to tubal infertility. However, the risk of tubal infertility due to CT infections is lower than PID incidence [76]. The proportion of tubal infertility among all causes of infertility varies from 40% in first-world countries to 85% in developing countries [1]. Undiagnosed and untreated chlamydial infections usually evolve to long-term persistent infections, in which chlamydial antigens chronically stimulate the host immune system. Abnormal humoral and cell-mediated immune responses and severe inflammation have been implicated in the development of immunopathological damage of fallopian tubes. Thus, the interaction between CT and the host becomes relevant for the illness outcome. However, the exact pathologic mechanism of CT-induced tubal damage and tubal infertility has not been elucidated yet.

In addition, acute and chronic maternal chlamydial infections constitute a significant risk factor for adverse pregnancy outcomes and newborns contagion. Untreated and persistent infections are strongly associated with ectopic pregnancy, which is the tubal development of the embryo and constitute the main cause of maternal mortality in the first trimester of pregnancy in developing countries. In addition, miscarriage, chrioamnionitis, low birth weight, stillbirth, premature rupture of membranes, and preterm birth are frequent pathological consequences of chlamydial infections [51,113,114]. Several mechanisms may contribute to the development of these pathologies, including direct fetal infection, placental damage, and severe puerperal maternal illness [120–124]. Nevertheless, the exact nature of chlamydial infection pathogenesis during pregnancy remains unexplained.

CT infections can also be vertically transmitted to newborns during labor, resulting in chlamydial conjunctivitis and/or pneumonia, which may possibly involve similar pathogenesis mechanisms to those occurring in the female genital tract.

Controversial reports point out CT as a risk factor for cervical carcinoma, independent of human papillomavirus [107]. It has been shown that CT interferes with multiple proapoptotic pathways to guarantee survival within host cells [125,126]. In addition, CT activates prosurvival signaling pathways for bacterial nutrient acquisition, expression of antiapoptotic factors, and synthesis of proinflammatory cytokines [127,128]. On the other hand, CT interferes with chromosome segregation and cytokinesis. In consequence, multinucleated cells and cells with aberrant number of chromosomes are often observed in cell cultures infected with CT [129]. Taken together, these findings suggest that persistent chlamydial infections might play a role in the development of cervical neoplasia. Further research is needed to shed light to this issue.

The high prevalence and incidence estimates worldwide, in conjunction to the diversity of clinical entities and long-term consequences of chlamydial infections, propel further research of the bacterial and host factors involved in the pathogenesis and damage to the reproductive system.

6. Important challenges: Prevention, diagnosis, and treatment of chlamydial infections

The widespread incidence and prevalence of sexually transmitted infections, especially among young population, made them a priority public-health concern worldwide. Screening, control programmes, and education in sexual behavioral aspects and contraception are fundamental for the prevention of chlamydial infections and their long-term sequelae, mainly PID and tubal infertility.

Routine screening allows the identification of asymptomatic carriers of CT and contributes to the early detection of chlamydial infections. Appropriated diagnostic services are required to obtain reliable results. The most confident tests for the detection of CT involve nucleid acid amplification techniques that are not available in all laboratories, especially in third-world countries. Nucleic acid amplification tests are more sensitive than culture or antigen tests.

Improvement in molecular diagnostics will lead to improvement in treatment and prevention of damage to reproductive tissues. It has been shown that screening is cost-effective even in low prevalence populations, due to the high costs of treatment of complications resulting from undiagnosed and untreated chlamydial infections [130]. The implement of additional targeted screening of women at risk will contribute to reduce the CT-associated infertility.

Additionally, clinicians should be aware about the latest therapeutic management of chlamydial cervicitis and PID. Different antibiotics such as azithromycin, doxycycline, ofloxacin, erythromycin, and amoxicillin may be useful for treating genital chlamydial infections [131]. The antibiotic selection depends on the characteristics of the drug itself like pharmacokinetics, half-life, and bioavailability, concentration in mucous membranes and genital tissues, development of gastrointestinal tract side effects, safe use in pregnancy, as well as, the characteristics of the host and the clinical course of chlamydial infection. The effectiveness of therapy relies on timely treating sex partners and to abstain from sexual intercourse until completing the whole antibiotic scheme.

Unceasing efforts are conducted for the development of a chlamydial vaccine. Nevertheless, until now, no effective chlamydial vaccines are available. The knowledge of bacterial factors involved in pathogenicity will help in addressing optimal vaccine design that prevents not only chlamydial infection but also progression to infertility.

Acknowledgements

The authors acknowledge CONICET (PIP), Foncyt (PICT 2116) and UNCuyo grants to M.T.D. for their support in research. They apologize to those investigators whose work could not be cited because of space constraints.

Author details

Agustín Luján, Silvina Fili and María Teresa Damiani*

*Address all correspondence to: meteresadamiani@gmail.com

Laboratory of Phagocytosis and Intracellular Transport, IHEM-CONICET, School of Medicine, University of Cuyo, Mendoza, Argentina

References

[1] World Health Organization. Prevalence and incidence of selected sexually transmitted infections, Chlamydia trachomatis, Neisseria gonorrhoeae, syphilis and Tricho-

monas vaginalis: Methods and results used by WHO to generate 2005 estimate. WHO. 2011;1–38.

[2] CDC. Incidence, Prevalence, and Cost of Sexually Transmitted Infections in the United States. CDC Fact Sheet. 2013;40(February):1–4.

[3] Stephens RS, Kalman S, Lammel C, Fan J, Marathe R, Aravind L, et al. Genome sequence of an obligate intracellular pathogen of humans: Chlamydia trachomatis. Science (Internet). 1998;282(5389):754–759.

[4] Hybiske K, Stephens RS. Mechanisms of Chlamydia trachomatis entry into nonphagocytic cells. Infect Immun. 2007;75(8):3925–3934.

[5] Cocchiaro JL, Valdivia RH. New insights into Chlamydia intracellular survival mechanisms. Cell Microbiol. 2009;11(11):1571–1878.

[6] Dautry-Varsat A, Subtil A, Hackstadt T. Recent insights into the mechanisms of Chlamydia entry. Cell Microbiol. 2005;7(12):1714–1722.

[7] Chen JC, Stephens RS. Chlamydia trachomatis glycosaminoglycan-dependent and independent attachment to eukaryotic cells. Microb Pathog. 1997;22(1):23–30.

[8] Abromaitis S, Stephens RS. Attachment and entry of chlamydia have distinct requirements for host protein disulfide isomerase. PLoS Pathog. 2009;5(4):1–12.

[9] Menozzi FD, Pethe K, Bifani P, Soncin F, Brennan MJ, Locht C. Enhanced bacterial virulence through exploitation of host glycosaminoglycans. Mol Microbiol. 2002;43(6):1379–1386.

[10] Su B, Karint M. Mitogen-activated gene expression protein kinase cascades and regulation of gene expression. Curr Opin Immunol. 1996;8(3):402–411.

[11] Fadel S, Eley A. Chlamydia trachomatis OmcB protein is a surface-exposed glycosaminoglycan-dependent adhesion. J Med Microbiol. 2007;56(1):15–22.

[12] Mölleken K, Schmidt E, Hegemann JH. Members of the Pmp protein family of Chlamydia pneumoniae mediate adhesion to human cells via short repetitive peptide motifs. Mol Microbiol. 2010;78(4):1004–1017.

[13] Engel J. Tarp and Arp: How Chlamydia induces its own entry. Proc Natl Acad Sci U S A. 2004;101(27):9947–9948.

[14] Lane BJ, Mutchler C, Al Khodor S, Grieshaber SS, Carabeo RA. Chlamydial entry involves TARP binding of guanine nucleotide exchange factors. PLoS Pathog. 2008;4(3):1–11.

[15] Jewett TJ, Miller NJ, Dooley CA, Hackstadt T. The conserved tarp actin binding domain is important for chlamydial invasion. PLoS Pathog. 2010;6(7):1–11.

[16] Damiani MT, Gambarte Tudela J, Capmany A. Targeting eukaryotic Rab proteins: A smart strategy for chlamydial survival and replication. Cell Microbiol. 2014;16(9): 1329–1338.

[17] Gambarte Tudela J, Capmany A, Romao M, Quintero C, Miserey-Lenkei S, Raposo G, Goud B, Damiani MT. The late endocytic Rab39a GTPase regulates the interaction between multivesicular bodies and chlamydial inclusions. J Cell Sci. 2015;128(16):3068–3081.

[18] Hybiske K, Stephens RS. Mechanisms of host cell exit by the intracellular bacterium Chlamydia. Proc Natl Acad Sci U S A. 2007;104(27):11430–11435.

[19] Beatty WL, Byrne GI, Morrison RP. Repeated and persistent infection with Chlamydia and the development of chronic inflammation and disease. Trends Microbiol. 1994;2(3):94–98.

[20] Bastidas RJ, Elwell CA, Engel JN, Valdivia RH. Chlamydial intracellular survival strategies. Cold Spring Harb Perspect Med. 2013;3(5): 1–20.

[21] Rzomp KA, Scholtes LD, Briggs BJ, Whittaker GR, Scidmore MA. Rab GTPases are recruited to chlamydial inclusions in both a species-dependent and species-independent manner. Infect Immun. 2003;71(10):5855–5870.

[22] Hackstadt T, Fischer ER, Scidmore MA, Rockey DD, Heinzen RA. Origins and functions of the chlamydial inclusion. Trends Microbiol. 1997;5(7):288–293.

[23] Fields KA, Hackstadt T. The chlamydial inclusion: Escape from the endocytic pathway. Annu Rev Cell Biol. 2002;18:221–245.

[24] Moore ER, Fischer ER, Mead DJ, Hackstadt T. The chlamydial inclusion preferentially intercepts basolaterally directed sphingomyelin-containing exocytic vacuoles. Traffic. 2008;9(12):2130–2140.

[25] Rejman Lipinski A, Heymann J, Meissner C, Karlas A, Brinkmann V, Meyer TF, et al. Rab6 and Rab11 regulate Chlamydia trachomatis development and golgin-84-dependent Golgi fragmentation. PLoS Pathog. 2009;5(10): 1–12.

[26] Capmany A, Damiani MT. Chlamydia trachomatis intercepts golgi-derived sphingolipids through a rab14-mediated transport required for bacterial development and replication. PLoS One. 2010;5(11): 1–17.

[27] Leiva N, Capmany A, Damiani MT. Rab11-Family of Interacting Protein 2 associates with chlamydial inclusions through its Rab-binding domain and promotes bacterial multiplication. Cell Microbiol. 2013;15(1):114–129.

[28] Beatty WL. Trafficking from CD63-positive late endocytic multivesicular bodies is essential for intracellular development of Chlamydia trachomatis. J Cell Sci. 2006;119(Pt 2):350–359.

[29] Cocchiaro J, Kumar Y, Fischer ER, Hackstadt T, Valdivia RH. Cytoplasmic lipid droplets are translocated into the lumen of the Chlamydia trachomatis parasitophorous vacuole. Proc Natl Acad Sci U S A. 2008;105(27):9379–9384.

[30] Saka HA, Valdivia R. Emerging roles for lipid droplets in immunity and host-pathogen interactions. Annu Rev Cell Dev Biol. 2012;28(1):411–437.

[31] Derré I, Swiss R, Agaisse H. The lipid transfer protein CERT interacts with the Chlamydia inclusion protein IncD and participates to ER-Chlamydia inclusion membrane contact sites. PLoS Pathog. 2011;7(6): 1–13.

[32] Elwell CA, Jiang S, Kim JH, Lee A, Wittmann T, Hanada K, et al. Chlamydia trachomatis co-opts gbf1 and cert to acquire host sphingomyelin for distinct roles during intracellular development. PLoS Pathog. 2011;7(9): 1–20.

[33] Robertson KD, Gu L, Rowe RK, Beatty WL. Inclusion biogenesis and reactivation of persistent Chlamydia trachomatis requires host cell sphingolipid biosynthesis. PLoS Pathog. 2009;5(11): 1–9.

[34] Clifton DR, Fields KA, Grieshaber SS, Dooley CA, Fischer ER, Mead DJ, et al. A chlamydial type III translocated protein is tyrosine-phosphorylated at the site of entry and associated with recruitment of actin. Proc Natl Acad Sci U S A. 2004;101(27): 10166–10171.

[35] Grieshaber S, Swanson JA, Hackstadt T. Determination of the physical environment within the Chlamydia trachomatis inclusion using ion-selective ratiometric probes. Cell Microbiol. 2002;4(5):273–283.

[36] Vandahl BBS, Stensballe A, Roepstorff P, Christiansen G, Birkelund S. Secretion of Cpn0796 from Chlamydia pneumoniae into the host cell cytoplasm by an autotransporter mechanism. Cell Microbiol. 2005;7(6):825–836.

[37] Trentmann O, Horn M, Van Scheltinga ACT, Neuhaus HE, Haferkamp I. Enlightening energy parasitism by analysis of an ATP/ADP transporter from chlamydiae. PLoS Biol. 2007;5(9):1938–1951.

[38] Derré I, Pypaert M, Dautry-Varsat A, Agaisse H. RNAi screen in Drosophila cells reveals the involvement of the tom complex in Chlamydia infection. PLoS Pathog. 2007;3(10):1446–1458.

[39] Mylonas I. Female genital Chlamydia trachomatis infection: Where are we heading? Arch Gynecol Obstet. 2012;285(5):1271–1285.

[40] Stephens RS, Sanchez-Pescador R, Wagar EA, Inouye C, Urdea MS. Diversity of Chlamydia trachomatis major outer membrane protein genes. J Bacteriol. 1987;169(9): 3879–3885.

[41] Baehr W, Zhang YX, Joseph T, Su H, Nano FE, Everett KD, et al. Mapping antigenic domains expressed by Chlamydia trachomatis major outer membrane protein genes. Proc Natl Acad Sci U S A. 1988;85(11):4000–4004.

[42] Millman K, Black CM, Johnson RE, Stamm E, Jones RB, Hook EW, et al. Population-based genetic and evolutionary analysis of Chlamydia trachomatis urogenital strain variation in the United States. J Bacteriol. 2004;186(8):2457–2465.

[43] Stothard DR, Boguslawski G, Jones RB. Phylogenetic analysis of the Chlamydia trachomatis major outer membrane protein and examination of potential pathogenic determinants. Infect Immun. 1998;66(8):3618–3625.

[44] Brown WJ, Rockey DD. Identification of an antigen localized to an apparent septum within dividing chlamydiae? Infect Immun. 2000;68(2):708–715.

[45] Nelson DE, Virok DP, Wood H, Roshick C, Johnson RM, Whitmire WM, et al. Chlamydial IFN-gamma immune evasion is linked to host infection tropism. Proc Natl Acad Sci U S A. 2005;102(30):10658–10663.

[46] Borges V, Nunes A, Ferreira R, Borrego MJ, Gomes JP. Directional evolution of chlamydia trachomatis towards niche-specific adaptation. J Bacteriol. 2012;194(22):6143–6153.

[47] Jeffrey BM, Suchland RJ, Quinn KL, Davidson JR, Stamm WE, Rockey DD. Genome sequencing of recent clinical Chlamydia trachomatis strains identifies loci associated with tissue tropism and regions of apparent recombination. Infect Immun. 2010;78(6):2544–2553.

[48] Dean D, Oudens E, Bolan G, Padian N, Schachter J. Major outer membrane protein variants of *Chlamydia trachomatis* are associated with severe upper genital tract infections and histopathology in San Francisco. J Infect Dis 1995;172(4):1013–1022.

[49] Brunham RC, Plummer FA, Stephens RS. Bacterial antigenic variation, host immune response, and pathogen-host coevolution. Infect Immun. 1993;61(6):2273–2276.

[50] Mascellino MT, Ciardi MR, Oliva A, Cecinato F, Hassemer MP, Borgese L. Chlamydia trachomatis detection in a population of asymptomatic and symptomatic women: Correlation with the presence of serological markers for this infection. New Microbiol. 2008;31(2):249–256.

[51] Domeika M, Domeika K, Paavonen J, Mårdh PA, Witkin SS. Humoral immune response to conserved epitopes of Chlamydia trachomatis and human 60-kDa heat-shock protein in women with pelvic inflammatory disease. J Infect Dis. 1998;177(3): 714–719.

[52] Swanborg RH, Boros DL, Whittum-Hudson JA, Hudson AP. Molecular mimicry and horror autotoxicus: Do chlamydial infections elicit autoimmunity? Expert Rev Mol Med. 2006;8(29):1–23.

[53] Linhares IM, Witkin SS. Immunopathogenic consequences of Chlamydia trachomatis 60 kDa heat shock protein expression in the female reproductive tract. Cell Stress Chaperones. 2010;15(5):467–473.

[54] Peña AS, Karimi O, Crusius JBA. A new avenue to investigate: The autophagic process. From Crohn's disease to Chlamydia. Drugs Today. 2009;45(Suppl. B):113–117.

[55] Carter JD, Inman RD, Whittum-Hudson J, Hudson AP. Chlamydia and chronic arthritis. Ann Med. 2011;44(8):1–9.

[56] Henderson IR, Nataro JP. Virulence functions of autotransporter proteins. Infect Immun. 2001;69(3):1231–1243.

[57] Subtil A, Blocker A, Dautry-Varsat A. Type III secretion system in Chlamydia species: Identified members and candidates. Microbes Infect. 2000;2(4):367–369.

[58] Betts HJ, Wolf K, Fields KA. Effector protein modulation of host cells: Examples in the Chlamydia spp. arsenal. Curr Opin Microbiol. 2009;12(1):81–87.

[59] Beeckman DSA, Vanrompay DCG. Zoonotic *Chlamydophila psittaci* infections from a clinical perspective. Clin Microbiol Infect. 2009;15(1):11–17.

[60] Hackstadt T, Scidmore MA, Shaw EI, Fischer ER. The Chlamydia trachomatis IncA protein is required for homotypic vesicle fusion. Cell Microbiol. 1999;1(2):119–130.

[61] Delevoye C, Nilges M, Dehoux P, Paumet F, Perrinet S, Dautry-Varsat A, et al. SNARE protein mimicry by an intracellular bacterium. PLoS Pathog. 2008;4(3): 1–14.

[62] Geisler WM, Suchland RJ, Whittington WL, Stamm WE. Quantitative culture of Chlamydia trachomatis: relationship of inclusion-forming units produced in culture to clinical manifestations and acute inflammation in urogenital disease. J Infect Dis. 2001;184(10):1350–1354.

[63] Jewett TJ, Fischer ER, Mead DJ, Hackstadt T. Chlamydial TARP is a bacterial nucleator of actin. Proc Natl Acad Sci U S A. 2006;103(42):15599–15604.

[64] Belland RJ, Scidmore MA, Dean D, Hogan D, Whitmire WM, McClarty G, et al. Chlamydia trachomatis cytotoxicity associated with complete and partial cytotoxin genes. Proc Natl Acad Sci U S A. 2001;98(24):13984–13989.

[65] Carlson JH, Hughes S, Hogan D, Cieplak G, Sturdevant DE, McClarty G, et al. Polymorphisms in the Chlamydia trachomatis cytotoxin locus associated with ocular and genital isolates. Infect Immun. 2004;72(12):7063–7072.

[66] Vora GJ, Stuart ES. A role for the glycolipid exoantigen (GLXA) in chlamydial infectivity. Curr Microbiol. 2003;46(3):217–223.

[67] Brade L, Nurminen M, Makela PH, Brade H. Antigenic properties of *Chlamydia trachomatis* lipopolysaccharide. Infect Immun. 1985;48(2):569–572.

[68] Omsland A, Sixt BS, Horn M, Hackstadt T. Chlamydial metabolism revisited: Interspecies metabolic variability and developmental stage-specific physiologic activities. FEMS Microbiol Rev. 2014;38(4):779–801.

[69] Wood H, Fehlner-Gardner C, Berry J, Fischer E, Graham B, Hackstadt T, et al. Regulation of tryptophan synthase gene expression in Chlamydia trachomatis. Mol Microbiol. 2003;49(5):1347–1359.

[70] Witkin SS, Jeremias J, Toth M, Ledger WJ. Cell-mediated immune response to the recombinant 57-kDa heat-shock protein of Chlamydia trachomatis in women with salpingitis. J Infect Dis. 1993;167(6):1379–1383.

[71] Kol A, Lichtman AH, Finberg RW, Libby P, Kurt-Jones EA. Cutting edge: Heat shock protein (HSP) 60 activates the innate immune response: CD14 is an essential receptor for HSP60 activation of mononuclear cells. J Immunol. 2000;164(1):13–17.

[72] LaVerda D, Albanese LN, Ruther PE, Morrison SG, Morrison RP, Ault KA, et al. Seroreactivity to Chlamydia trachomatis Hsp10 correlates with severity of human genital tract disease. Infect Immun. 2000;68(1):303–309.

[73] Kinnunen A, Molander P, Morrison R, Lehtinen M, Karttunen R, Tiitinen A, et al. Chlamydial heat shock protein 60-specific T cells in inflamed salpingeal tissue. Fertil Steril. 2002;77(1):162–166.

[74] Jha R, Srivastava P, Salhan S, Finckh A, Gabay C, Mittal A, et al. Spontaneous secretion of interleukin-17 and -22 by human cervical cells in Chlamydia trachomatis infection. Microbes Infect. Elsevier Masson SAS; 2011;13(2):167–178.

[75] Spear GT, Kendrick SR, Chen HY, Thomas TT, Bahk M, Balderas R, et al. Multiplex immunoassay of lower genital tract mucosal fluid from women attending an urban STD clinic shows broadly increased IL1ß and lactoferrin. PLoS One. 2011;6(5):1–7.

[76] Low N, Egger M, Sterne JAC, Harbord RM, Ibrahim F, Lindblom B, et al. Incidence of severe reproductive tract complications associated with diagnosed genital chlamydial infection: The Uppsala Women's Cohort Study. Sex Transm Infect. 2006;82(3): 212–218.

[77] Agrawal T, Vats V, Salhan S, Mittal A. Mucosal and peripheral immune responses to chlamydial heat shock proteins in women infected with Chlamydia trachomatis. Clin Exp Immunol. 2007;148(3):461–468.

[78] Srivastava P, Jha R, Bas S, Salhan S, Mittal A. In infertile women, cells from Chlamydia trachomatis infected sites release higher levels of interferon-gamma, interleukin-10 and tumor necrosis factor-alpha upon heat-shock-protein stimulation than fertile women. Reprod Biol Endocrinol. 2008;6:20.

[79] Mascellino MT, Margani M, Oliva A. Helicobacter pylori: Determinant and markers of virulence. Dis Markers. 2009;27(3-4):137–156.

[80] Darville T, Hiltke TJ. Pathogenesis of genital tract disease due to Chlamydia trachomatis. J Infect Dis. 2010;201(S2):114–125.

[81] Morrison SG, Su H, Caldwell HD, Morrison RP. Immunity to murine Chlamydia trachomatis genital tract reinfection involves B cells and CD4+ T cells but not CD8+ T cells. Infect Immun. 2000;68(12):6979–6987.

[82] Holland MJ, Bailey RL, Conway DJ, Culley F, Miranpuri G, Byrne GI, et al. T helper type-1 (Th1)/Th2 profiles of peripheral blood mononuclear cells (PBMC); responses to antigens of Chlamydia trachomatis in subjects with severe trachomatous scarring. Clin Exp Immunol. 1996;105(3):429–435.

[83] Horne AW, Stock SJ, King AE. Innate immunity and disorders of the female reproductive tract. Reproduction. 2008;135(6):739–749.

[84] Lal JA, Malogajski J, Verweij SP, De Boer P, Ambrosino E, Brand A, et al. Chlamydia trachomatis infections and subfertility: Opportunities to translate host pathogen genomic data into public health. Public Health Genomics. 2013;16(1-2):50–61.

[85] Ingalls RR, Rice PA, Qureshi N, Takayama K, Juey Shin Lin, Golenbock DT. The inflammatory cytokine response to Chlamydia trachomatis infection is endotoxin mediated. Infect Immun. 1995;63(8):3125–3130.

[86] Prebeck S, Kirschning C, Dürr S, da Costa C, Donath B, Brand K, et al. Predominant role of toll-like receptor 2 versus 4 in Chlamydia pneumoniae-induced activation of dendritic cells. J Immunol. 2001;167(6):3316–3323.

[87] Heine H, Müller-Loennies S, Brade L, Lindner B, Brade H. Endotoxic activity and chemical structure of lipopolysaccharides from Chlamydia trachomatis serotypes E and L2 and Chlamydophila psittaci 6BC. Eur J Biochem. 2003;270(3):440–450.

[88] Welter-Stahl L, Ojcius DM, Viala J, Girardin S, Liu W, Delarbre C, et al. Stimulation of the cytosolic receptor for peptidoglycan, Nod1, by infection with Chlamydia trachomatis or Chlamydia muridarum. Cell Microbiol. 2006;8(6):1047–1057.

[89] Walker J, Tabrizi SN, Fairley CK, Chen MY, Bradshaw CS, Twin J, et al. Chlamydia trachomatis incidence and re-infection among young women – Behavioural and microbiological characteristics. PLoS One. 2012;7(5):1–9.

[90] Price MJ, Ades AE, de Angelis D, Welton NJ, Macleod J, Turner K, et al. Incidence of Chlamydia trachomatis infection in women in England: Two methods of estimation. Epidemiol Infect. 2014;142(3):562–576.

[91] Bender N, Herrmann B, Andersen B, Hocking JS, van Bergen J, Morgan J, et al. Chlamydia infection, pelvic inflammatory disease, ectopic pregnancy and infertility: Cross-national study. Sex Transm Infect. 2011;87(7):601–608.

[92] Hall JV, Schell M, Dessus-Babus S, Moore CG, Whittimore JD, Sal M, et al. The multifaceted role of oestrogen in enhancing Chlamydia trachomatis infection in polarized human endometrial epithelial cells. Cell Microbiol. 2011;13(8):1183–1199.

[93] Borth N, Massier J, Franke C, Sachse K, Saluz HP, Hänel F. Chlamydial protease CT441 interacts with SRAP1 co-activator of estrogen receptor and partially alleviates its co-activation activity. J Steroid Biochem Mol Biol. 2010;119(1–2):89–95.

[94] Sonnex C. Influence of ovarian hormones on urogenital infection. Sex Transm Infect. 1998;74(1):11–19.

[95] Agrawal T, Vats V, Wallace PK, Salhan S, Mittal A. Role of cervical dendritic cell subsets, co-stimulatory molecules, cytokine secretion profile and beta-estradiol in development of sequalae to Chlamydia trachomatis infection. Reprod Biol Endocrinol. 2008;6:46.

[96] Wan C, Latter JL, Amirshahi A, Symonds I, Finnie J, Bowden N, et al. Progesterone Activates Multiple Innate Immune Pathways in Chlamydia trachomatis-Infected Endocervical Cells. Am J Reprod Immunol. 2014;71(2):165–177.

[97] Beagley KW, Gockel CM. Regulation of innate and adaptive immunity by the female sex hormones oestradiol and progesterone. FEMS Immunol Med Microbiol. 2003;38(1):13–22.

[98] Kaushic C, Zhou F, Murdin AD, Charles R, Zhou FAN. Effects of estradiol and progesterone on susceptibility and early immune responses to Chlamydia trachomatis infection in the female reproductive tract. Infect Immun.2000 Jul;68(7):4207–4216.

[99] Macleod J, Salisbury C, Low N, McCarthy A, Sterne JAC, Holloway A, et al. Coverage and uptake of systematic postal screening for genital Chlamydia trachomatis and prevalence of infection in the United Kingdom general population: Cross sectional study. BMJ. 2005;330(7497):940.

[100] Wiesenfeld HC, Hillier SL, Krohn MA, Landers DV, Sweet RL. Bacterial vaginosis is a strong predictor of Neisseria gonorrhoeae and Chlamydia trachomatis infection. Clin Infect Dis. 2003;36(5):663–668.

[101] Korn AP, Hessol NA, Padian NS, Bolan GA, Donegan E, Landers DV, et al. Risk factors for plasma cell endometritis among women with cervical Neisseria gonorrhoeae, cervical Chlamydia trachomatis, or bacterial vaginosis. Am J Obstet Gynecol. 1998;178(5):987–990.

[102] Da Silva CS, Adad SJ, De Souza MAH, Barcelos ACM, Terra APS, Murta EFC. Increased frequency of bacterial vaginosis and Chlamydia trachomatis in pregnant women with human papillomavirus infection. Gynecol Obstet Invest. 2004;58(4):189–193.

[103] Quintero CA, Tudela JG, Damiani MT. Rho GTPases as pathogen targets: Focus on curable sexually transmitted infections. Small GTPases. 2015;(May):1–11.

[104] Gong Z, Luna Y, Yu P, Fan H. Lactobacilli inactivate Chlamydia trachomatis through lactic acid but not H2O2. PLoS One. 2014;9(9):e107758.

[105] Richmond SJ, Sparling PF. Genital chlamydial infections. Am J Epidemiol. 1976;103(5):428–435.

[106] Batteiger BE, Tu W, Ofner S, Pol B Van Der, Diane R, Orr DP, et al. Repeated Chlamydia trachomatis genital infections in adolescent women. J Infect Dis. 2011;201(1): 42–51.

[107] Paavonen J, Eggert-Kruse W. Chlamydia trachomatis: Impact on human reproduction. Hum Reprod Update. 1999;5(5):433–447.

[108] Lewis D, Newton DC, Guy RJ, Ali H, Chen MY, Fairley CK, et al. The prevalence of Chlamydia trachomatis infection in Australia: A systematic review and meta-analysis. BMC Infect Dis. 2012;12(1):113.

[109] Bé Bé Ar C, De Barbeyrac B. Genital Chlamydia trachomatis infections. Clin Microbiol Infect. 2009;15:4–10.

[110] Haggerty CL, Gottlieb SL, Taylor BD, Low N, Xu F, Ness RB. Risk of sequelae after Chlamydia trachomatis genital infection in women. J Infect Dis. 2010;(2):S134–S155.

[111] Chernesky MA, Lee H, Schachter J, Burczak JD, Stamm WE, McCormack WM, et al. Diagnosis of Chlamydia trachomatis urethral infection in symptomatic and asymptomatic men by testing first-void urine in a ligase chain reaction assay. J Infect Dis. 1994;170(5):1308–1311.

[112] Hillis SD, Joesoef R, Marchbanks PA, Wasserheit JN, Cates W, Westrom L. Delayed care of pelvic inflammatory disease as a risk factor for impaired fertility. Am J Obstet Gynecol. Mosby; 1993;168(5):1503–1509.

[113] Martin DH, Koutsky L, Eschenbach DA, Daling JR, Alexander ER, Benedetti JK, et al. Prematurity and perinatal mortality in pregnancies complicated by maternal Chlamydia trachomatis infections. JAMA. 1982;247(11):1585–1588.

[114] Gravett MG. Independent associations of bacterial vaginosis and Chlamydia trachomatis infection with adverse pregnancy outcome. JAMA. 1986;256(14):1899.

[115] Gencay M, Koskiniemi M, Saikku P, Puolakkainen M, Raivio K, Koskela P, et al. Chlamydia trachomatis seropositivity during pregnancy is associated with perinatal complications. Clin Infect Dis. 1995;21:424–426.

[116] Oakeshott P, Kerry S, Aghaizu A, Atherton H, Hay S, Taylor-Robinson D, et al. Randomised controlled trial of screening for Chlamydia trachomatis to prevent pelvic inflammatory disease: The POPI (prevention of pelvic infection) trial. BMJ. 2010;340:c1642.

[117] Herzog SA, Althaus CL, Heijne JC, Oakeshott P, Kerry S, Hay P, et al. Timing of progression from Chlamydia trachomatis infection to pelvic inflammatory disease: A mathematical modelling study. BMC Infect Dis. 2012;12(1):187.

[118] Price MJ, Ades AE, De Angelis D, Welton NJ, MacLeod J, Soldan K, et al. Risk of pelvic inflammatory disease following Chlamydia trachomatis infection: Analysis of prospective studies with a multistate model. Am J Epidemiol. 2013;178(3):484–492.

[119] Paavonen J, Lehtinen M. Immunopathogenesis of chlamydial pelvic inflammatory disease: The role of heat-shock proteins. Infect Dis Obs Gynecol. 1994;2(3):105–110.

[120] Khader SA, Gopal R. IL-17 in protective immunity to intracellular pathogens. Virulence. 2010;1(5):423–427.

[121] Agrawal T, Bhengraj AR, Vats V, Salhan S, Mittal A. Expression of TLR 2, TLR 4 and iNOS in cervical monocytes of Chlamydia trachomatis-infected women and their role in host immune response. Am J Reprod Immunol. 2011;66(6):534–543.

[122] Gupta R, Vardhan H, Srivastava P, Salhan S, Mittal A. Modulation of cytokines and transcription factors (T-Bet and GATA3) in CD4 enriched cervical cells of Chlamydia trachomatis infected fertile and infertile women upon stimulation with chlamydial inclusion membrane proteins B and C. Reprod Biol Endocrinol. 2009;7:84.

[123] Balasubramaniam ES, Van Noorden S, El-Bahrawy M. The expression of interleukin (IL)-6, IL-8, and their receptors in fallopian tubes with ectopic tubal gestation. Fertil Steril. 2012;98(4):898–904.

[124] Lewis ME, Belland RJ, Abdel Rahman YM, Beatty WL, Aiyar AA, Zea AH, et al. Morphologic and molecular evaluation of Chlamydia trachomatis growth in human endocervix reveals distinct growth patterns. Front Cell Infect Microbiol. 2014;4:71.

[125] Fan T, Lu H, Hu H, Shi L, McClarty GA, Nance DM, et al. Inhibition of apoptosis in chlamydia-infected cells: Blockade of mitochondrial cytochrome c release and caspase activation. J Exp Med. 1998;187(4):487–496.

[126] Rajalingam K, Al-younes H, Müller A, Meyer TF, Szczepek AJ, Rudel T, et al. Epithelial cells infected with Chlamydophila pneumoniae are resistant to apoptosis. Infect Immun. 2001 Dec;69(12):7880–7888.

[127] Buchholz KR, Stephens RS. The extracellular signal-regulated kinase/mitogen-activated protein kinase pathway induces the inflammatory factor interleukin-8 following Chlamydia trachomatis infection. Infect Immun. 2007;75(12):5924–5929.

[128] Rajalingam K, Sharma M, Lohmann C, Oswald M, Thieck O, Froelich CJ, et al. Mcl-1 is a key regulator of apoptosis resistance in Chlamydia trachomatis-infected cells. PLoS One. 2008;3(9) :1–11.

[129] Grieshaber SS, Grieshaber NA, Miller N, Hackstadt T. Chlamydia trachomatis causes centrosomal defects resulting in chromosomal segregation abnormalities. Traffic. 2006;7(8):940–949.

[130] Puolakkainen M, Hiltunen-Back E, Reunala T, Suhonen S, Lähteenmäki P, Lehtinen M, et al. Comparison of performances of two commercially available tests, a PCR assay and a ligase chain reaction test, in detection of urogenital Chlamydia trachomatis infection. J Clin Microbiol. 1998;36(6):1489–1493.

[131] Horner PJ. Azithromycin antimicrobial resistance and genital Chlamydia trachomatis infection: Duration of therapy may be the key to improving efficacy. Sex Transm Infect. 2012;88(3):154–156.

Chapter 10

Staphylococcal Infection and Infertility

Liyun Shi, Huanhuan Wang and Zhe Lu

Additional information is available at the end of the chapter

http://dx.doi.org/10.5772/62663

Abstract

Staphylococcus sp. is not only a commensal bacterium but also a major human pathogen that causes a wide range of clinical infections, such as skin and soft tissue infection, pleuropulmonary and osteoarticular infection, and endocarditis as well as life-threatening systemic infections. More evidence is currently emerging to show that *Staphylococcus,* particularly *Staphylococcus aureus,* can colonize the reproductive systems and affect their structure and function. Staphylococcal infection has become one of the most common causes of infertility in both males and females. This chapter focuses on the epidemiology, pathophysiology, clinical manifestations, and treatment of staphylococcal infection and infertility.

Keywords: *Staphylococcus,* infection, infertility

1. Introduction

Bacterial infection in reproductive organs is one of the most common causes of infertility in both male and female patients. It is also associated with sexually transmitted infections and adverse pregnancy outcomes. Infection with different microorganisms, such as chlamydia, mycoplasma, and certain bacteria, may lead to various clinical manifestations of human reproductive function. *Staphylococcus* sp., although a commensal bacterium, is a leading cause of skin and soft tissue infections and life-threatening systemic infections. More evidence is currently emerging to support the vaginal colonization of *Staphylococcus* sp. and its involvement in heterosexual transmission and infertility, but the knowledge is relatively scarce. In this chapter, genital staphylococcal infection and its relationship with infertility are discussed in detail.

2. Overview of staphylococcal infection

2.1. The staphylococci

Bacteria in the genus *Staphylococcus* are referred to Gram-positive spherical bacteria that widely affect man and other mammals. The bacteria are about 0.5–1.0 μm in diameter and grow in clusters, pairs, and occasionally in short chains. Staphylococci are divided into two groups based on their ability to clot blood plasma. The coagulase-positive staphylococci constitute the most pathogenic species *Staphylococcus aureus*. The coagulase-negative staphylococci (CNS) comprise over 30 other species, most of which are commensals of skin without causing infections. However, the incidence of infections of *Staphylococcus epidermidis*and other CNS has currently been rising. Among the known staphylococci, *S. aureus* is the most important human pathogen and causes a wide range of clinical infections [1]. It colonizes mainly the nasal passages, but also the other anatomical locales, such as skin, oral cavity, and gastrointestinal tract. Critically, *S. aureus* has been proved to be one of the most prevalent organisms in male and female genital tract, and its implication in the pathogenesis of reproductive diseases and infertility has attracted increasing attention [2]. In addition, the CNS stains such as *S. epidermidis* and *Staphylococcus haemolyticus* are also listed as the bacteria that can occupy and associated with male infertility.

2.2. The pathogenesis of *Staphylococcus aureus*

S. aureus is the leading cause of bacterial infections affecting an enormous population worldwide. By invading the bloodstream, lower respiratory tract, and skin and soft tissue, *S. aureus* can potentially cause some of the most severe hospital-associated and community-acquired illnesses. *S. aureus* produces a myriad of virulence factors that allow the organism to gain entry into tissues, attach to host cells, and secret exoproteins and toxins. The known virulence factors include lipoteichioic acid (LTA), toxic shock syndrome toxin-1 (TSST-1), staphylococcal enterotoxin A (SEA), and staphylococcal enterotoxin B. In addition, *S. aureus* expresses a cohort of special factors that indirectly exert pathogenic effects through interfering with host defense mechanisms. This category involves capsular polysaccharide, protein A, and leukocidin. The classical Panton and Valentine (PV) leukocidin is considered as a contributing factor for necrotizing skin infections due to its leukotoxic activity [3]. Recently, a novel strategy was invented whereby *S. aureus* successfully escapes neutrophil-mediated defensive machinery and establishes its invasion and infection. In this case, *S. aureus* secretes the nuclease and adenosine synthase to convert neutrophil extracellular traps (NETs) to deoxyadenosine, which triggers the caspase-3-triggered death of immune cells [4].

2.3. The host defense against staphylococcal infection

Neutrophils represent the host's first line of defense against invasion by *S. aureus* and a critical determinant in the outcome of staphylococcal infections. Following the uptake of bacteria, neutrophils typically undergo accelerated apoptosis and are cleared by macrophages through efferocytosis. This process results in eradication of the microbe and recovery of inflammation.

The pathogen recognition pattern receptor, toll-like receptor (TLR2), is proved to be the dominant receptor for *S. aureus*. TLR2 on the surface of innate immune cells recognizes the components of the bacterial cell wall such as teichoic acid, LTA, and PGN-embedded lipopeptides [5]. TLR2 then dimerizes with either TLR1 or TLR6 and recruits the adaptor proteins, such as TIRAP and MyD88, and the serine/threonine kinases IRAK-1 and IRAK-4 to initiate the subsequent signaling. The signaling cascade ultimately leads to the activation of the transcription factor nuclear factor-kappa B (NF-κB) and mitogen-activated protein kinases (MAPKs), which promotes the production of proinflammatory cytokines such as tumor necrosis factor (TNF)-α, interleukin (IL)-1β, IL-6, and IL-12p70 and chemokines such as (C-C motif) ligand (CCL)2, CCL3, and CCL4. Besides TLR2, C-type lecin receptors (CLRs) can also bind to surface sugars of *S. aureus* and enhance the phagocytic ability of antigen-presenting cells (APCs) [6]. The cytokines and chemokines released by the innate immune cells and/or the infected tissue cells have important roles in combating infection of *S. aureus*. They can recruit the innate immune cells to site of infection and activate the immune cells to phagocytose and kill the microbes. However, the extensive infiltration of inflammatory cells and the copious secretion of proinflammatory mediators may also cause tissue damage and immunopathology if the inflammation is unresolved.

When innate immune mechanisms are not sufficient to clear the bacterial infection, an adaptive immunity against *S. aureus*, such as T helper (Th)1 and Th17, and humoral antibody responses, might be required [7]. The production of IL-1 and IL-17A, upon activation of Th1 or Th17 cells, is presumably conductive to the abscess formation at site of infection. Abscessification is regarded as a hallmark of *S. aureus* infections and is essential for the clearance of bacteria through phagocytosis and oxidative burst. On the other hand, Th1 response during *S. aureus* infections is frequently associated with the activity of staphylococcal superantigens (SAgs). For example, TSS has been found to activate roughly 20% of T cells and trigger massive proliferation of T cells and production of cytokines [8]. A strong proinflammatory/Th1 response was also ascribed to the effect of SEA, which is another staphylococcal SAg.

2.4. Clinical manifestations of staphylococcal infection

Manifestations of staphylococcal infections usually depend on the type of infection, the site, the route, and the microbial dose. Common types of infections include skin infections (e.g. folliculitis, furuncles, impetigo, wound infections, and scalded skin syndrome), soft-tissue infections (e.g. pyomyositis, septic bursitis, and septic arthritis), toxic shock syndrome, purpura fulminans, endocarditis, osteomyelitis, pneumonia, food poisoning, and urinary tract infection [1, 9]. Despite associated with such a wide spectrum of clinical manifestations, *S. aureus* is still a commensal bacterium. Approximately 30% of the human population is colonized with this microbe [10]. However, with a growing number of health care–associated and antibiotic-resistant strain–driven infections, the pathogenic staphylococcal infection has significantly increased during the past two decades. In particular, the dramatic rising of antibiotic-resistant strains has become a serious threat to public health. The term MRSA refers to methicillin-resistant *S. aureus* with the potential to resist all β-lactam antibiotics such as penicillins and cephalosporins. Resistance is usually conferred by the acquisition of a non-native gene encoding a penicillin-binding protein (PBP2a) that has significantly lower affinity for β-lactams [11]. In addition to MRSA, the vancomycin-intermediate/resistant *S. aureus* (VISA/VRSA) strain has also been reported in staphylococcal infection, particularly in some cases of enterococcal infection.

3. Epidemiology of genitourinary staphylococcal infection

Barring the role of a few bacteria such as *Chlamydia* whose impact on fertility has been well established, the significance of other bacteria in infertility is controversial. An epidemiological research revealed that the prevalence of bacterial vaginosis (BV) as 70.34% among infertile women. Previously, the categories of organisms with the potential to cause bacterial infection in female reproductive system have involved *Gardnerella vaginalis, Mobiluncus* sp., *Bacteroide* sp., *Prevotella* sp., and *Mycoplasma* sp. [12]. In general, Gram-positive bacteria were significantly higher in number than the Gram-negative bacteria. Series of epidemiological studies have revealed that *Staphylococcus* is among the top bacterium detected from reproductive organs and is closely related with infertility. For example, Momoh et al. [13] reported a prevalence rate of 38.7% *S. aureus* from high vaginal swab and endocervical swabs and a prevalence of 75% from semen cultures of infertile couples. Another investigation identified *S. aureus* as the most prevalent vaginal pathogen (57.33%) among local infertile women, followed by *Escherichia coli* (25.33%) [14].

Parallel to the situation in females, abnormal presence of *Staphylococcus* sp. has been increasingly evidenced in the genitourinary system of male patients with fertile problem. In a study of a total of 140 sperm samples collected from the University of Benin Teaching Hospital, *S. aureus* (28.3%) and *S. saprohyticus* (13.0%) were the most common pathogens found and have negative effects on sperm motility and morphology [15]. The commonest bacteria isolated from 160 men attending infertility clinics in South-eastern Nigeria were *Proteus* sp., *S. aureus,* and *E. coli,* and most of the detected strains were resistant to antibiotics assessed[16]. Besides the *S. aureus,* other staphylococci are also commonly found in infertile male patients. *S. epidermidis* was found to be one of the most common bacteria in 295 infertile males at the Hospital Juárez de México, and the bacteria profoundly affected the sperm motility, pH, morphology, and viscosity [17].

In healthy women of child-bearing age, the protective mucosa in the vagina is populated with microflora typically dominated by lactobacilli, and their dominance over pathogenic anaerobes is positively associated with vaginal health. Thanks to the biological antagonism provided by a healthy vaginal microbiota, opportunistic microorganisms are in very low numbers in normal vagina. It is proven that lactobacilli provide a constant acidic pH value and maintain the appropriate concentration of hydrogen peroxide in the genital environment. While under the condition of BV, the concentration of lactobacilli reduces but of some pathogenic bacteria, especially anaerobes or microaerophiles, increase [18]. BV represents the most common vaginal syndrome that affects fertile, premenopausal, and pregnant women, with an incidence rate ranging from 20% to 50% [19, 20]. BV is not caused by one specific pathogenic microorganism but rather by an imbalance of vaginal microbiota. *Staphylococcus* sp., as a kind of amphimicrobian, has been established as one of the specific pathogenic bacteria related to BV. BV is frequently disregarded because the symptoms are often absent or insignificant. However, this vaginal disorder has already become the most common lower genital tract disorder among women of reproductive age and the most prevalent cause of vaginal discharge and malodour.

Genitourinary MRSA carriage and infection are not rare. A retrospective study was previously conducted on 57 pregnant women positive for MRSA over a 4.5-year period. The data showed that skin and soft tissue infection accounted for 96% of cases and recurrent infection occurred in 58% of the women [21]. Vaginal colonization with *S. aureus* and MRSA was further valuated by Chen *et al.*, who reported that 507 *S. aureus* isolates (17.1%) were obtained from vaginal cultures of 2963 pregnant women, of which 14 (2.8%) were MRSA [22]. In addition, MRSA has become the predominant pathogen that causes the surgically managed infections in the genitourinary area. *S. aureus*, along with *E. coli*, *Streptococci*, and *Trichomonas vaginalis*, forms the abnormal vaginal flora that contributes to the onset of aerobic vaginitis. These pathogenic bacteria substantially alter the vaginal lactate concentration and increase the levels of inflammatory cytokines such as IL-6, IL-1β and leukemia inhibitory factor (LIF) in the vaginal fluid. Two methicillin-sensitive stains of *S. aureus* (MNPE and CDC587) have been documented to induce the expression of IL-8 in human vaginal epithelial cells [23]. Alterations in vaginal microbiology have been associated with many pathological conditions such as endometritis, miscarriage, premature labor, and infertility [24]. Moreover, the flora and cytokines imbalance has implicated in the pathogenesis of pelvic inflammatory disease (PID) and cervicitis and is also a risk factor for urinary tract infection and sexually transmitted disease (STD) [25].

4. Staphylococcal infection and male infertility

Urogenital tract infections in males are one of the significant etiological factors in infertility. The infection of bacteria such as *Staphylococcus* sp. has been detected at the male reproductive tract. Staphylococcal infection in male reproductive organs and accessory glands may exert detrimental effect on sperm activity. Previous studies indicated that staphylococci not only affect the sperm activity but also impact the secretory capacity of the epididymis, seminal vesicles, and prostate [26]. In fact, staphylococci have been identified as one of the most common strains that can be detected in the male reproductive system. However, the percentages of males that get infected with staphylococci vary with the different isolation methods and procedures used in different studies. It has been demonstrated that *S. aureus* infection significantly interferes with semen quality and activity. It deteriorates the volume of semen and the concentration of sperm as well as the motility, morphology, and vitality of sperm. Therefore, a causative relationship may exist between staphylococcal infection and male infertility. A previous study reported a 20.6% infection of *S. aureus* in the semen samples from males with fertility problems. More importantly, *S. aureus* infection was found to be closely related to poor semen quality and reduced sperm motility [27]. Also, an investigation by a

Poland group associated *S. aureus* infection with abnormal semen parameters or other surogenital tract infection [28].

Besides these prospective studies, several *in vitro* studies also support the effect of *Staphylococcus* on sperm activity and its relation with infertility. It was revealed that infection of the normal human ejaculated spermatozoa with *S. haemolyticus* profoundly impacted the architecture and integrity of the sperm plasma membrane. Bacterial infection serves as a contributing factor for severe injury of sperm membrane stability and mitochondrial activity with potential consequences of male fertility [29]. In addition, exposure of ejaculated spermatozoa to *S. haemolyticus* was found to trigger a simultaneous decrease in the percentage of sperm with normal $\Delta\Psi m$ and an increase in the proportion of sperm with Annexin V staining, indicative of apoptotic cells. The data suggested a determinant role of staphylococcal infection in sperm fate [30]. Despite the above findings, the role for staphylococci in male infertility has remained somewhat controversial. A previous study showed that, although *Staphylococcus* sp. was the most common bacteria isolated in 299 asymptomatic men undergoing fertility evaluation, the bacterial counts were not correlated with semen parameters [31].

In an effort to understand the mechanism whereby staphylococci modulate sperm activity, investigators currently identified some of the key molecules that have profound effect on sperm activity. Kaur and Prabha *et al.* firstly identified sperm agglutinating factor (SAF). Based on the observation that *S. aureus* can adhere to the sperm head as well as sperm tail and agglutinate mouse spermatozoa, the group finally isolated a protein with a molecular weight of approximately 57 kDa from *S. aureus* and implicated the protein in control of sperm motility and survival. Moreover, SAF potentially affects various sperm parameters such as Mg^{2+}-dependent ATPase activity, acrosome status, and apoptosis. In support of this, a profound morphological alteration occurs in the spermatozoa upon binding with SAF, as detected with scanning electron microscopy. Also, SAF has a spermicidal effect at high concentrations and may have the potential to function as active ingredient of a vaginal contraceptive. Further studies indicate that the interaction of SAF with spermatozoa is receptor mediated, and the receptor has been isolated and purified from human spermatozoa. This sperm surface receptor component showed homology to glutamate decarboxylase and major histocompatibility complex (MHC) class I molecule [32]. Intriguingly, the receptor was shown to be able to counteract the detrimental effects of SAF on sperm parameters and alleviate SAF-induced infertility in mice [33]. In addition, Prabha *et al.* isolated the SAF from an *E. coli* strain. This kind of SAF also leads to sperm agglutination, the compromised Mg^{2+}-dependent ATPase activity, and spermatozoa apoptosis.

In 2009, another protein with sperm regulatory effect, named sperm immobilization factor (SIF), was identified from *S. aureus*. SIF is a protein with the molecular weight of approximately 20 kDa. Similar to SAF, SIF causes multiple defects in the head, midpiece, neck, and tail region of human spermatozoa [34]. It can completely inhibit Mg^{2+} ATPase activity of spermatozoa at the concentration of 100 μg/ml and reduce calcium ionophore–induced acrosome reaction. The interaction between SIF and spermatozoa is also ligand-receptor dependent. The analysis by matrix-assisted laser desorption ionization–time of flight (MALDI-TOF) showed that the receptor shares sequence similarity with MHC class II antigen. Interestingly, SIF has been

http://dx.doi.org/10.5772/62663

found to impede motile bacteria, in addition to sperm, such as *E. coli, Pseudomonas aeruginosa,* and *Proteus mirabilis.* The molecular mimicry of SIF receptor has been confirmed between spermatozoa and bacteria [35].

In addition to the effector molecules mentioned above, some novel mechanisms responsible for the staphylococcal regulation of sperm have now been discovered. A recent study on the semen of 589 infertile males indicated that other virulence genes in *S. aureus,* such as hlg (33.3%), scn (23.3%), cna (20%), hlb (20%), and clfA (18.3%), were possibly responsible for spermatozoal immobilization [36]. Berktas et al. raised another point of view that, rather than the direct interaction between bacteria and sperm, the alteration in genital microenvironment or ver-consumption of energy by high dose of bacterium led to the loss of sperm motility [37].

5. Staphylococcal infection and female infertility

Bacterial infection in female reproductive system, such as staphylococcal infection, can profoundly affect all the phases of a woman's life in relation to the period of pre-pregnancy, fertilization, pregnancy, and reproduction. It has been demonstrated that BV is the most common lower genital tract disorder among women of reproductive age. In particular, staphylococcal infection is presumed to be a contributing factor for the adverse pregnancy outcomes and female infertility. Staphylococcal infection causes malodorous vaginal discharge and is causally associated with sexually transmitted infections. Also, it has been implicated in the development of endometritis (endometriosis), another crucial factor to female infertility.

5.1. Inflammatory response and hypothalamic endocrine

An immune/inflammatory challenge is considered as an important factor that impinges the reproduction process in animals and humans [38]. It can affect reproduction at the level of the hypothalamus, pituitary gland, or gonads. Nonetheless, the major impact is thought to occur within the brain or the pituitary gland [39]. Bacterial endotoxins can trigger the release of cytokines and other immune mediators in the hypothalamus, where the luteinizing hormone (LH)-releasing hormone and gonadotropin-releasing hormone (GnRH) neurons are located [40]. Numerous *in vitro* and *in vivo* studies showed that the immune stress and the subsequent action of proinflammatory cytokines have a profound impact on the secretory activity of GnRH and LH neurons in the hypothalamus [41]. These interconnections between the immune and the neuroendocrine systems are suggested to be based on the mutual sharing of receptors and mediators.

As described above, staphylococcal infection either in peripheral or directly in vagina can arouse strong immune/inflammatory reaction systematically or locally. The released cytokines and chemokines then act on the pituitary gland and reproductive organs, which may finally lead to menoxenia, irregular ovulation, and infertility. Evidences have shown that staphylococcal infection generates a large quantity of cytokines in female reproductive system. These mediators have an important role in the control of reproductive neuroendocrine, ovarian physiology, fetal implantation and development, and placenta function. Previous study revealed a correlation between BV, elevated IL-1β and IL-8, and idiopathic infertility, suggesting that abnormal vaginal flora and the vaginal inflammatory response may be responsible for the idiopathic infertility in women undergoing *in vitro* fertilization [42].

5.2. Premature ovarian failure

Female mammals are born with a finite number of oocytes that gradually decreases during prepubertal development and adult life [43]. Each oocyte is encircled by somatic granulosa cells (GCs) to form the basic functioning unit of the ovary—the follicle. The size of the oocytes at birth and the rate of endowment depletion dominate the ovarian functional lifespan. On the other hand, programmed cell death (apoptosis) has been considered one of the most prevalent mechanisms that contribute to the age-related exhaustion of oocytes. Therefore, a precise balance has to be achieved between prosurvival and proapoptotic molecules to maintain the final destiny of the follicle [44, 45].

It is well recognized that immune/inflammatory response participates in many aspects of reproductive physiology, such as ovulation, menstruation, and implantation. Recent studies suggest that the inflammatory stress caused by staphylococcal infection may also affect ovarian reserve and cyclicity in women. Proinflammatory reaction, such as its correspondent neurotransmitter secretion, inflammatory gene transcription, and signaling pathway activation, was thought to play essential roles in the process. Moreover, the production of neurotransmitter, such as sphingolipid ceramide, further acts as a second messenger to promote age-related apoptosis of oocytes. Evidence showed that lower ceramide levels observed in acid sphingomyelinase-deficient mice resulted in a larger postnatal pool of oocytes compared with their wild-type counterparts. Conversely, Bax-null female mice exhibited to extend the ovarian lifespan [46]. These data may provide novel perspectives on the regulation of oocyte dynamics by bacterial infection and link the critical biological processes such as infection, inflammation, cell survival, and female fertility.

5.3. Bacterial vaginosis and endometritis

BV is a polymicrobial syndrome mainly due to an imbalance of vaginal microbiota. Colonization and proliferation of staphylococci is supposed to be one of the reasons for the increase in pathogenic bacteria, anaerobic bacteria, or microaerophiles. During the pathogenesis of BV, the overgrowth of anaerobes promotes the production of noxious substances, such as polyamines and other compounds. These metabolic products may further trigger the release of proinflammatory cytokines IL-1β and IL-8 and thus cause tissue damage and physiological imbalance [47]. BV can directly affect congenital formation and female fertility as an ascending dissemination of the related bacteria species proved to cause tubal factor infertility.

Another complication accompanied by vaginal staphylococcal infection is chronic endometritis (CE), a local inflammatory disease characterized by unusual plasmacytic infiltration in the endometrial stromal areas [48]. CE frequently happens in the later stage of the infection or under repeated infection. It tends to be neglected in gynecologic practice because of its less apparent symptom and the requirement of time-consuming histopathologic examinations. In most cases, the diagnosis is made based on gynecological indications, such as abnormal uterine bleeding (AUB) and infertility [49]. In a study on 64 CE patients and 28 healthy women, the biochemical analysis revealed that IL-6, IL-1β, and TNF-α levels were markedly higher in menstrual effluents of women with CE when compared with control subjects [50]. It is suggested that the infection and inflammation alter the endometrial cytokine profiles, which may further impair endometrial function and lead to menstrual abnormalities and reduced embryo receptivity [51]. Moreover, the proteomic analysis identified the key signaling pathways involved in inflammation and oxidative stress are closely related with carcinogenetic processes. These studies associate the onset of CE with female infertility, obstetric and neonatal abnormity, and complications. The altered endometrial gene expression may explain the impaired endometrial receptivity and endometrial hyperplastic lesions observed in women affected by CE [52].

5.4. Abnormal fetal implantation

In rodents and humans, implantation is the first coordinated encounter between mother and baby. The abnormal implantation and placentation may lead to various dysfunctions throughout the pregnancy. Pre-eclampsia (PE) is a pregnancy-induced disorder characterized by hypertension and proteinuria. It is estimated to affect about 8% of pregnancies and is thought to be unique to humans [53]. The etiology of PE still remains poorly understood, but abnormal placentation is proved to be a major reason for this disease. In addition, local infection and immune responses are critically involved in the process of implantation [54]. Increased placental secretion of proinflammatory cytokines as well as the angiogenic regulators has been implicated in the widespread maternal endothelial dysfunction and the development of PE. It has been shown that cytokines produced within the uterine microenvironment can alter trophoblast action [55], impair implantation, and placenta vascularization, which may account for the recurrent miscarriage in women [56]. Elevated circulating IL-15 levels, proportional to severity of diseases, have been detected in the serum of PE mothers when compared with healthy controls [57]. Also, IL-11 is also proved to be a contributing factor for the impaired trophoblast invasion, spiral artery remodeling, and altered placental labyrinth morphology. These functional abnormities further lead to the development of PE-like features, such as elevated systolic blood pressure (SBP), proteinuria, and kidney glomerular pathology. Another proinflammatory cytokine, interferon (IFN)-γ, was also elevated in plasma, circulating leukocytes, and decidua of patients with PE [58]. Besides this, decidual natural killer (dNK) cells, the predominant immune cell, coincide with the decidualization at the maternal-fetal interface in human and mice. All of these studies point to a critical role of immune/inflammatory response during the implanting and placental development. More importantly, vaginal *Staphylococcus* infection, an infectious agent frequently observed in the uterus, may participate in the development of implantation disorder presumably by the induction of local immune reaction.

6. Therapy

Antibiotic strategy is considered the most potential therapeutic methods against staphylococcal infection and the resultant infertility. However, the emergence of antibiotic resistance has dramatically increased in the past two decades and becomes a serious threat to the worldwide public health. According to the National Healthcare Safety Network (NHSN) and Centers for Disease Control and Prevention, *S. aureus* and *Enterococcus* are the two most commonly reported pathogens, accounting for 15.6% and 13.9% of health care–associated infections, respectively. In particular, *S. aureus* is notorious for its ability to acquire the resistance to any antibiotic during the treatment of infection-associated infertility.

6.1. Methicillin

The introduction of penicillin in the early 1940s significantly reduced fatal invasive staphylococcal infection. However, the resistant strains, mostly *S. aureus* strains, emerged rapidly. These strains possess a plasmid-encoding enzyme, penicillinase, which can irreversibly hydrolyze the β-lactam, thus acquiring the drug resistance. Methicillin is a narrow-spectrum β-lactam antibiotic of the penicillin class. It can effectively block the synthesis of bacterial cell walls by inhibiting the peptidic cross-linkage between the linear peptidoglycan polymer chains. Therefore, the antibiotic destroys the integrity of the cell wall and selectively kills Gram-positive bacteria. Compared with penicillin, methicillin harbors an orthodimethoxyphenyl group attached to the side chain of the β-lactam, which, in turn, forms a steric effect to prevent penicillinase from hydrolyzing the β-lactam. Even though, the first strain of MRSA, with an altered PBP2a to reduced affinity for the β-lactam, was reported two years later [59]. Now, MRSA refers to any strain of *S. aureus* that has developed resistance to β-lactam antibiotics such as the penicillins (methicillin, dicloxacillin, nafcillin, oxacillin, etc.) and the cephalosporins. Resistance is generally conferred by the acquisition of the mecA gene, which encodes a PBP2a. Due to the significantly decreased affinity for β-lactams, MRSA strains restore the ability of cell wall biosynthesis to continue even in the presence of typically inhibitory concentrations of antibiotic [11].

6.2. Vancomycin

Vancomycin belongs to the glycopeptide antibiotic class and is effective in treatment of serious infections caused by *Staphylococcus*. It is one of the main resources for combating infections caused by MRSA but is not recommended to treat the disease caused by methicillin-sensitive *S. aureus* (MSSA). Vancomycin is a complex compound consisting of a branched tricyclic glycosylated peptide and is a rare example of a halo-organic natural compound containing two covalently bonded chlorine atoms. The bactericidal activity of vancomycin is associated with its ability to bind at the D-Ala-D-Ala dipeptide terminus of the nascent peptidoglycan in Gram-positive bacteria and thereby to inhibit the peptidoglycan synthesis [60]. Common side effects associated this antibiotic involve pain in the area of injection and allergic reactions, and problems with hearing, low blood pressure, or bone marrow suppression occasionally occur. The strain with the reduced susceptibility to vancomycin (VISA) was first described in 1996, and the alteration of the D-Ala-D-Ala dipeptide was supposed to be the main reason underlying this resistance.

6.3. Linezolid

Linezolid has been used for treatment of serious infections caused by Gram-positive bacteria that are resistant to other antibiotics such as MRSA. Its spectrum of activity is similar to that of vancomycin, a well-established antibiotic for MRSA infections. Either linezolid or vancomycin has been recommended by the US guidelines as the first-line treatment for hospital-acquired (nosocomial) MRSA pneumonia [61]. Mechanistically, linezolid binds to the 50s subunit of the bacterial ribosome through interaction with the central loop of the 23S rRNA and thus impedes the growth of bacteria by disrupting their production of proteins. Point mutation of 23S rRNA is the most common mechanism of linezolid resistance [62]. The common side effects of linezolid include diarrhea, headache, nausea, vomiting, rash, constipation, altered taste perception, and discoloration of the tongue, although they happen relatively rarely.

6.4. Daptomycin

Daptomycin is the first cyclic lipopeptide approved for clinical use in 2003. It is a calcium-dependent antibiotic comprising a lipid molecule conjugated with anionic peptide. Daptomycin interacts with the cytoplasmic membrane in a calcium-dependent, leading to the cell membrane depolarization, ion loss, and cell death [63]. Many antibiotic-resistant strains, such as MRSA and VRSA, were found to be effectively inhibited by daptomycin. Till 2008, the first case of daptomycin resistance was reported, and the underlying mechanism is currently still not very clear [64]. However, the mutation of the mprF gene, which encodes lysyl-phosphatidyl glycerol (LPG) synthetase, might be related to the occurrence of resistant strains. LPG can catalyze the coupling of lysine to PG and transfer the lysyl-PG to the outer leaflet of the membrane. In this way, LPG increases the positive charge and thus reduces the binding of Ca^{2+}-bound daptomycin to bacterial membranes [65].

Besides the routinely used antibiotics mentioned above, numerous new antibiotics are developed to serve as the alternatives in treating staphylococcal infection and the associated infertility. For example, teicoplanin or quinupristin/dalfopristin has been widely used with daptomycin to treat Gram-positive bacterial infection. Some of the potential antibiotics, such as oritavancin and iclaprim, are currently in the early stages of clinical development, and other promising candidates, such as ceftobiprole, dalbavancin, and telavancin, are still being developed [66].

Author details

Liyun Shi[1*], Huanhuan Wang[2] and Zhe Lu[2]

*Address all correspondence to: shi_liyun@msn.com

1 Department of Microbiology and Immunology, Nanjing University of Chinese Medicine, Nanjing, China

2 Department of Basic Medical Science, School of Medicine, Hangzhou Normal University, Hangzhou, China

References

[1] Lowy FD. *Staphylococcus aureus* infections. N Engl J Med. 1998;339:520–532.

[2] Guinan ME, Dan BB, Guidotti RJ, Reingold AL, Schmid GP, Bettoli EJ, Lossick JG, Shands KN, Kramer MA, Hargrett NT, Anderson RL, Broome CV. Vaginal colonization with *Staphylococcus aureus* in healthy women: a review of four studies. Ann Intern Med. 1982;96:944–947. DOI:10.7326/0003-4819-96-6-944

[3] Pauli NT, Kim HK, Falugi F, Huang M, Dulac J, Henry Dunand C, Zheng NY, Kaur K, Andrews SF, Huang Y, DeDent A, Frank KM, Charnot-Katsikas A, Schneewind O, Wilson PC. *Staphylococcus aureus* infection induces protein A-mediated immune evasion in humans. J Exp Med. 2014;211:2331–2339. DOI:10.1084/jem.20141404

[4] Thammavongsa V, Missiakas DM, Schneewind O. *Staphylococcus aureus* degrades neutrophil extracellular traps to promote immune cell death. Science 2013;342:863–866. DOI:10.1126/science.1242255

[5] Takeuchi O, Akira S. Pattern recognition receptors and inflammation. Cell 2010;140:805–820. DOI:10.1016/j.cell.2010.01.022

[6] Figdor CG, van Kooyk Y, Adema GJ. C-type lectin receptors on dendritic cells and Langerhans cells. Nat Rev Immunol. 2002;2:77–84. DOI:10.1038/nri723

[7] Miller LS, Cho JS. Immunity against *Staphylococcus aureus* cutaneous infections. Nat Rev Immunol. 2011;11:505–518. DOI:10.1038/nri3010

[8] McCormick JK, Yarwood JM, Schlievert PM. Toxic shock syndrome and bacterial superantigens: an update. Annu Rev Microbiol. 2001;55:77–104.

[9] Tong SY, Davis JS, Eichenberger E, Holland TL, Fowler VG Jr. Staphylococcus aureus infections: epidemiology, pathophysiology, clinical manifestations, and management. Clin Microbiol Rev. 2015;28:603–661. DOI:10.1128/CMR.00134-14

[10] Wertheim HF, Melles DC, Vos MC, van Leeuwen W, van Belkum A, Verbrugh HA, Nouwen JL. The role of nasal carriage in *Staphylococcus aureus* infections. Lancet Infect Dis. 2005;5:751–762.

[11] Peacock SJ, Paterson GK. Mechanisms of methicillin resistance in *Staphylococcus aureus*. Annu Rev Biochem. 2015;84:577–601. DOI:10.1146/annurev-biochem-060614-034516

[12] Hillier SL. Diagnostic microbiology of bacterial vaginosis. Am J Obstet Gynecol. 1993;169:455–459.

[13] Momoh ARM, Orhue PO, Okolo PO, Odaro D, Momoh AA. The antibiogram types of auto-agglutinating *Staphylococcus aureus* strains isolated from the semen samples of males with infertility problems in Edo state, Nigeria. E3 J Med Res. 2012;1:17–24.

[14] Ghiasi M, Fazaeli H, Kalhor N, Sheykh-Hasan M, Tabatabaei-Qomi R. Assessing the prevalence of bacterial vaginosis among infertile women of Qom city. Iran J Microbiol. 2014;6:404–408.

[15] Isaiah IN, Nche BT, Nwagu IG, Nnanna II. Current studies on bacterospermia the leading cause of male infertility: a protégé and potential threat towards mans extinction. N Am J Med Sci. 2011;3:562–564. DOI:10.4297/najms.2011.3559

[16] Uneke CJ, Ugwuoru CD. Antibiotic susceptibility of urogenital microbial profile of infertile men in South-eastern Nigeria. Andrologia 2010;42:268–273. DOI:10.1111/j.1439-0272.2009.00988.x

[17] Huerta M, Cervera Aguilar R, Hernández I, Ayala AR. Frequency and etiology of seminal infections in the study of infertile couples. Ginecol Obstet Mex. 2002;70:90–94.

[18] Mastromarino P, Vitali B, Mosca L. Bacterial vaginosis: a review on clinical trials with probiotics. New Microbiol. 2013;36:229–238.

[19] Allsworth JE, Peipert JF. Prevalence of bacterial vaginosis: 2001–2004 National Health and Nutrition Examination Survey data. Obstet Gynecol. 2007;109:114–120. DOI:10.1016/S0920-5861(96)00164-2

[20] Koumans EH, Sternberg M, Bruce C, McQuillan G, Kendrick J, Sutton M, Markowitz LE. The prevalence of bacterial vaginosis in the United States, 2001–2004; associations with symptoms, sexual behaviors, and reproductive. Sex Transm Dis. 2007;34:864–869.

[21] Laibl VR, Sheffield JS, Roberts S, McIntire DD, Trevino S, Wendel GD Jr. Clinical presentation of community-acquired methicillin-resistant *Staphylococcus aureus* in pregnancy. Obstet Gynecol. 2005;106:461–465.

[22] Chen KT, Huard RC, Della-Latta P, Saiman L. Prevalence of methicillin-sensitive and methicillin-resistant *Staphylococcus aureus* in pregnant women. Obstet Gynecol. 2006;108:482–487. DOI:10.1097/01.AOG.0000227964.22439.e3

[23] Donders GG, Vereecken A, Bosmans E, Dekeersmaecker A, Salembier G, Spitz B. Definition of a type of abnormal vaginal flora that is distinct from bacterial vaginosis: aerobic vaginitis. BJOG 2002;109:34–43. DOI:10.1111/j.1471-0528.2002.00432.x

[24] Koumans EH, Markowitz LE, Hogan V. Indications for therapy and treatment recommendations for bacterial vaginosis in nonpregnant and pregnant women: a synthesis of data. Clin Infect Dis. 2002;35:S152–S172.

[25] Harmanli OH, Cheng GY, Nyirjesy P, Chatwani A, Gaughan JP. Urinary tract infections in women with bacterial vaginosis. Obstet Gynecol. 2000;95:710–712.

[26] Marconi M, Pilatz A, Wagenlehner F, Diemer T, Weidner W. Impact of infection on the secretory capacity of the male accessory glands. Int Braz J Urol. 2009;35:299–308.

[27] Onemu SO, Ibeh IN. Studies on the significance of positive bacterial semen cultures in male fertility in Nigeria. Int J Fertil Womens Med. 2001;46:210–214.

[28] Filipiak E, Marchlewska K, Oszukowska E, Walczak-Jedrzejowska R, Swierczynska-Cieplucha A, Kula K, Slowikowska-Hilczer J. Presence of aerobic micro-organisms and their influence on basic semen parameters in infertile men. Andrologia 2015;47:826–831. DOI:10.1111/and.12338

[29] Fraczek M, Piasecka M, Gaczarzewicz D, Szumala-Kakol A, Kazienko A, Lenart S, Laszczynska M, Kurpisz M. Membrane stability and mitochondrial activity of human-ejaculated spermatozoa during in vitro experimental infection with *Escherichia coli, Staphylococcus haemolyticus* and *Bacteroides ureolyticus*. Andrologia 2012;44:315–329. DOI:10.1111/j.1439-0272.2012.01283.x

[30] Fraczek M, Hryhorowicz M, Gaczarzewicz D, Szumala-Kakol A, Kolanowski TJ, Beutin L, Kurpisz M. Can apoptosis and necrosis coexist in ejaculated human spermatozoa during in vitro semen bacterial infection? J Assist Reprod Genet 2015;32:771–779. DOI:10.1007/s10815-015-0462-x

[31] Rodin DM, Larone D, Goldstein M. Relationship between semen cultures, leukospermia, and semen analysis in men undergoing fertility evaluation. Fertil Steril 2003;79(Suppl. 3):1555–1558.

[32] Kaur K, Prabha V. Impairment by sperm agglutinating factor isolated from *Escherichia coli*: receptor specific interactions. Biomed Res Int. 2013;2013:548497. DOI: 10.1155/2013/548497

[33] Kaur S, Prabha V. Receptor mediated amelioration of the detrimental effects of sperm agglutinating factor on sperm parameters. Andrology 2013;1:624–631. DOI: 10.1111/j.2047-2927.2013.00088.x

[34] Prabha V, Gupta T, Kaur S, Kaur N, Kala S, Singh A. Isolation of a spermatozoal immobilization factor from *Staphylococcus aureus* filtrates. Can J Microbiol. 2009;55:874–878. DOI:10.1139/w09-032

[35] Prabha V, Chaudhary N, Kaur S. Molecular mimicry between spermatozoa and bacteria. J Urol. 2011;186:2442–2447. DOI:10.1016/j.juro.2011.07.084

[36] Li B, Yang X, Ye JZ, Chen HL, Hou YB, Du J, Zhou TL. Spermatozoal immobilization ability and virulence genes of *Staphylococcus aureus* isolated from the semen of infertile men. Zhonghua Nan Ke Xue. 2015;21:881–886.

[37] Berktas M, Aydin S, Yilmaz Y, Cecen K, Bozkurt H. Sperm motility changes after coincubation with various uropathogenic microorganisms: an in vitro experimental study. Int Urol Nephrol. 2008;40:383–389. DOI:10.1007/s11255-007-9289-4

[38] Herman AP, Krawczynska A, Bochenek J, Dobek E, Herman A, Tomaszewska-Zaremba D. LPS-induced inflammation potentiates the IL-1beta-mediated reduction of

LH secretion from the anterior pituitary explants. Clin Dev Immunol. 2013;2013:926937. DOI:10.1155/2013/926937

[39] Herman AP, Tomaszewska-Zaremba D. Effect of endotoxin on the expression of GnRH and GnRHR genes in the hypothalamus and anterior pituitary gland of anestrous ewes. Anim Reprod Sci. 2010;120:105–111. DOI:10.1016/j.anireprosci.2010.03.011

[40] Igaz P, Salvi R, Rey JP, Glauser M, Pralong FP, Gaillard RC. Effects of cytokines on gonadotropin-releasing hormone (GnRH) gene expression in primary hypothalamic neurons and in GnRH neurons immortalized conditionally. Endocrinology 2006;147:1037–1043.

[41] Refojo D, Arias P, Moguilevsky JA, Feleder C. Effect of bacterial endotoxin on in vivo pulsatile gonadotropin secretion in adult male rats. Neuroendocrinology 1998;67:275–281.

[42] Spandorfer SD, Neuer A, Giraldo PC, Rosenwaks Z, Witkin SS. Relationship of abnormal vaginal flora, proinflammatory cytokines and idiopathic infertility in women undergoing IVF. J Reprod Med. 2001;46:806–810.

[43] Broekmans FJ, Soules MR, Fauser BC. Ovarian aging: mechanisms and clinical consequences. Endocr Rev. 2009;30:465–493. DOI:10.1210/er.2009-0006

[44] Tilly JL. Apoptosis and ovarian function. Rev Reprod. 1996;1:162–172.

[45] Hussein MR. Apoptosis in the ovary: molecular mechanisms. Hum Reprod. 2005;11:162–177.

[46] Uri-Belapolsky S, Shaish A, Eliyahu E, Grossman H, Levi M, Chuderland D, Ninio-Many L, Hasky N, Shashar D, Almog T, Kandel-Kfir M, Harats D, Shalgi R, Kamari Y. Interleukin-1 deficiency prolongs ovarian lifespan in mice. Proc Natl Acad Sci USA. 2014;111:12492–12497. DOI:10.1073/pnas.1323955111

[47] Romero R, Chaiworapongsa T, Kuivaniemi H, Tromp G. Bacterial vaginosis, the inflammatory response and the risk of preterm birth: a role for genetic epidemiology in the prevention of preterm birth. Am J Obstet Gynecol. 2004;190:1509–1519.

[48] Kitaya K, Matsubayashi H, Yamaguchi K, Nishiyama R, Takaya Y, Ishikawa T, Yasuo T, Yamada H. Chronic endometritis: potential cause of infertility and obstetric and neonatal complications. Am J Reprod Immunol. 2016;75:13–22. DOI:10.1111/aji.12438

[49] Gilmore H, Fleischhacker D, Hecht JL. Diagnosis of chronic endometritis in biopsies with stromal breakdown. Hum Pathol. 2007;38:581–584. DOI:10.1016/j.humpath.2006.09.002

[50] Tortorella C, Piazzolla G, Matteo M, Pinto V, Tinelli R, Sabba C, Fanelli M, Cicinelli E. Interleukin-6, interleukin-1beta, and tumor necrosis factor alpha in menstrual ef-

fluents as biomarkers of chronic endometritis. Proc Natl Acad Sci USA. 2014;112:15928–15933. DOI:10.1073/pnas.1515076112

[51] Maybin JA, Critchley HO, Jabbour HN. Inflammatory pathways in endometrial disorders. Mol Cell Endocrinol. 2011;335:42–51. DOI:10.1016/j.mce.2010.08.006

[52] Di Pietro C, Cicinelli E, Guglielmino MR, Ragusa M, Farina M, Palumbo MA, Cianci A. Altered transcriptional regulation of cytokines, growth factors, and apoptotic proteins in the endometrium of infertile women with chronic endometritis. Am J Reprod Immunol. 2013;69:509–517. DOI:10.1111/aji.12076

[53] Sibai B, Dekker G, Kupferminc M. Pre-eclampsia. Lancet 2005;365:785–799.

[54] Erlebacher A. Immunology of the maternal-fetal interface. Annu Rev Immunol. 2013;31:387–411. DOI:10.1146/annurev-immunol-032712-100003

[55] Dimitriadis E, White CA, Jones RL, Salamonsen LA. Cytokines, chemokines and growth factors in endometrium related to implantation. Hum Reprod. 2005;11:613–630. DOI:10.1093/humupd/dmi023

[56] Toth B, Haufe T, Scholz C, Kuhn C, Friese K, Karamouti M, Makrigiannakis A, Jeschke U. Placental interleukin-15 expression in recurrent miscarriage. Am J Reprod Immunol. 2010;64:402–410. DOI:10.1111/j.1600-0897.2010.00879.x

[57] Sones JL, Lob HE, Isroff CE, Davisson RL. Role of decidual natural killer cells, interleukin-15, and interferon-gamma in placental development and preeclampsia. Am J Physiol Regul Integr Comp Physiol. 2014;307:R490–R492. DOI:10.1152/ajpregu.00176.2014

[58] Murphy SP, Tayade C, Ashkar AA, Hatta K, Zhang J, Croy BA. Interferon gamma in successful pregnancies. Biol Reprod. 2009;80:848–859. DOI:10.1095/biolreprod.108.073353

[59] Seybold U, Kourbatova EV, Johnson JG, Halvosa SJ, Wang YF, King MD, Ray SM, Blumberg HM. Emergence of community-associated methicillin-resistant *Staphylococcus aureus* USA300 genotype as a major cause of health care-associated blood stream infections. Clin Infect Dis. 2006;42:647–656.

[60] Levine DP. Vancomycin: a history. Clin Infect Dis. 2006;42(Suppl. 1):S5–S12.

[61] American Thoracic Society & Infectious Diseases Society of America. Guidelines for the management of adults with hospital-acquired, ventilator-associated, and health care-associated pneumonia. Am J Respir Crit Care Med. 2005;171:388–416. DOI:10.1164/rccm.200405-644ST

[62] Mendes RE, Deshpande LM, Jones RN. Linezolid update: stable in vitro activity following more than a decade of clinical use and summary of associated resistance mechanisms. Drug Resist. 2014;17:1–12. DOI:10.1016/j.drup.2014.04.002

[63] Patel D, Husain M, Vidaillac C, Steed ME, Rybak MJ, Seo SM, Kaatz GW. Mechanisms of in-vitro-selected daptomycin-non-susceptibility in *Staphylococcus aureus*. Int J Antimicrob Agents. 2011;38:442–446. DOI:10.1016/j.ijantimicag.2011.06.010

[64] Hobbs JK, Miller K, O'Neill AJ, Chopra I. Consequences of daptomycin-mediated membrane damage in Staphylococcus aureus. J Antimicrob Chemother. 2008;62:1003–1008. DOI:10.1093/jac/dkn321

[65] Jones T, Yeaman MR, Sakoulas G, Yang SJ, Proctor RA, Sahl HG, Schrenzel J, Xiong YQ, Bayer AS. Failures in clinical treatment of *Staphylococcus aureus* infection with daptomycin are associated with alterations in surface charge, membrane phospholipid asymmetry, and drug binding. Antimicrob Agents Chemother. 2008;52:269–278.

[66] Vuong C, Yeh AJ, Cheung GY, Otto M. Investigational drugs to treat methicillin-resistant *Staphylococcus aureus*. Expert Opin Investig Drugs. 2016;25:73–93. DOI: 10.1517/13543784.2016.1109077

Chapter 11

HIV Infection and Infertility

Thana Khawcharoenporn and Beverly E. Sha

Additional information is available at the end of the chapter

http://dx.doi.org/10.5772/62390

Abstract

Human immunodeficiency virus (HIV) infection has become a chronic and manageable disease since the availability of combination antiretroviral therapy (cART). Persons living with HIV are living longer with better quality of life. Given that worldwide many HIV-infected individuals are in the reproductive age, fertility and reproductive desire have emerged as clinically important issues among this population. Biological changes caused by HIV, including systemic illnesses, stress, and weight loss, may affect the function of reproductive organs and result in infertility. Newly diagnosed HIV infection may cause psychological trauma and decrease in sexual drive and sexual activity. Several HIV/acquired immune deficiency syndrome (AIDS)-related comorbidities have been reported to be associated with infertility. These include orchitis, acute epididymitis, and pelvic inflammatory disease caused by opportunistic pathogens and coinfections with sexually transmitted infections (STIs) acquired through a similar route of transmission as HIV. The common STIs caused by *Neisseria gonorrhoeae, Chlamydia trachomatis, Ureaplasma urealyticum, Treponema pallidum,* herpes simplex virus-2, and *Trichomonas vaginalis* can damage the reproductive system and cause infertility. Hypogonadism especially in men with AIDS is one of the important endocrine disorders that causes infertility. Although cART provides significant benefits in reducing morbidity and mortality among HIV-infected persons, some antiretroviral drugs, including nucleoside reverse transcriptase inhibitors, are toxic to cellular mitochondria and may affect the mitochondrial biogenesis of sperm and oocytes. HIV-infected individuals may have limited access to reproductive care given the severity of their disease, cost of care, stigmatization, and lack of specific HIV infection/infertility knowledge among their providers.

In the post–cART era, reproductive care has become an important issue to be co-managed with HIV care. Reproductive care includes not only comprehensively managing HIV infection but also minimizing the risk of horizontal HIV transmission in serodiscordant couples, providing suitable options for unprotected timed intercourse, intrauterine insemination with partner or donor sperm, in vitro fertilization with intracytoplasmic sperm injection (IVF/ICSI), embryo donation, and adoption. This chapter reviews potential effects of HIV infection, related opportunistic infections, and physical and psychological comorbidities on fertility; the impact of cART on fertility; and the management of reproductive issues among HIV-infected individuals.

Keywords: HIV, AIDS, Infection, Infertility

1. Introduction

There were approximately 37 million people living with human immunodeficiency virus (PLWHIV) globally at the end of 2014.[1] The course of HIV infection has changed from a deadly disease to a chronic and manageable disease since the introduction of combination antiretroviral therapy (cART) in the 1990s. The estimated life expectancy of a 20-year-old PLWHIV has increased from 30 years during 1996–1999 to 46 years during 2006–2008 according to the UK Collaborative HIV Cohort Study.[2] The increased life expectancy along with improved quality of life has led to increase in reproductive desire among this population.[3] Fertility of PLWHIV can be affected by HIV infection and associated infections. Infections can physically impact the anatomical structure and biological function of the reproductive system, whereas stress and psychiatric disorders related to HIV infection may lessen sexual drive and frequency of sexual intercourse. In addition, socioeconomic factors including limited financial means, difficulty accessing HIV care, and stigmatization can contribute to social withdrawal and reduced reproductive potential among PLWHIV. Management of reproductive health along with cART has become a necessary component of comprehensive HIV care in the post–cART era. The etiologies and epidemiology of HIV-related infertility, factors that may impact fertility, and management options and considerations for infertility among HIV-infected individuals are reviewed in this chapter.

2. Epidemiology of HIV-related infertility

The data on the magnitude and burden of HIV-related infertility derive mostly from studies conducted among HIV-infected women. A previous study using data from case–control studies and theoretical predictions from a model of the proximate determinants of fertility and HIV incidence in African countries demonstrated the 25–40% lower rate of fertility among HIV-infected women compared to HIV-negative women.[4] In a prospective cohort study from the United States during 1994–2002, women with HIV were less likely to conceive than uninfected women (pregnancy rates 7.4 vs.15.2 per 100 person-years, respectively).[5] Using demographic and health surveys between 2003 and 2007, the Joint United Nations Program on HIV/AIDS (UNAIDS) estimated that the global age-specific fertility ratio for HIV-infected women in the reproductive age group of 20–44 years is 0.53 to 0.76 compared to that of women without HIV.[6] A survey study conducted at HIV fertility clinics in the United Kingdom demonstrated a 40% prevalence of tubal factor infertility among HIV-infected women.[7] Despite the infertility in women living with HIV, pregnancy rates among this population have

http://dx.doi.org/10.5772/62390

increased steadily over the past 10 years to between 4 and 6 pregnancies per 100 person-years, varying by region due to the advances in HIV treatment and mother-to-child transmission prevention.[8] This may reflect an increase in reproductive desire and/or unexpected pregnancies and indicate the need for reproductive health care, fertility management, and family planning along with HIV comprehensive care among PLWHIV.

3. HIV effects on fertility

There are several factors associated with HIV infection that can potentially affect fertility in PLWHIV. These factors can be categorized into biological factors, psychological factors, and social factors (Figure 1).

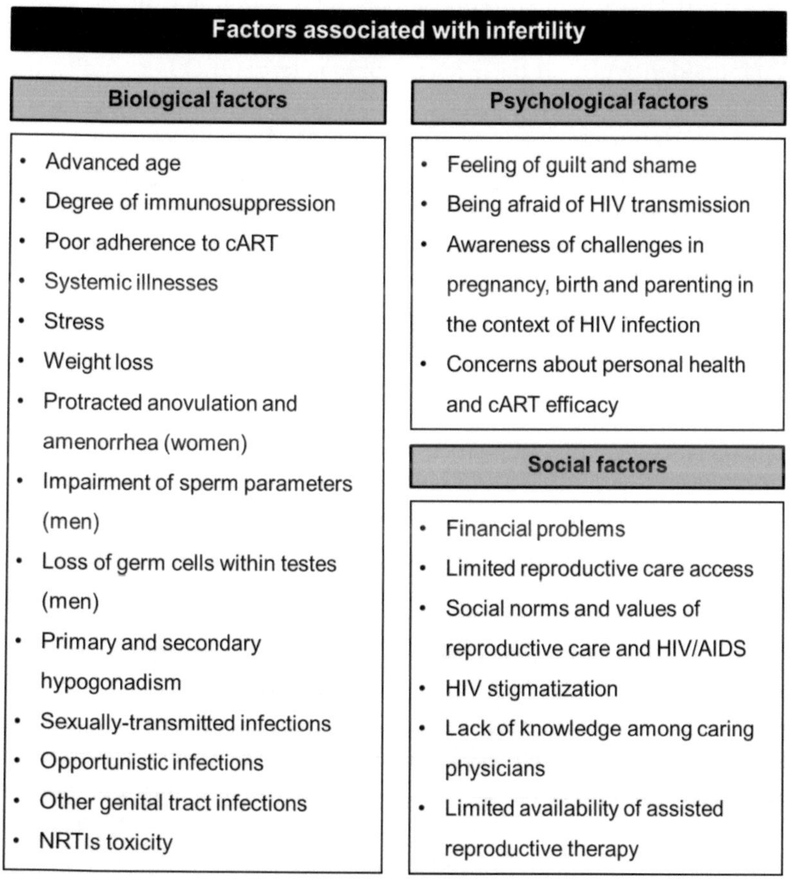

Note: AIDS, acquired immune deficiency syndrome; cART, combination antiretroviral therapy; HIV, human immunodeficiency virus; NRTIs, nucleoside reverse transcriptase inhibitors.

Figure 1. Factors associated with infertility among people living with human immunodeficiency virus

3.1. Biological factors

Demographic characteristics that have been reported to be associated with low rates of pregnancy among HIV-infected women include advanced age, white ethnicity (compared to black ethnicity), having CD4 cell count of less than 100 cells/mm^3, and poor adherence to cART. [8-10] Systemic illnesses from HIV and its related comorbidities, stress, and weight loss generally impact the reproductive potential of both sexes.[3] HIV-infected women are more likely than non-HIV-infected women to have protracted anovulation and amenorrhea.[11-14] The number of ovulatory cycles was found to correlate with the severity of immunosuppression and having an AIDS diagnosis. Although there have been no reports of ovarian aging or failure,[15] HIV-infected women may have reduced ovarian reserve.[16] In HIV-infected men, impairment of sperm parameters affecting fertility has been described. The impairment includes lower ejaculation volume, sperm count, and progressive motility (defined as the percent of sperm with forward motility) despite normal morphology compared to non-HIV-infected men.[17-19] Sperm concentration levels, total count, and motility were found to positively correlate with the height of the CD4 cell count, indicating the adverse effect of worsening immunodeficiency on these sperm parameters.[19] Other studies demonstrated that the semen of HIV-infected men was more viscous and contained fewer motile sperm but more round cells.[20] In addition, a study of testicular specimens from autopsy samples (1981–1998) revealed progressive loss of germ cells within the testes with prolonged survival with AIDS.[21] Although recent data indicate that cART significantly decreased total sperm count and progressive motility and increased the proportion of abnormal sperm forms,[22] these adverse effects are balanced by the overwhelming benefits of cART for immune reconstitution, morbidity and mortality reduction, and overall improvement of sperm characteristics associated with higher CD4 cell counts.

3.1.1. Hypogonadism and HIV/AIDS

Hypogonadism was recognized as a relatively common condition early in the HIV epidemic and characterized by a low level of testosterone among HIV-infected men. Hypogonadism can be categorized into primary hypogonadism, which is a disorder of the testes, and secondary hypogonadism, which is a disorder of the pituitary or hypothalamus. Hypogonadism can be associated with various signs and symptoms, including muscle wasting, weight loss, low bone mineral density, and decreased libido.[23] During the early course of HIV disease, men tend to have normal serum testosterone levels. As the disease progresses to AIDS, low serum testosterone levels become more frequent, particularly in those with more advanced immunosuppression (e.g., CD4 cell count less than 100 cells/mm^3). Early in the HIV epidemic, 30–50% of symptomatic HIV-infected men had low total serum testosterone levels, which significantly correlated with weight loss and CD4 cell depletion.[24-26] The prevalence of hypogonadism in HIV-infected men has decreased with cART initiation occurring at earlier stages of HIV infection. Effective HIV therapy can normalize testosterone levels over time.[27] Most cases of decreased testosterone levels in HIV-infected men are related to secondary hypogonadism.[24, 28] Other characteristics that have been reported to be associated with low testosterone levels include older age, a detectable HIV RNA level of greater than 10,000 copies/

mL, injection drug use, hepatitis C coinfection, high body mass index, and insulin resistance. [28-31] In addition, several medications commonly used among HIV-infected individuals can affect testosterone levels through varied mechanisms. Systemic glucocorticoids and megestrol acetate can cause hypogonadism by suppressing the hypothalamic–pituitary–gonadal axis, whereas a high dose of ketoconazole (at least 400 mg per day) directly inhibits steroidogenesis. Psychotropic medications can cause hyperprolactinemia and testosterone deficiency, whereas chronic use of alcohol, opiates, and marijuana can impair testosterone production.[32, 33]

Primary hypogonadism	Secondary hypogonadism
Congenital abnormalities	**Congenital abnormalities**
· Klinefelter's syndrome	· Congenital GnRH deficiency
· Other chromosomal abnormalities (e.g., 46, XY/XO; 47, XYY)	· Leptin or leptin receptor mutation
· Mutation in the FSH and LH receptor genes	· Gonadotropin subunit mutations
· Cryptorchidism	
· Disorders of androgen biosynthesis	
· Myotonic dystrophy	
· Congenital anorchia	
· Varicocele	
Acquired diseases	**Acquired diseases**
· Infectious orchitis	· Hyperprolactinemia
· Radiation	· Gonadal steroids
· Alkylating and antineoplastic agents	· Glucocorticoids
· Ketoconazole	· Continuous opiate administration
· Glucocorticoids	· Critical illness
· Dibromochloropropane	· Chronic systemic illness
· Trauma	· Anorexia nervosa
· Testicular torsion	· Diabetes mellitus
· Bilateral orchiectomy	· Obesity
· Autoimmune damage	· Pituitary adenoma
· Chronic systemic diseases	· Metastatic tumor damaging pituitary gland
· Cirrhosis	· Sarcoidosis
· Chronic kidney disease	· Hemochromatosis
· Idiopathic	· Tuberculous meningitis
	· Pituitary apoplexy
	· Trauma
	· Idiopathic

Note: FSH, follicle-stimulating hormone; GnRH, gonadotropin-releasing hormone; LH, luteinizing hormone.

Table 1. Causes of hypogonadism in males

HIV-infected men with symptomatic hypogonadism may present with loss of facial and body hair, decreased muscle mass and strength, diminished libido, impotence, testicular atrophy, gynecomastia, depression, low energy, and poor concentration.[34] Diagnosis of hypogonadism is made based on a clinical suspicion and low serum testosterone levels (generally less than 300 ng/dL). The screening test of choice is the serum total testosterone concentration (free plus protein-bound fractions). However, in some cases, the total testosterone levels may be normal, whereas the free levels may be low because of the higher sex hormone-binding globulin levels among HIV-infected persons. Thus, in a patient with suspected testosterone deficiency and serum total testosterone concentration in the lower half of the normal range (less than 500 ng/dL), the free testosterone levels should be assessed.[34] Testosterone levels should not be evaluated during an acute illness because of the transient decline of androgen levels related to the acute event. To distinguish between primary and secondary hypogonadism, follicle-stimulating hormone (FSH) and luteinizing hormone (LH) levels need to be measured. The elevated FSH and LH levels suggest primary hypogonadism, whereas normal or low levels of FSH and LH are consistent with secondary hypogonadism. Further evaluation should be geared toward diagnosing the possible causes of primary and secondary hypogonadism in HIV-infected men as detailed in Table 1.

3.1.2. Comorbid diseases and HIV/AIDS

3.1.2.1. Sexually Transmitted Infections (STIs)

The impact of STIs on fertility among PLWHIV depends on the local prevalence of the STIs. Given the common route of transmission of causative agents and immunosuppressive status caused by HIV, STIs tend to be more prevalent, to be more severe, to take longer to resolve, and to be more prone to treatment failure in HIV-infected persons compared to the general population. Common causative pathogens for STIs among PLWHIV include bacteria, such as *Neisseria gonorrhoeae, Chlamydia trachomatis, Ureaplasma urealyticum, Mycoplasma hominis, Mycoplasma genitalium, Treponema pallidum, Haemophilus ducreyi,* and *Klebsiella granulomatis*; viruses, such as hepatitis B and C viruses, herpes simplex virus (HSV), and human papillomavirus (HPV); and protozoa, such as *Trichomonas vaginalis*. The underlying pathogenesis for STI-related infertility is direct damage and subsequent anatomical and functional abnormalities of the genital organs, including the testes and epididymis in men and cervix, uterus, fallopian tubes, and ovaries in women. A previous study demonstrated that the DNA of STI pathogens was detected in semen of 45 of 241 asymptomatic men seeking an infertility investigation (19%) and was associated with a decrease in sperm concentration, motile sperm concentration, total sperm count, and neutral alpha glucosidase concentration.[35]

Gonorrhea is a STI caused by *N. gonorrhea* and commonly manifests as urethritis in both sexes and pelvic inflammatory disease in women. The reported complications related to fertility of gonorrhea include urethral strictures and subsequent impairment of testicular functions in men.[36] Similarly, *C. trachomatis* can cause urethritis in both sexes and pelvic inflammatory disease in females. Epidemiologic data suggest that *C. trachomatis* may be associated with tubal obstruction and subsequent infertility in women.[37] The impact of Mycoplasma, that is, *U.*

http://dx.doi.org/10.5772/62390

urealyticum, M. hominis, and *M. genitalium*, on fertility is uncertain. *U. urealyticum* may cause infertility through its effects on sperm chromatin and DNA, whereas *M. genitalium* can attach to spermatozoa and can be transported to the female genital tract.[38, 39] Syphilis is caused by *T. pallidum* and is more prevalent among PLWHIV. Orchitis, epididymitis, and testicular mass have been reported as manifestations of syphilis in HIV-infected men.[40, 41] Although *H. ducreyi* and *K. granulomatis* do not directly affect the reproductive tract, they both cause ulcers and lymphadenopathy around the genital area, which may affect reproductive potential.

Chronic viral hepatitis B and C can cause impairment in sperm concentration, motility, morphology, and viability, whereas HPV primarily affects sperm motility.[42] The presence of HSV DNA in semen has been associated with decreased sperm concentration and reduced motility.[43] In HIV-infected women, chronic HPV infection increases the risk of cervical cancer development and possibly leads to infertility. An important protozoan *T. vaginalis* is the cause of vaginitis, endometritis, adnexitis, and pyosalpinx in women, which can lead to infertility and preterm birth and low birth weight of the newborn.[44] In men, it is associated with complications including urethritis, prostatitis, epididymitis, and infertility through inflammatory damage or interference with sperm function.[44]

3.1.2.2. Opportunistic Infections (OIs)

HIV-infected persons are at increased risk for opportunistic infections (OIs) depending on their degree of immunosuppression. Tuberculosis is a common OI in HIV-tuberculosis endemic locales and its prevalence is higher among PLWHIV compared to non-HIV-infected persons, regardless of the CD4 cell count. Genital tract infection caused by *Mycobacterium tuberculosis* contributes to infertility and poorer reproductive health outcomes in both sexes.[3] Salmonellosis, toxoplasmosis, and cryptococcosis can manifest as disseminated infections involving the genital organs. Although cytomegalovirus (CMV) can cause orchitis and epididymitis in HIV-infected men, there are no data on its effect on sperm characteristics.[42] Candidiasis is frequently reported among HIV-infected persons with CD4 cell counts less than 200 cells/mm^3. It is the cause of balanitis in men and vaginitis and cervicitis in women, which may affect fertility.

3.1.2.3. Other infections

Other infectious causes of orchitis in both HIV-infected and non-HIV-infected men include bacteria, such as *Escherichia coli, Klebsiella pneumoniae, Pseudomonas aeruginosa, Staphylococcus* spp., and *Streptococcus* spp., and viruses, such as mumps, varicella, coxsackievirus, and echovirus.[45] These infections may also contribute to infertility.

3.1.3. Antiretroviral agents

Nucleoside reverse transcriptase inhibitors (NRTIs) remain key components of recommended cART regimens. They inhibit HIV-1 reverse transcriptase, which reduces viral replication and improves disease control. However, these medications also inhibit mitochondrial DNA (mtDNA) synthesis and cause a decrease in polypeptides involved in electron transport, which can result in cell injury.[46] The degree of mitochondrial toxicity is specific to each NRTI. Theoretically, an HIV-infected person's fertility may be affected by NRTI use via the damage to mitochondrial biogenesis of gametes.[3] This is supported by the mtDNA depletion observed in sperm and oocytes of HIV-infected patients taking NRTIs and in low oocyte mtDNA in patients with ovarian insufficiency.[47-49] Data from epidemiologic studies are conflicting regarding the impact of cART on fertility. A prospective cohort from the United States reported the lower likelihood of conception associated with antiretroviral therapy among HIV-infected women,[5] whereas a more recent study from Africa demonstrated significantly higher pregnancy rates among HIV-infected women on cART compared to those not on cART.[50] However, these two studies were conducted in different settings and time, and specific behavioral and biological mechanisms were not explored. Zidovudine (azidothymidine, AZT) is the NRTI drug that has been studied the most. In animal studies, AZT has been shown to suppress cell division in the preimplantation mouse embryo, causing reduction in inner cell mass proliferation, greater number of resorptions, and fewer fetuses.[51, 52] A previous study demonstrated that exposure to NRTI transplacentally caused significant fetal mitochondrial damage in experimental monkeys.[53] Unfortunately, there have been no studies examining fertility effect of NRTIs in humans.

3.2. Psychological factors

Decrease in sexual activity after a new diagnosis of HIV infection is usually observed and may be accompanied by the feeling of guilt and shame and aggravated by the stigma related to HIV infection.[54] Individuals recently diagnosed with HIV infection reported to have decreased desire for or interest in sex relations. They also reported to use condom more consistently during sexual intercourse to avoid transmission of HIV to their partners.[55] Previous studies indicated that HIV-infected women often chose to avoid pregnancy.[56, 57] However, another study revealed that high-risk behaviors, unplanned pregnancies, and pregnancy termination remain prevalent among this population.[58] In the pre–cART era, there was a significant increase in the pregnancy termination rate from 3.5 to 6.3 per 100 women-years following a new HIV diagnosis in the United Kingdom and Ireland[56] and 47% of pregnancies were voluntarily terminated following a new HIV diagnosis in an Australian study.[57] The reasons for pregnancy termination may include challenges of pregnancy, birth and parenting in the context of HIV infection, concerns about increased risks of complications related to pregnancy and delivery, and risk of HIV transmission to the newborn. A previous study reported that unplanned pregnancy, lower CD4 cell count, and having an HIV-infected current partner were factors associated with the decision to terminate a pregnancy.[59] Following the introduction of cART with overall improvement in health and immune status of HIV-infected women, the rates of elective pregnancy termination after a HIV diagnosis were 22%-26% decreased from the pre–cART period.[60, 61] With the success of cART in preventing mother-to-child HIV transmission, HIV infection was reported to have no effect on desire for pregnancy among young urban African Americans aged 15–24 years.[62] Reproductive desire among PLWHIV may now be associated with personal health, cART, concern about HIV transmission, and social factors. Some HIV-infected persons have an increased desire for children as a way of concealing their HIV-infected status and improving their feelings of self-worth. Others stated that their HIV diagnosis increased their desire for children at an earlier age and some chose to have children following advances in HIV care.[63-65]

3.3. Social factors

The HIV/AIDS epidemic has a significant impact on the economic and political stability of a nation. Awareness of HIV/AIDS at the population level may affect the age of sexual debut, frequency of sexual intercourse, safer sex and contraceptive practices, perceived value of marriage, social norms, and fertility intentions and choices of PLWHIV.[3] The dramatic improvement in the life expectancy of PLWHIV and reduction in HIV transmission rates following treatment of the infected partner have changed ethical considerations regarding childbearing in HIV-infected individuals. Early in the HIV/AIDS epidemic, pregnancy in HIV-infected women was considered morally problematic, whereas recently, the Ethics Committee of the American Society for Reproductive Medicine stated that it is ethical for health care providers to assist PLWHIV who seek pregnancy when optimal precautions to prevent HIV transmission are utilized.[66] Despite more opportunities for access to reproductive care, PLWHIV still face multiple obstacles. First, the severity of their disease, level of immunosuppression, presence of OIs, and other comorbid diseases may impair their fertility. Second, their HIV provider may have limited knowledge to counsel them on reproductive health issues, and infertility specialists may have limited expertise in providing care for HIV-infected persons. Third, HIV stigmatization could potentially preclude them from establishing reproductive care. Finally, assisted fertility therapy (AFT) is technically complicated in regard to HIV transmission prevention and costliness and may not be available in all settings.[3]

4. Fertility management

Fertility management for PLWHIV should be comprehensive and involve cART, specific management for factors associated with infertility, and AFT while minimizing the risk of horizontal and vertical transmission of HIV.

4.1. Combination antiretroviral therapy

With advances in the development of antiretroviral agents, cART has become more potent and effective, more tolerable and convenient to administer, and less toxic. Current guidelines recommend that PLWHIV should receive cART when they are willing and able to commit to treatment and understand the benefits and risks of therapy and the importance of adherence, regardless of the CD4 cell count level.[67] The benefits of early cART among persons with a CD4 cell count above 500 cells/mm^3 were demonstrated in a recent large-scale randomized trial that showed a reduction in mortality, AIDS-related events, and non–AIDS-related events in those started on cART immediately versus waiting until the CD4 cell count fell below 350 cells/mm^3.[68] The currently recommended initial cART regimens consist of a backbone of two NRTIs and any one drug from the following drug classes: non-NRTI, protease inhibitor with a booster, or integrase inhibitor with or without a booster.[67, 69, 70] The initial cART regimens recommended by different consensus guidelines are shown in Table 2. A patient-specific regimen from these lists will be chosen based on convenience of administration, adverse reactions, local availability, cost, and health plan coverage. The goals of cART are immunologic response, defined as an increase in CD4 cell count, and virologic response, defined as HIV RNA suppression below the lower limit of detection. By extending life expectancy and improving overall health, immunity, and quality of life from cART, cART is expected to improve fertility outcomes. Achieving a sustained virologic response is particularly important to reduce the risk of HIV horizontal and vertical transmission during conception attempts, pregnancy, and delivery.

DHHS 2015	EACS 2015	WHO 2013
ABC + 3TC + DTG	ABC + 3TC + DTG	TDF + FTC/3TC + EFV
TDF + FTC + DTG	TDF + FTC + DTG	
TDF + FTC + EVG/c or TAF + FTC + EVG/c	TDF + FTC + EVG/c	
TDF + FTC + RAL	TDF + FTC + RAL	
TDF + FTC + DRV/r	TDF + FTC + DRV/r	
	TDF + FTC + RPV	

Note: 3TC, lamivudine; ABC, abacavir; DHHS, the U.S. Department of Health and Human Services; DRV/r, ritonavir-boosted darunavir; DTG, dolutegravir; EACS, European AIDS Clinical Society; EFV, efavirenz; EVG/c, cobicistat-boosted elvitegravir; FTC, emtricitabine; RAL, raltegravir; RPV, rilpivirine; TAF, tenofovir alafenamide; TDF, tenofovir disoproxil fumarate; WHO, World Health Organization.

Table 2. Recommended first-line combination antiretroviral therapy regimens based on consensus guidelines

4.2. Specific management for factors associated with infertility

4.2.1. Management of biological factors

Immunosuppression and wasting syndrome can be improved by cART. In addition, PLWHIV who are taking cART with sustained immunologic and virologic responses will have reduced incidences of OIs, such as tuberculosis, salmonellosis, toxoplasmosis, cryptococcosis, CMV infection, and candidiasis. NRTIs selected for the backbone of a cART regimen should have the least toxicity on mitochondria to minimize the impact on oocytes and sperm. These "safer" NRTIs include tenofovir, abacavir, lamivudine, and emtricitabine.[67, 69, 70] Good general health and less physical stress are associated with normal ovulation and menstrual cycles in HIV-infected women, whereas cART improves overall sperm parameters among HIV-infected men. STIs, OIs, and other infections should be promptly diagnosed and treated to prevent damage to the genital organs. It is important that sex partners of patients with STIs should be counseled, tested, and treated accordingly.

Hypogonadism should be recognized early, correctly diagnosed, and treated in HIV-infected men. Testosterone treatment is indicated in men with low serum concentrations of testosterone and any of the following signs or symptoms including low libido and/or hypogonadal symptoms, low bone mineral density, low body mass, or weight loss despite virologic response to cART. Prior to initiation of testosterone replacement therapy, patients should be evaluated for coexisting depression and psychosocial stressors along with baseline laboratory studies including complete blood count, a metabolic panel, lipid panel, and a prostate-specific antigen (PSA). Long-term effects of suppression of the hypothalamic–pituitary–gonadal axis, promoting malignancy of the prostate gland and cardiovascular diseases, in those older than 60 years should be carefully monitored. Patients with a history of prostate cancer, a palpable prostate nodule, or an elevated PSA should not be prescribed testosterone replacement therapy.[34, 71] The routes of testosterone administration should be based on the patient's preference and include transdermal patch, gel, and intramuscular injection. For injections, the initial dose is 200 mg every 2 weeks or 100 mg every week. The dose can be titrated based on testosterone levels measured midway between injections aiming for the mid-normal reference range. Testosterone replacement therapy should continue as long as there are symptomatic benefits and no adverse effects.

4.2.2. *Management of psychological and social factors*

Knowledge about HIV and its epidemiology, routes of transmission, clinical course, long-term prognosis, and benefit of cART is critical to PLWHIV in reducing HIV transmission to their sexual partners and improvinge their adherence and outcomes. A previous study demonstrated that increased reproductive intention was associated with patient optimism regarding cART efficacy.[72] To overcome the challenges in pregnancy, birth, and parenting, PLWHIV should be informed about the recent advances in antenatal, perinatal, and postnatal care to prevent HIV transmission to their newborns. Family planning counseling should be provided to prepare them for child rearing and to cope with any problems they may face. Issues on reproductive care access for PLWHIV are very new for many developing countries, because the main goals for HIV care in these countries are currently improving access to HIV testing and treatment. Financial burdens, medical coverage, and availability of centers that can provide AFT need to be considered when developing and implementing local, regional, and national policies or guidelines for the reproductive care of PLWHIV. In the meantime, physicians who care for PLWHIV should update their knowledge to optimally assess and manage fertility issues among persons with HIV infection. HIV stigmatization may be reduced by campaigns and specific interventions that are appropriate and feasible for each locale.

4.3. Assisted fertility therapy

Relevant issues to be considered regarding fertility treatment in PLWHIV include risk of HIV horizontal transmission in serodiscordant heterosexual couples and methods to reduce HIV transmission. Generally, the rate of HIV heterosexual transmission is approximately 1 per

500 to 1 per 1,000 episodes of unprotected sexual intercourse.[3] However, the risk of transmission can increase significantly if there are genital tract infections from STIs or OIs, trauma with sex, lack of male circumcision, and high plasma HIV RNA levels in seropositive persons.[73, 74] Thus, a thorough evaluation is needed before AFT. History including a detailed history of their HIV infection and any associated complications, recent CD4 cell counts and HIV RNA levels, past and current cART regimens, history of antiretroviral drug resistance, ongoing HIV risk behaviors, and fertility problems should be obtained. Physical examination should focus on signs relevant to causes of infertility, genital organs, and Pap smear in women. An HIV-infected partner should be treated with cART until HIV RNA suppression has been achieved prior to AFT. Partners who have STIs need to be treated to reduce transmission risks of HIV and STI-associated pathogens. Trauma during sexual intercourse should be avoided or minimized, and safer sex practices should be encouraged outside the conception attempts. Proposed algorithm for fertility management among HIV-infected couples is shown in Figure 2.

Post-exposure prophylaxis (PEP) with cART in uninfected partners may be used after the unprotected sexual intercourse (conception attempt). Although there have not been well-designed studies in human that assess the efficacy of this intervention, the benefits of HIV transmission reduction have been shown in an animal study and a retrospective study of health care workers exposing to body fluids of HIV-infected persons.[75, 76] The recommended PEP regimens that are also safe if the pregnancy does occur are combined tenofovir, emtricitabine, and ritonavir-boosted atazanavir, ritonavir-boosted darunavir, or raltegravir.[77] PEP should be initiated as soon as possible after HIV exposure but within 48 hours and should be continued for 28 days. Because of its demonstrated efficacy, tenofovir–emtricitabine (TDF/FTC) once daily for pre-exposure prophylaxis (PrEP) administered to the seronegative partner is now the preferred approach to reduce the risk of HIV transmission among serodiscordant couples. Among heterosexual couples, pericoital tenofovir vaginal gel was the first PrEP intervention that showed a 39% efficacy at reducing HIV acquisition among high-risk South African women.[78] Several other randomized controlled trials have demonstrated the benefit of PrEP at reducing HIV acquisition among HIV-negative at-risk individuals including 1) the iPrEx study that demonstrated 44% reduction in the incidence of HIV among men who have sex with men taking daily oral TDF/FTC,[79] 2) the Partners-PrEP study that demonstrated 75% and 67% reduction in the incidence of HIV among serodiscordant couples taking daily oral TDF or TDF/FTC, respectively, in Africa,[80] and 3) the TDF2 study that demonstrated 62% reduction in the incidence of HIV among heterosexual men and women taking daily oral TDF/FTC in Botswana.[81] Pharmacokinetic data suggest that PrEP should begin at least 1 week before unprotected sex for optimal benefit. The uninfected partners who choose to take PEP and/or PrEP need to be regularly screened and monitored for HIV infection and adverse effects of the drugs in PEP and/or PrEP regimens.[67, 77]

In regards to limiting risk of HIV vertical transmission, cART given to HIV-infected women antenatally and avoiding breastfeeding can reduce the rate of transmission from 25–40% to less than 1%.[67] Invasive procedures, such as amniocentesis, chorionic villus sampling, and use of fetal scalp electrodes, should be avoided in HIV-infected women because these can

http://dx.doi.org/10.5772/62390

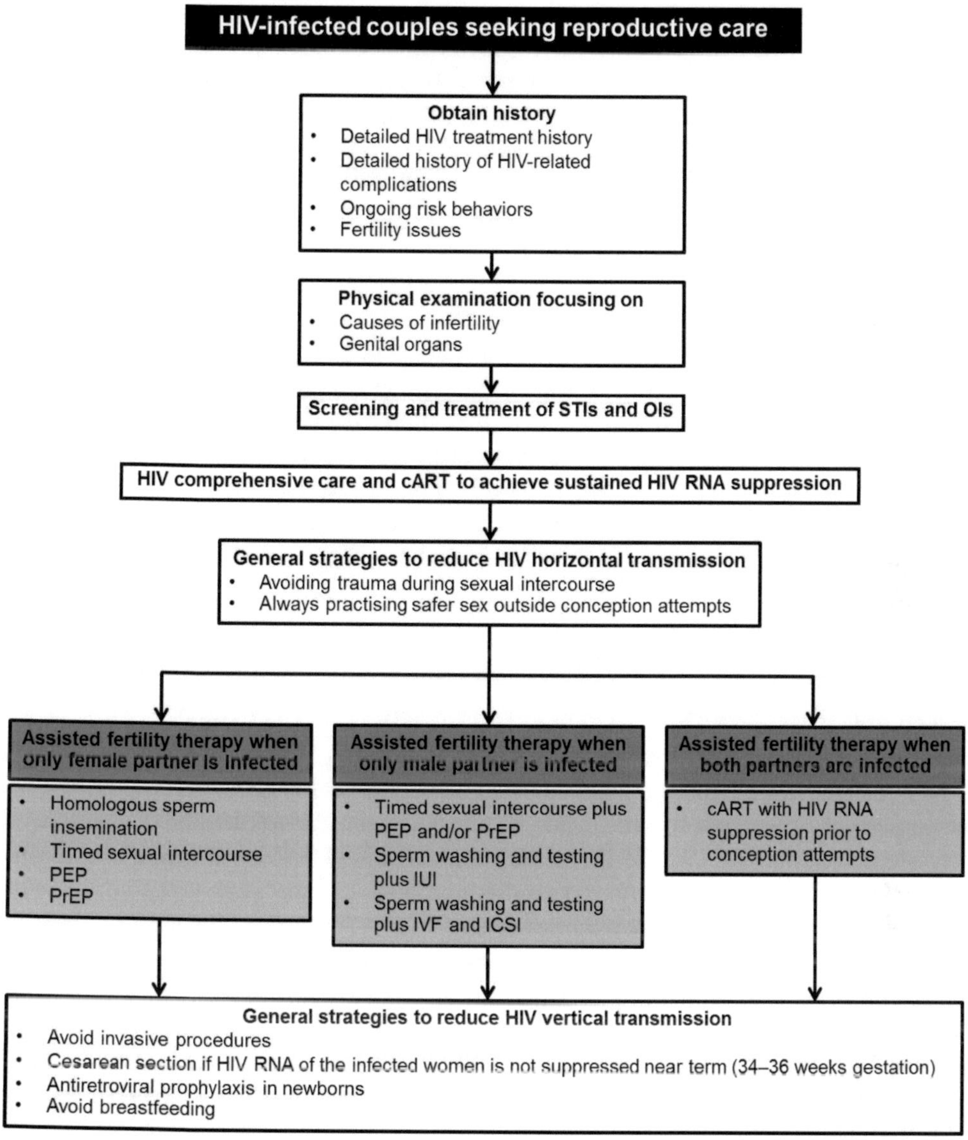

Note: cART, combination antiretroviral therapy; HIV, human immunodeficiency virus; ICSI, intracytoplasmic sperm injection; IUI, intrauterine insemination; IVF, in vitro fertilization; OIs, opportunistic infections; PEP, post-exposure prophylaxis; PrEP, pre-exposure prophylaxis; RNA, ribonucleic acid; STIs, sexually transmitted infections.

Figure 2. Proposed algorithm of fertility management in HIV-infected couples

increase the risk of fetal/infant exposure to maternal body fluids. Cesarean section instead of normal vaginal delivery can further reduce the risk of maternal-infant transmission in HIV-infected pregnant women whose HIV RNA has not been suppressed following cART. United States guidelines use a HIV RNA level of >1,000 copies/mL at 34–36 weeks gestation as a threshold for recommending Cesarean section, whereas European guidelines recommend a threshold of >50 copies/mL.[67, 69] Women who achieve virologic suppression near term can proceed with vaginal delivery without increased transmission risk. Antiretroviral prophylactic regimens for newborns of HIV-infected mothers should be prescribed based on the risk of transmission. In general, AZT is recommended for the first 4–6 weeks of life with additional medications added if the mother did not achieve viral suppression. HIV-infected mothers should not breastfeed their babies due to the risk of transmission via breast milk.

4.3.1. *AFT when only the female partner is infected*

If a woman is HIV infected and her male partner is uninfected, HIV transmission can be avoided by using homologous insemination with the male partner's sperm. However, if this option is not feasible, such as the desire to become pregnant naturally, couples should limit unprotected sexual intercourse to the time of ovulation (timed intercourse) using ovulation kits or basal body temperature monitoring to predict ovulation. These measures allow couples to limit the number of unprotected sexual encounters. In addition, the HIV-infected women should be on cART with a suppressed viral load. The male partner may choose to take PEP and/or PrEP to reduce the risk of HIV transmission; however, these options are not as safe as homologous insemination.[82]

4.3.2. *AFT when only the male partner is infected*

Conception between an HIV-infected man and his HIV-uninfected female partner is more complicated. The risk of HIV transmission can be reduced by using timed intercourse when the HIV-infected man's plasma HIV RNA is undetectable on cART. However, the HIV transmission of timed intercourse in this setting has been reported to be associated with inconsistent condom use outside the conception attempt.[83] Thus, the practice of timed intercourse alone to prevent HIV transmission to the female partner is not generally recommended in this setting.[82] Additional PEP and/or PrEP may be used to reduce HIV transmission. A study of serodiscordant couples, in which the woman was treated with oral tenofovir taken shortly before and after each unprotected sexual encounter, showed that none of the women became infected with HIV and pregnancy rates reached 75% after 12 attempts.[84] Based on available data, once-daily TDF/FTC for the women would generally be recommended throughout the conception period in countries where resources are available for PrEP.

Sperm preparation and testing prior to intrauterine insemination (IUI) have been described as methods to reduce the chance of HIV transmission to the uninfected female partner. The sperm preparation involves a three-step process.[3, 82] First, the liquefied semen is filtered through a Percoll gradient. Next, the isolated spermatozoa are washed to eliminate seminal plasma and hyperosmotic gradient media. Finally, a modified swim-up method recovers highly motile spermatozoa from leukocytes. After this process, the final sperm specimen is tested by polymerase chain reaction assays for the presence of HIV. If this final specimen tests negative, it is used for insemination. In men with severe dyspermia, the final swim-up step that removes infected leukocytes cannot be performed and thus the semen should be tested for HIV DNA. Utilizing this process, 1,600 inseminations were performed in 513 HIV-uninfected women and resulted in 228 pregnancies. At 1-year follow-up, none of the children older than 3 months of age and none of the mothers became HIV infected.[85] In addition, studies reviewing world-wide data in 2004 and data from several centers demonstrated no HIV transmission to the uninfected female partners who were inseminated using sperm washing and IUI.[86, 87]

There have been recent data supporting the use of IVF/ICSI to reduce HIV transmission to uninfected women. A 10-year retrospective study of 181 serodiscordant couples undergoing IVF/ICSI, in which sperm was prepared using a modified density-gradient centrifugation and the swim-up method, revealed no HIV infection among the uninfected women and their 170 children.[88] Another study from the Center for Reproductive Assisted Techniques for HIV in Europe reported no evidence of seroconversion in any uninfected partners or children on follow-up.[86] Unfortunately, these techniques are generally prohibitively expensive. Although the data on efficacy and safety of the AFT techniques are encouraging, the potential risk of HIV transmission is not completely eliminated and more studies are required. Until then, serodiscordant couples should also be counseled about other safer options, including using donor sperm, donor embryo, adoption, or not having children.[82] If couples want to have their own biological children, they should be informed about available risk reduction techniques and the availability of centers that can provide effective methods of sperm preparation and testing. Fertility centers should use approved study protocols with informed consent and provide appropriate follow-up of sexual partners and their children.

4.3.3. *AFT when both partners are infected*

While HIV seroconcordant couples do not have the same concerns about HIV transmission as do HIV serodiscordant couples, the risk of transmission of different strains of HIV between each other or superinfection exists. HIV superinfection in seroconcordant couples has been reported to increase the risk of HIV RNA rebound and decrease in CD4 cell count following immune reactivation.[89] The best way to minimize the risk of superinfection and optimize reproductive outcomes for couples and their offspring is to use cART to achieve HIV RNA suppression in both partners prior to conception attempts.

4.4. Healthcare workers and cross-contamination risks

Healthcare workers are at risk of exposure to blood-borne pathogens, including HIV through patient care. However, if standard universal precautions to prevent the transmission of infectious diseases are followed, the risk of acquiring these pathogens is very small and is not sufficient to deny reproductive services to PLWHIV. To date, there have been no reports of occupational HIV transmission to health care workers performing AFT, suggesting that the risk of transmission is extremely low. Theoretical concerns about contaminating other gametes and embryos stored in the same laboratory from cross-contamination have been raised. To date, no such event has been reported. To avoid this risk, it is recommended that samples from HIV-infected persons be processed in a separate laboratory or designated space within the main laboratory and to use a dedicated storage tank.[82]

5. Conclusions

Reproductive issues have become more relevant among PLWHIV who are living longer and are staying healthier on cART. Fertility outcomes of PLWHIV have been improving for the past decade, although they remain inferior to those of the general population. HIV can impact fertility in many ways that involve biological, psychological, and social factors. Assessing and managing fertility issues in HIV-infected individuals and couples involve the use of cART, diagnosing and correcting causes of infertility, and AFT, which has become more effective and safer. Further studies are needed to address the efficacy and safety of AFT techniques as well as the complex social and ethical challenges of fertility issues of HIV-infected persons. Healthcare workers caring for PLWHIV should be knowledgeable in both HIV infection and reproductive health because they may now be legally and ethically obligated to provide reproductive care and assistance to this population.

Author details

Thana Khawcharoenporn[1*] and Beverly E. Sha[2]

*Address all correspondence to: thanak30@yahoo.com

1 Division of Infectious Diseases, Faculty of Medicine, Thammasat University, Pathumthani, Thailand

2 Division of Infectious Diseases, Rush University Medical Center, Chicago, IL, USA

References

[1] UNAIDS. Fact Sheet 2015. Available at: www.unaids.org/en/resources/campaigns/HowAIDSchangedeverything/factsheet. Accessed 16 December 2015.

[2] May M, Gompels M, Delpech V, Porter K, Post F, Johnson M, et al. Impact of late diagnosis and treatment on life expectancy in people with HIV-1: UK Collaborative HIV Cohort (UK CHIC) Study. BMJ 2011; 343: d6016. doi: 10.1136/bmj.d6016.

[3] Kushnir VA, Lewis W. Human immunodeficiency virus/acquired immunodeficiency syndrome and infertility: emerging problems in the era of highly active antiretrovirals. Fertil Steril 2011; 96: 546–553.

[4] Zaba B, Gregson S. Measuring the impact of HIV on fertility in Africa. AIDS 1998; 12 Suppl 1: S41–S50.

[5] Massad LS, Springer G, Jacobson L, Watts H, Anastos K, Korn A, et al. Pregnancy rates and predictors of conception, miscarriage and abortion in US women with HIV. AIDS 2004; 18: 281–286.

[6] Chen WJ, Walker N. Fertility of HIV-infected women: insights from demographic and health surveys. Sex Transm Infect 2010; 86: ii22–ii27.

[7] Frodsham LC, Boag F, Barton S, Gilling-Smith C. Human immunodeficiency virus infection and fertility care in the United Kingdom: demand and supply. Fertil Steril 2006; 85: 285–289.

[8] Westreich D, Maskew M, Rubel D, MacDonald P, Jaffray I, Majuba P. Incidence of pregnancy after initiation of antiretroviral therapy in South Africa: a retrospective clinical cohort analysis. Infect Dis Obstet Gynecol 2012; 2012: 917059.

[9] Huntington SE, Thorne C, Bansi LK, Anderson J, Newell ML, Taylor GP, et al. Predictors of pregnancy and changes in pregnancy incidence among HIV-positive women accessing HIV clinical care. AIDS 2013; 27: 95–103.

[10] Lancaster KE, Kwok C, Rinaldi A, Byamugisha J, Magwali T, Nyamapfeni P, et al. Incident pregnancy and pregnancy outcomes among HIV-infected women in Uganda and Zimbabwe. Int J Gynaecol Obstet 2015; 131: 255–259.

[11] Chirgwin KD, Feldman J, Muneyyirci-Delale O, Landesman S, Minkoff H. Menstrual function in human immunodeficiency virus-infected women without acquired immunodeficiency syndrome. J Acquir Immune Defic Syndr Hum Retrovirol 1996; 12: 489–94.

[12] Cejtin HE, Kalinowski A, Bacchetti P, Taylor RN, Watts DH, Kim S, et al. Effects of human immunodeficiency virus on protracted amenorrhea and ovarian dysfunction. Obstet Gynecol 2006; 108: 1423–1431.

[13] Ellerbrock TV, Wright TC, Bush TJ, Dole P, Brudney K, Chiasson M. Characteristics of menstruation in women infected with HIV. Obstet Gynecol 1996; 87: 1030–1034.

[14] Harlow SC, Schuman P, Cohen M, Ohmit SE, Cu-Uvin S, Lin X, et al. Effect of HIV infection on menstrual cycle length. J Acquir Immune Defic Syndr 2000; 24: 68–75.

[15] Seifer DB, Golub ET, Lambert-Messerlian G, Springer G, Holman S, Moxley M, et al. Biologic markers of ovarian reserve and reproductive aging: application in a cohort study of HIV infection in women. Fertil Steril 2007; 88: 1645–1652.

[16] Coll O, Fiore S, Floridia M, Giaquinto C, Grosch-Wörner I, Guiliano M, et al. Pregnancy and HIV infection: a European consensus on management. AIDS 2002; 16 Suppl 2: S1–S18.

[17] White DJ, Mital D, Taylor S, St John JC. Sperm mitochondrial DNA deletions as a consequence of long term highly active antiretroviral therapy. AIDS 2001; 15: 1061–1062.

[18] Bujan L, Sergerie M, Moinard N, Martinet S, Porte L, Massip P, et al. Decreased semen volume and spermatozoa motility in HIV-1-infected patients under antiretroviral treatment. J Androl 2007; 28: 444–452.

[19] Nicopoullos JD, Almeida PA, Ramsay JW, Gilling-Smith C. The effect of human immunodeficiency virus on sperm parameters and the outcome of intrauterine insemination following sperm washing. Hum Reprod 2004; 19: 2289–2297.

[20] Crittenden JA, Handelsman DJ, Stewart GJ. Semen analysis in human immunodeficiency virus infection. Fertil Steril 1992; 57: 1294–1299.

[21] Shevchuk MM, Pigato JB, Khalife G, Armenakas NA, Fracchia JA. Changing testicular histology in AIDS: its implication for sexual transmission of HIV. Urology 1999; 53: 203–208.

[22] Nicopoullos JD, Almeida P, Vourliotis M, Gilling-Smith C. A decade of the sperm-washing programme: correlation between markers of HIV and seminal parameters. HIV Med 2011; 12: 195–201.

[23] Wanke CA, Silva M, Knox TA, Forrester J, Speigelman D, Gorbach SL. Weight loss and wasting remain common complications in individuals infected with human immunodeficiency virus in the era of highly active antiretroviral therapy. Clin Infect Dis 2000; 31: 803–805.

[24] Dobs AS, Dempsey MA, Ladenson PW, Polk BF. Endocrine disorders in men infected with human immunodeficiency virus. Am J Med 1988; 84: 611–616.

[25] Raffi F, Brisseau JM, Planchon B, Rémi JP, Barrier JH, Grolleau JY. Endocrine function in 98 HIV-infected patients: a prospective study. AIDS 1991; 5: 729–733.

[26] Christeff N, Gharakhanian S, Thobie N, Rozenbaum W, Nunez EA. Evidence for changes in adrenal and testicular steroids during HIV infection. J Acquir Immune Defic Syndr 1992; 5: 841–846.

[27] Dubé MP, Parker RA, Mulligan K, Tebas P, Robbins GK, Roubenoff R, et al. Effects of potent antiretroviral therapy on free testosterone levels and fat-free mass in men in a prospective, randomized trial: A5005s, a substudy of AIDS Clinical Trials Group Study 384. Clin Infect Dis 2007; 45: 120–126.

[28] Klein RS, Lo Y, Santoro N, Dobs AS. Androgen levels in older men who have or who are at risk of acquiring HIV infection. Clin Infect Dis 2005; 41: 1794–1803.

[29] Araujo AB, O'Donnell AB, Brambilla DJ, Simpson WB, Longcope C, Matsumoto AM, et al. Prevalence and incidence of androgen deficiency in middle-aged and older men: estimates from the Massachusetts Male Aging Study. J Clin Endocrinol Metab 2004; 89: 5920–5926.

[30] Grossmann M, Gianatti EJ, Zajac JD. Testosterone and type 2 diabetes. Curr Opin Endocrinol Diabetes Obes 2010; 17: 247–256.

[31] Zitzmann M. Testosterone deficiency, insulin resistance and the metabolic syndrome. Nat Rev Endocrinol 2009; 5: 673–681.

[32] Misra M, Papakostas GI, Klibanski A. Effects of psychiatric disorders and psychotropic medications on prolactin and bone metabolism. J Clin Psychiatry 2004; 65: 1607–1618.

[33] Cooper OB, Brown TT, Dobs AS. Opiate drug use: a potential contributor to the endocrine and metabolic complications in human immunodeficiency virus disease. Clin Infect Dis 2003; 37 Suppl 2: S132–S136.

[34] Bhasin S, Cunningham GR, Hayes FJ, Matsumoto AM, Snyder PJ, Swerdloff RS, et al. Testosterone therapy in men with androgen deficiency syndromes: an Endocrine Society clinical practice guideline. J Clin Endocrinol Metab 2010; 95: 2536–2559.

[35] Bezold G, Politch JA, Kiviat NB, Kuypers JM, Wolff H, Anderson DJ. Prevalence of sexually transmissible pathogens in semen from asymptomatic male infertility patients with and without leukocytospermia. Fertil Steril 2007; 87: 1087–1097.

[36] Ochsendrof FR. Sexually transmitted infections: impact on male fertility. Andrologia 2008; 40: 72–75.

[37] Eggert-Kruse W, Gerhard I, Näher H, Tilgen W, Runnebaum B. Chlamydial infection —a female and/or male infertility factor? Fertil Steril 1990; 53: 1037–1043.

[38] Reichart M, Kahane I, Bartoov B. In vivo and in vitro impairment of human and ram sperm nuclear chromatin integrity by sexually transmitted *Ureaplasma urealyticum* infection. Biol Reprod 2000; 63: 1041–1048.

[39] Svenstrup HF, Fedder J, Abraham-Peskir J, Birkelund S, Christiansen G. *Mycoplasma genitalium* attaches to human spermatozoa. Hum Reprod 2003; 18: 2103–2109.

[40] Michelson HE. Syphilis of the epididymis. JAMA 1919; 73: 1431–1433.

[41] Varma R, Baithun S, Alexander S, Goh BT. Acute syphilitic interstitial orchitis mimicking testicular malignancy in an HIV-1 infected man diagnosed by *Treponema pallidum* polymerase chain reaction. Int J STD AIDS 2009; 20: 65–66.

[42] Garolla A, Pizzol D, Bertoldo A, Menegazzo M, Barzon L, Foresta C. Sperm viral infection and male infertility: focus on HBV, HCV, HIV, HPV, HSV, HCMV, and AAV. J Reprod Immunol 2013; 100: 20–29.

[43] Neofytou E, Sourvinos G, Asmarianaki M, Spandidos DA, Makrigiannakis A. Prevalence of human herpes virus types 1-7 in the semen of men attending an infertility clinic and correlation with semen parameters. Fertil Steril 2009; 91: 2487–2494.

[44] Fichorova RN. Impact of *T. vaginalis* infection on innate immune responses and reproductive outcome. J Reprod Immunol 2009; 83: 185–189.

[45] Brookings C, Goldmeier D, Sadeghi-Nejad H. Sexually transmitted infections and sexual function in relation to male fertility. Korean J Urol 2013; 54: 149–156.

[46] Lewis W, Day BJ, Copeland WC. Mitochondrial toxicity of NRTI antiviral drugs: an integrated cellular perspective. Nat Rev Drug Discov 2003; 2: 812–22.

[47] Pavili L, Daudin M, Moinard N, Walschaerts M, Cuzin L, Massip P, et al. Decrease of mitochondrial DNA level in sperm from patients infected with human immunodeficiency virus-1 linked to nucleoside analogue reverse transcriptase inhibitors. Fertil Steril 2010; 94: 2151–2156.

[48] Lopez S, Coll O, Durban M, Hernandez S, Vidal R, Suy A, et al. Mitochondrial DNA depletion in oocytes of HIV-infected antiretroviral-treated infertile women. Antivir Ther 2008; 13: 833–838.

[49] May-Panloup P, Chretien MF, Jacques C, Vasseur C, Malthiery Y, Reynier P. Low oocyte mitochondrial DNA content in ovarian insufficiency. Hum Reprod 2005; 20: 593–597.

[50] Myer L, Carter RJ, Katyal M, Toro P, El-Sadr WM, Abrams EJ. Impact of antiretroviral therapy on incidence of pregnancy among HIV-infected women in Sub-Saharan Africa: a cohort study. PLoS Med 2010; 7: e1000229.

[51] Toltzis P, Mourton T, Magnuson T. Effect of zidovudine on preimplantation murine embryos. Antimicrob Agents Chemother 1993; 37: 1610–1613.

[52] Toltzis P, Marx CM, Kleinman N, Levine EM, Schmidt EV. Zidovudine-associated embryonic toxicity in mice. J Infect Dis 1991; 163: 1212–1218.

[53] Gerschenson M, Nguyen V, Ewings EL, Ceresa A, Shaw JA, St Claire MC, et al. Mitochondrial toxicity in fetal *Erythrocebus patas* monkeys exposed transplacentally to zidovudine plus lamivudine. AIDS Res Hum Retroviruses 2004; 20: 91–100.

[54] Delvaux T, Nöstlinger C. Reproductive choice for women and men living with HIV: contraception, abortion and fertility. Reprod Health Matters 2007; 15: 46–66.

[55] Agboghoroma CO, Giwa-Osagie OF. Management of infertility in HIV infected couples: a review. Afr J Reprod Health 2012; 16: 13–20.

[56] Stephenson JM, Griffioen A. The effect of HIV diagnosis on reproductive experience. Study Group for the Medical Research Council Collaborative Study of Women with HIV. AIDS 1996; 10: 1683–1687.

[57] Thackway SV, Furner V, Mijch A, Cooper DA, Holland D, Martinez P, et al. Fertility and reproductive choice in women with HIV-1 infection. AIDS 1997; 11: 663–667.

[58] Wilson TE, Massad LS, Riester KA, Barkan S, Richardson J, Young M, et al. Sexual, contraceptive, and drug use behaviors of women with HIV and those at high risk for infection: results from the Women's Interagency HIV Study. AIDS 1999; 13: 591–598.

[59] Floridia M, Tamburrini E, Tibaldi C, Anzidei G, Muggiasca ML, Meloni A, et al. Voluntary pregnancy termination among women with HIV in the HAART era (2002–2008): a case series from a national study. AIDS Care 2010; 22: 50–53.

[60] Townsend CL, Cortina-Borja M, Peckham CS, Tookey PA. Trends in management and outcome of pregnancies in HIV-infected women in the UK and Ireland, 1990–2006. BJOG 2008; 115: 1078–1086.

[61] Bongain A, Berrebi A, Mariné-Barjoan E, Dunais B, Thene M, Pradier C, et al. Changing trends in pregnancy outcome among HIV-infected women between 1985 and 1997 in two southern French university hospitals. Eur J Obstet Gynecol Reprod Biol 2002; 104: 124–128.

[62] Finocchario-Kessler S, Sweat MD, Dariotis JK, Anderson JR, Jennings JM, Keller JM, et al. Childbearing motivations, pregnancy desires, and perceived partner response to a pregnancy among urban female youth: does HIV-infection status make a difference? AIDS Care 2012; 24: 1–11.

[63] Craft SM, Delaney RO, Bautista DT, Serovich JM. Pregnancy decisions among women with HIV. AIDS Behav 2007; 11: 927–935.

[64] Nattabi B, Li J, Thompson SC, Orach CG, Earnest J. A systematic review of factors influencing fertility desires and intentions among people living with HIV/AIDS: implications for policy and service delivery. AIDS Behav 2009; 13: 949–968.

[65] Squires KE, Hodder SL, Feinberg J, Bridge DA, Abrams S, Storfer SP, et al. Health needs of HIV-infected women in the United States: insights from the women living positive survey. AIDS Patient Care STDS 2011; 25: 279–285.

[66] Ethics Committee of the American Society for Reproductive Medicine. Human immunodeficiency virus and infertility treatment. Fertil Steril 2010; 94: 11–15.

[67] Department of Health and Human Services. Guidelines for the use of antiretroviral agents in HIV-1-infected adults and adolescents. Available at: http://aidsinfo.nih.gov/guidelines. Accessed 3 January 2016.

[68] Lundgren JD, Babiker AG, Gordin F, Emery S, Grund B, Sharma S, et al. Initiation of antiretroviral therapy in early asymptomatic HIV infection. N Engl J Med 2015; 373: 795–807.

[69] European AIDS Clinical Society. The European Guidelines for treatment of HIV-infected adults in Europe. Available at: www.eacsociety.org/guidelines/eacs-guidelines/eacs-guidelines.html. Accessed 3 January 2016.

[70] World Health Organization. Consolidated guidelines on the use of antiretroviral drugs for treating and preventing HIV infection. Available at: www.who.int/hiv/pub/guidelines/arv2013/download/en/. Accessed 3 January 2016.

[71] Basaria S, Coviello AD, Travison TG, Storer TW, Farwell WR, Jette AM, et al. Adverse events associated with testosterone administration. N Engl J Med 2010; 363: 109–122.

[72] Kaida A, Lima VD, Andia I, Kabakyenga J, Mbabazi P, Emenyonu N, et al. The WHOMEN's Scale (Women's HAART Optimism Monitoring and EvaluatioN Scale v. 1) and the association with fertility intentions and sexual behaviours among HIV-positive women in Uganda. AIDS Behav 2009; 13: S72–S81.

[73] Galvin SR, Cohen MS. The role of sexually transmitted diseases in HIV transmission. Nat Rev Microbiol 2004; 2: 33–42.

[74] Laga M, Nzila N, Goeman J. The interrelationship of sexually transmitted diseases and HIV infection: implications for the control of both epidemics in Africa. AIDS 1991; 5: S55–S63.

[75] Otten RA, Smith DK, Adams DR, Pullium JK, Jackson E, Kim CN, et al. Efficacy of postexposure prophylaxis after intravaginal exposure of pig-tailed macaques to a human-derived retrovirus (human immunodeficiency virus type 2). J Virol 2000; 74: 9771–9775.

[76] Cardo DM, Culver DH, Ciesielski CA, Srivastava PU, Marcus R, Abiteboul D, et al. A case-control study of HIV seroconversion in healthcare workers after percutaneous exposure. Centers for Disease Control and Prevention Needlestick Surveillance Group. N Engl J Med 1997; 337: 1485–1490.

[77] Kuhar DT, Henderson DK, Struble KA, Heneine W, Thomas V, Cheever LW, et al. Updated US Public Health Service guidelines for the management of occupational exposures to human immunodeficiency virus and recommendations for postexposure prophylaxis. Infect Control Hosp Epidemiol 2013; 34: 875–892.

[78] Abdool Karim Q, Abdool Karim SS, Frohlich JA, Grobler AC, Baxter C, Mansoor LE, et al. Effectiveness and safety of tenofovir gel, an antiretroviral microbicide, for the prevention of HIV infection in women. Science 2010; 329: 1168–1174.

[79] Grant RM, Lama JR, Anderson PL, McMahan V, Liu AY, Vargas L et al. Preexposure chemoprophylaxis for HIV prevention in men who have sex with men. N Engl J Med 2010; 363: 2587–2599.

[80] Baeten JM, Donnell D, Ndase P, Mugo NR, Campbell JD, Wangisi J et al. Antiretroviral prophylaxis for HIV prevention in heterosexual men and women. N Engl J Med 2012; 367: 399–410.

[81] Thigpen MC, Kebaabetswe PM, Paxton LA, Smith DK, Rose CE, Segolodi TM, et al. Antiretroviral preexposure prophylaxis for heterosexual HIV transmission in Botswana. N Engl J Med 2012; 367: 423–434.

[82] Ethics Committee of American Society for Reproductive Medicine. Human immunodeficiency virus (HIV) and infertility treatment: a committee opinion. Fertil Steril 2015; 104: e1–e8.

[83] Mandelbrot L, Heard I, Henrion-Geeant E, Henrion R. Natural conception in HIV-negative women with HIV-infected partners. Lancet 1997; 349: 850–851.

[84] Vernazza PL, Graf I, Sonnenberg-Schwan U, Geit M, Meurer A. Preexposure prophylaxis and timed intercourse for HIV-discordant couples willing to conceive a child. AIDS 2011; 25: 2005–2008.

[85] Semprini AE, Levi-Setti P, Ravizza M, Pardi G. Assisted conception to reduce the risk of male-to-female sexual transfer of HIV in serodiscordant couples: an update [abstract]. Presented at the 1998 Symposium on AIDS in Women, Sao Paulo, Brazil, September 14–15, 1998.

[86] Bujan L, Hollander L, Coudert M, Gilling-Smith C, Vucetich A, Guibert J, et al. Safety and efficacy of sperm washing in HIV-1 serodiscordant couples where the male is infected: results from the European CREAThE network. AIDS 2007; 21: 1909–1914.

[87] Kambin S, Batzer F. Assisted reproductive technology in HIV serodiscordant couples. Sex Reprod Menopause 2004; 2: 92–100.

[88] Sauer MV, Wang JG, Douglas NC, Nakhuda GS, Vardhana P, Jovanovic V, et al. Providing fertility care to men seropositive for human immunodeficiency virus: reviewing 10 years of experience and 420 consecutive cycles of in vitro fertilization and intracytoplasmic sperm injection. Fertil Steril 2009; 91: 2455–2460.

[89] Smith DM, Richman DD, Little SJ. HIV superinfection. J Infect Dis 2005; 192: 438–444.

Chapter 12

Metabolic Adaptation of Isocitrate Lyase in the Yeast Pathogen *Candida albicans*

Doblin Sandai

Additional information is available at the end of the chapter

http://dx.doi.org/10.5772/62406

Abstract

The *ICL1* gene, which encodes the glyoxylate cycle enzyme isocitrate lyase (Icl1), is required for the growth of *Candida albicans* on non-fermentable carbon sources and for this yeast to be virulent. The aim of this study is to test the stability of the Icl1 enzyme in response to glucose. Glucose was found to trigger the degradation of the *ICL1* but the CaIcl1 was not destabilized by glucose. When CaIcl1 was expressed in *Saccharomycess cerevisiae*, it was not degraded in response to glucose, suggesting that CaIcl1 has lost the molecular signal that triggers destabilization in response to glucose. However, when ScIcl1 was expressed in *C. albicans* it was rapidly degraded in response to glucose indicating that *C. albicans* has retained the molecular apparatus for glucose-accelerated degradation of target proteins. ScIcl1 degradation was slowed in Ca*ubi4/ubi4* in which ubiquitin-mediated protein turnover is reduced. Furthermore, the addition of putative ubiquitination site to the carboxyl-terminus of CaIcl1 led to the glucose-accelerated degradation of this protein. *C. albicans* has retained the apparatus for ubiquitin-mediated degradation of target protein in response to glucose. However, CaIcl1 has lost the Ubi-site that mediate glucose accelerated protein degradation, thereby allowing *C. albicans* to simultaneously assimilate alternative carbon sources and glucose.

Keywords: Glyoxylate cycle, isocitrate lyase (Icl1), metabolic adaptation, virulence, pathogenicity

1. Introduction

Candida albicans is a major fungal pathogen of humans causes superficial and deep-seated candidiasis infections [1, 2]. *C. albicans* is an opportunistic pathogen residing as a commensal in the oral cavity and gastrointestinal and urogenital tracts of many individuals [3, 4]. The severity of candidiasis ranges from superficial mucosal infections to systemic or disseminated infections. In healthy individuals, *C. albicans* is relatively harmless. However, immunocompromised patients can get disseminated candidiasis in deep tissues that are difficult to diagnose and can result in death [5, 6].Treatment involves the use of antifungals such as fluconazole, amphotericin B and caspofungin [7, 8]. However, these treatments are not always successful [9].

This chapter addresses the metabolic adaptation of isocitrate lyase (ICL1) of this fungal pathogen in humans. This topic is important for studying the pathogenicity of *C. albicans* because this medically important fungus must grow to cause infections, and to grow it must assimilate carbon. *C. albicans* can occupy various diverse niches in humans, and many of these niches contain a range of different carbon sources. The question arises whether this pathogen is able to exploit this range of carbon sources if glucose happens to be present. This would not be the case in the model yeast *Saccharomycess cerevisiae* because various forms of glucose regulation inhibit the assimilation of alternative carbon sources in this model yeast [10 - 13]. Therefore, this first compares the impact of glucose on the assimilation of alternative carbon sources in these two yeasts and then examines whether molecular mechanisms exist in *C. albicans* to promote the rapid turnover of target proteins in response to glucose. Hence, this section focusses on commensalism, *C. albicans* infections, and antifungal therapies.

Candida infections have been reported for virtually every tissue of the human body, and they can be classified according to different criteria [14]. Superficial infections affect the skin and mucous membranes [15]. In contrast, invasive candidiases include candidemia, acute or chronic haematogenously disseminated candidiasis (infections of the bloodstream), and deep-seated infections of the internal organs [16].

C. albicans has evolved to become an effective commensal organism [17]. In the state of commensalism, *Candida* species live as relatively harmless members of the microflora of healthy individuals causing no discernible disease. *Candida* species are "carried" in the oral cavity, the GI tract, the anus and groin of healthy individuals, and also in the vaginal canal and vulva of healthy women [14, 18]. *Candida* is carried by the most of healthy individuals and can attain surprisingly high densities without symptoms of disease [19]. *C. albicans* is found in stools of about 50% healthy people in addition to the many bacteria that usually inhabit the GI tract [20]. The proliferation of pathogenic microorganisms such as *Candida* is inhibited partly by the growth of harmless bacteria in these niches [21]. The symbiosis of these microorganisms depends on the amount of mucus, the peristaltic behaviour of the bowel and the presence of specific host antibodies and on the capacity of these microbes to adhere to epithelial cells [20].

C. albicans is the most virulent *Candida* species; among the *Candida* species, *C. albicans* is the most commonly isolated yeasts from susceptible hosts [22 - 24]. Multiple risk factors play a role in increasing likelihood of *C. albicans* undergoing the transition from harmless commensal to a virulent pathogen. These risk factors include injuries or traumatic surgery; the presence of indwelling devices, such as catheters or prosthetic devices; antibiotic treatment, which reduces the competitiveness of bacterial species in host niches; and age, with new born babies or aged individuals displaying increased risk of infection [14, 24, 25].

Candidemia is defined as the isolation of *Candida* from at least one blood culture specimen. This type of infection is mainly acquired as the result of neutropenia, injuries caused by recent surgery or the presence of indwelling devices. Also the use of broad-spectrum antibiotics

http://dx.doi.org/10.5772/62406

represents another significant risk factor [16]. *Candida* not only often infects the livers of patients during systemic candidiasis but can also thrive in their spleen, brain or kidney [26].

C. albicans skin infections mostly occur in warm and moist niches such as the armpit, the perineum and skin folds. Similarly, *Candida* is a common cause of nappy (diaper) rash in infants, and it particularly affects obese and elderly adults, as well as the inframammary region of women. Itching and burning are the common symptoms of these types of infections [15]. Most women suffer from oral and vaginal infections (thrush) at least once in their life time [27]. Also, HIV and AIDS -patients suffered from oral thrush before the advent of the highly active anti-retroviral treatment (HAART), which includes a protease inhibitor that also inhibits an important virulence attribute of *C. albicans*- secreted aspartyl protease [28].

There are three main classes of clinically useful antifungal drugs: the polyenes, the azoles and the echinocandins. Amphotericin B is the main drug in the polyene family. It is thought to perturb the functionality of the fungal plasma membrane via interactions with ergosterol [29]. Unfortunately, the clinical utility of Amphotericin B is limited because it can cause nephrotoxicity in patients.

The azoles are an expanding family of compounds, as exemplified by the classic drug flucoazole. They target ergosterol synthesis, and hence the fungal plasma membrane [29]. Additional antifungal agents are being developed. These include triazoles such as posaconazole, ravuconazole and voriconazole. This strengthens the choice of azoles, which is the most successful antifungal class in the clinic since the late 1960s. Voriconazole is a broad spectrum drug that is fungicidal against some isolates of filamentous species [30]. Posaconazole also inhibits a broad spectrum of fungi, and has shown promising effects against Coccidioides in preclinical studies [31]. Meanwhile, ravuconazole has a long plasma half-life in humans that might improve its efficacy [32].

Echinocandins such as caspofungin, anidulafungin and micafungin target cell wall β-1 3-glucan synthesis [29]. The development of echinocandins represented a major advance in antifungal drug development because they targeted a new area of fungal cell biology -the cell wall [29]. *C. albicans* cells can become tolerant to echinocandin treatment via activation of the cell wall rescue pathway leading to elevated chitin synthesis [33].

2. Effect of glucose on alternative carbon sources in *Candida albicans*

The assimilation of carbon sources is fundamentally important for the growth of *C. albicans* and for the establishment of infections in the human host. As described earlier, to grow, a microbe must be able to assimilate carbon [34]. For most yeasts, glucose is generally a preferred carbon source and for *S. cerevisiae* the chosen mode of metabolism is often fermentative in the presence of excess glucose. This uses the Embden-Meyerhof or glycolytic pathway, resulting in the formation of ethanol. In the absence of glucose, *S. cerevisiae* adapts to utilise the alternative carbon sources that are available and switching to non-fermentable carbon metabolism.

Likewise, *C. albicans* alters the expression of its metabolic functions to facilitate cell survival [35]. *C. albicans* adjusts its metabolism to growth in biofilms by up-regulating amino acid biosynthesis genes [36]. When exposed to human neutrophils or cultured macrophages, *C. albicans* also up-regulates amino acid biosynthesis genes and displays a shift from fermentative to non-fermentative metabolism [35, 37, 38]. Importantly, the utilisation of non-fermentable carbon sources requires gluconeogenesis and the glyoxylate cycle [39]. Furthermore, the glyoxylate cycle is required for fungal virulence [40]. These examples illustrate the metabolic flexibility of this pathogen and the relevance of metabolic adaptation pathogenicity [41].

Our understanding of the physiology of *C. albicans* has been largely based on presumptions that the central carbon metabolism in *S. cerevisiae* and *C. albicans* is similar. In these fungi, the pathways of central carbon metabolism, including glycolysis, gluconeogenesis, the pentose phosphate pathway, the tricarboxylic acid (TCA) cycle and glyoxylate cycle, are highly conserved [14, 42]. However, metabolic differences do exist between *C. albicans* and *S. cerevisiae*, the most obvious of which relates to their patterns of sugar utilisation [41]. For example, *S. cerevisiae* belongs to the group that is called Crabtree-positive yeasts which have the ability to produce ethanol even in the presence of oxygen. In contrast, *C. albicans* is designated as a Crabtree-negative yeast [43] because it retains respiratory capacity in the presence of excess glucose [44].

As described earlier, pathways of alternative carbon assimilation in *S. cerevisiae* are subject of glucose repression study. The genetics of glucose repression have been studied, and the regulatory elements that drive this regulation have been described in *S. cerevisiae* [10, 12, 45, 46, 47]. These include co-regulatory mechanisms that act on common elements within the promoter sequences of gluconeogenic and glyoxylate cycle genes. The carbon source regulator elements (CSRE) in the promoters of the *S. cerevisiae PCK1, FBP1, MLS1* and *ACR1* are required for their transcriptional induction in the absence of glucose [48 - 52]. In addition the promoters of the *S. cerevisiae ICL1, MLS1* and *FBP1* genes contain binding sites for the transcription repressor Mig1 [53]. Mig1 represses the transcription of these genes in the presence of glucose, and the activity of Mig1 is being regulated by Snf1 (AMP kinase) signalling.

Transcript profiling of glucose responses in *C. albicans* and *S. cerevisiae* has shown that both yeasts are sensitive to very low levels of glucose [54, 55]. In *S. cerevisiae* and *C. albicans*, glycolytic genes were up-regulated and gluconeogenic and TCA cycle genes were down-regulated even when only 0.01% glucose was added to the growth medium. Yin *et al.* [54] also showed that *S. cerevisiae* ribosomal protein genes also respond to glucose but that they were less sensitive to glucose than the metabolic genes mentioned above. In *S. cerevisiae*, ribosomal protein gene expression was up-regulated following glucose addition at concentrations above 0.1% [54, 56].

Therefore addition of glucose to *S. cerevisiae* cells growing on alternative carbon sources causes a rapid shift from non-fermentative to fermentative metabolism, in part through tight regulation of gene transcription. Glucose also regulates metabolic activity in *S. cerevisiae* at post-transcriptional levels. Glucose triggers the accelerated decay of gluconeogenic mRNA (*PCK1, FBP1*) [54]. Furthermore, glucose triggers the catabolite inactivation and degradation of gluconeogenic and glyoxylate cycle enzymes in *S. cerevisiae.* Fructose-1,6-bisphophatase (FBPase) is expressed when yeast cells are grown on non-fermentable carbon sources. When the cells are then transferred to a glucose-containing medium, the cells rapidly degrade FBPase to inactivate gluconeogenic activity. This was shown by immunoprecipitation and Western blotting [57]. These authors found that the ubiquitin-conjugating enzyme Ubc8p contributes to glucose-induced ubiquitination of FBPase and that this ubiquitination proceeds the catabolite degradation of the enzyme via the proteasome [58], three other gluconeogenic and glyoxylate cycle enzymes were identified as additional targets of the catabolite inactivation machinery [59]. In addition, it was discovered that an amino-terminal proline residue is essential for the rapid degradation of FBPase in response to glucose. FBPase phosphorylation was not necessary for degradation to occur [59]. This amino-terminal ubiquitination target site on FBPase essentially functions as an autonomous, primary degradation signal.

We reasoned that glucose responses might have diverged significantly between *C. albicans* and *S. cerevisiae*. Our rationale was that the relaxation of glucose repression would confer an evolutionary advantage upon a yeast such as *C. albicans* by allowing this pathogen to continue to assimilate alternative carbon sources even when small amounts of glucose are present *in vivo*. This section describes the testing of this working hypothesis through comparison of the effects of glucose upon gluconeogenic and glyoxylate cycle gene expression in *C. albicans* and *S. cerevisiae*.

To understand carbon assimilation in *C. albicans*, growth on selected alternative carbon sources was first defined. Therefore analogous growth experiments were carried out for both *S. cerevisiae* and *C. albicans* in media containing glucose or alternative carbon sources. Lactic acid was chosen as one alternative carbon source because it is a three-carbon molecule of physio logical relevance found in various host niches and in the bloodstream after exercise [60]. Also Aberdeen Fungal Group Laboratory has generated a considerable body of data on cells grown on lactate [54, 55].

Yeast cells were grown overnight in media containing 2% lactate or 2% (2% each or 1% + 1%) both glucose and lactate. These cells were then harvested and used to inoculate fresh media of the same composition and grown for 10 hours. Glucose and ethanol levels and growth absorbance (at OD_{340}) were measured.

As expected, both yeasts grew better on media containing glucose plus lactate, than on lactate alone. *C. albicans* grew faster than *S. cerevisiae* on both media under these conditions. However, both yeasts displayed similar rates of glucose consumption and different ethanol accumulation under these conditions. Glucose was utilised rapidly by both *S. cerevisiae* and *C. albicans*. Ethanol levels in glucose plus lactate cultures significantly increased in *S. cerevisiae*, but they remained similar during glucose assimilation by *C. albicans*. This indicated that most glucose was not fermented to ethanol under the experimental conditions examined in *C. albicans* (minimal medium; 30°C; 200 rpm).

The fatty acid i.e. oleic acid was chosen as the second alternative carbon source for analysis. A fatty acid was chosen because lipids represent a rich source of carbon in the host, *C. albicans* is known to secrete lipases [61], and *C. albicans* is known to induce fatty acid β-oxidation genes following phagocytosis by macrophages [62].

Once again, analogous growth experiments were carried out for both *S. cerevisiae* and *C. albicans* in media containing oleic acid or glucose plus oleic acid. Yeasts cells were grown overnight in media containing 0.2% oleic acid or 2% glucose plus oleic acid, and these cells were used to inoculate fresh media containing the same amount of carbon sources. Growth was monitored for 10 hours. Once again, glucose and ethanol levels and absorbance (OD_{340}) were measured.

Both yeasts grew on oleic acid or on oleic acid plus glucose. As expected more growth was observed for both yeasts on the glucose containing medium compared with the medium containing oleic acid alone. *C. albicans* grew more efficiently than *S. cerevisiae* on both media. Once again, the rates of glucose consumption and ethanol production were different for both yeasts. Both yeasts consumed glucose rapidly, but ethanol levels were accumulated significantly throughout the experiment in *S. cerevisiae*. This suggested that most glucose was not fermented to ethanol under these conditions in *C. albicans*. Less ethanol was generated during growth on oleic acid (about 2 mg/ml or 0.02%) compared to during growth on lactic acid (about 4 mg/ml or 0.04%).

Previous work by Yin *et al.* [54] using Northern blotting and transcriptomic analyses showed that transcripts encoding the gluconeogenic enzymes (*FBP1* and *PCK1*) are repressed by glucose in *S. cerevisiae*. To reconfirm this report and to compare it with the glucose responses of *C. albicans* more directly in this study, we first examined the responses of *S. cerevisiae* glyoxylate cycle (*ScICL1*) and gluconeogenic mRNAs (*ScPCK1*) using the following experimental approach.

S. cerevisiae cells were grown to mid-exponential phase in a minimal medium containing lactate or oleic acid as the sole carbon source and lactate + glucose and oleic acid + glucose. The levels of the *S. cerevisiae ICL1* and *PCK1* mRNAs were measured relative to the housekeeping β-actin gene (*ScACT1*), following the addition of glucose to a final concentration of 2%. Samples were collected and frozen immediately in liquid nitrogen for RNA extraction. *S. cerevisiae ICL1, PCK1* and *ACT1* primers [63] were then designed, and the expression of these genes was quantified using Syber green quantitative real-time polymerase chain reaction (qRT-PCR).

ScICL1 mRNA levels showed a dramatic decrease within 30 minutes of glucose addition to cells growing on lactate or oleic acid. Similarly, *ScPCK1* mRNA levels declined after glucose addition to cells growing on lactate or oleic acid media. This strong repression occurred 30 minutes after glucose addition. These results confirmed that in *S. cerevisiae*, the *ICL1* and *PCK1* transcripts are strongly repressed by glucose [54]. At least for the *PCK1* mRNA, this repression is mediated by transcriptional repression and accelerated mRNA degradation [54].

Aberdeen Fungal Group Laboratory has also described the global transcriptional responses of *C. albicans* to low (0.01%), medium (0.1%) and high (1%) glucose concentrations by microarray analysis [55]. The data indicated that a total of 347 *C. albicans* genes were up-regulated, and 344 genes were down-regulated in response to at least one of the glucose concentrations examined. There are170 of these genes that were up-regulated and 180 genes that were down-regulated by 0.01% glucose, indicating that about half of glucose-regulated genes are responsive to low glucose levels. Therefore, the authors concluded that like *S. cerevisiae*, *C. albicans* is exquisitely sensitive to glucose, responding to concentrations as low as 0.01%. Hence, at the start of this study, an aim was to confirm the impact of glucose on specific mRNAs that encode enzymes required for the assimilation of alternative carbon sources. The transcripts encoding the glyoxylate cycle enzyme isocitrate lyase (*CaICL1*) and the gluconeogenic enzyme phosphoenolpyruvate carboxykinase (*CaPCK1*) were the main focus here.

C. albicans cells were grown to mid-exponential phase in media containing lactate or oleic acid as the sole carbon source using the same procedures described for *S. cerevisiae* by Yin *et al.* [54]. Glucose was then added to a final concentration of 2%; samples were taken for RNA analysis at various times thereafter; the levels of the *CaICL1, CaPCK1* and *CaACT1* mRNAs were measured by qRT-PCR. The relative expression of *CaICL1* (compared with the internal *CaACT1* control) was high in lactate- and oleic acid-grown cells compared with the cells that were exposed to glucose. The *CaICL1* mRNA was strongly down-regulated within 60 minutes after glucose addition under both of these growth conditions. The *CaPCK1* mRNA was expressed at relatively high levels in lactate- and oleic acid-grown cells, and was also strongly down-regulated within 60 minutes of glucose addition. These results confirmed that in both *S. cerevisiae* and *C. albicans*, the *ICL1* and *PCK1* genes are strongly repressed by glucose [63].

The next step is to test the effects of glucose on the expression levels of the CaIcl1 and CaPck1 proteins in *C. albicans* and to compare this response with the corresponding situation *S. cerevisiae.* In *S. cerevisiae,* the effects of glucose on fructose-1,6-bisphosphatase (FBPase) have been intensively studied and it was reported that the FBPase protein (ScFbp1) is rapidly degraded upon the addition of glucose [58]. Also it has been reported that the levels of cytosolic malate dehydrogenase, fructose-1,6-bisphosphatase, isocitrate lyase and phosphoenolpyruvate carboxykinase are all low in *S. cerevisiae* after glucose addition [59]. Therefore, as a starting point, we tested for ourselves whether Icl1 and Pck1 decline in *S. cerevisiae* upon glucose addition.

To achieve this, the *S. cerevisiae ICL1* coding region was tagged at its 3′-end with Myc_9 and the *PCK1* coding region was tagged with HA6. Control Western blots with these tagged strains and their untagged parental strains demonstrated that ScIcl1-Myc_9 and ScPck1-HA6 were expressed during growth on non-fermentable carbon sources [63].

After confirming the validity of the ScIcl1-Myc_9 and ScPck1-HA6 tagging, the next step is to examine the effects of glucose upon the stability of these proteins following glucose addition to *S. cerevisiae* cells. Therefore, the epitope-tagged *S. cerevisiae* strains were grown on lactate or oleic acid, and then glucose was added to a final concentration of 2%. All experiments were performed on exponentially growing cells. Samples were prepared at various times thereafter, and the levels of the ScIcl1-Myc_9 and ScPck1-HA6 proteins were measured by Western blotting. Clearly, glucose addition led to the degradation of ScIcl1 and ScPck1. These results confirmed that in *S. cerevisiae* Icl1 and Pck1 are degraded in response to glucose. Interestingly, the degradation of ScPck1 appears to start about 2 hours after glucose addition, whereas ScIcl1 degradation starts earlier. This might reflect differences in the mechanisms of glucose-activated degradation of these proteins, via ubiquitin-mediated or vacuole-mediated pathways, as described by Regelmann *et al.* [64].

Having confirmed that glucose addition to cells growing on non-fermentable carbon sources leads to the degradation of Icl1 and Pck1 in *S. cerevisiae,* the next step is to test the effects of glucose upon the corresponding enzymes in *C. albicans.*

C. albicans strains expressing Myc$_3$-tagged Icl1 or Myc$_3$-tagged Pck1 were then used in an analogous experimental design to our previous *S. cerevisiae* protein analysis. *C. albicans* cells were grown in media containing non-fermentable carbon sources (lactate or oleic acid) as sole carbon sources, and then 2% glucose was added while cells were in the exponential growth phase. Cells were then harvested at various time periods, and their proteins were extracted for Western blotting. Proteins were loaded in equal amounts onto the SDS/PAGE gels, and expression of the Myc$_3$-tagged CaIcl1 and CaPck1 proteins was detected with anti-Myc antibodies and the images quantified using a phosphorimager.

The *C. albicans* Icl1 protein was expressed during growth on lactate or oleic acid. Interestingly, CaIcl1 was not destabilised by the addition of 2% glucose. Indeed, CaIcl1 protein levels were not significantly different from the control even after 4 hours. Likewise, CaPck1 expression levels were relatively high during growth on lactate or oleic acid, and CaPck1 was also not destabilised by glucose addition. These data suggested that glucose does not affect the stability of the CaIcl1 and CaPck1 proteins. This behaviour of *C. albicans* was in direct contrast to that observed in *S. cerevisiae,* in which the Icl1 and Pck1 proteins were destabilised by glucose [63].

Carbon assimilation is essential for the generation of new biomass (i.e. growth). Therefore, the growth of *C. albicans* in the immunocompromised host depends upon the assimilation of available carbon sources *in vivo,* and the fungus must adjust its metabolism to the microenvironments it occupies in the host [41].

Previous reports have suggested that *S. cerevisiae* might provide a reasonable metabolic paradigm for *C. albicans* as reviewed by Brown [41]. Certainly, many of the pathways of central metabolism are conserved in fungi, including the glycolytic, gluconeogenic and pentose phosphate pathways and the TCA and glyoxylate cycles [14, 42]. Pathways for the generation of storage and cell wall carbohydrates are also conserved. Furthermore, the pathways of amino acid, lipid and nucleotide catabolism and anabolism appear to be conserved. However, significant metabolic differences do exist between *C. albicans* and *S. cerevisiae,* as revealed by their different patterns of sugar utilisation. In fact, differences in the patterns of carbohydrate assimilation are used routinely to distinguish *C. albicans* from other microbes in the clinic [65, 66]. Also, significant differences in the regulation of carbon metabolism are emerging for *C. albicans* and *S. cerevisiae* [67, 68]. Based on these observations, we tested whether there are metabolic differences in carbon assimilation between these fungi. The approach here was to measure the effects of glucose upon the assimilation by *S. cerevisiae* and *C. albicans* of radiolabelled lactic or oleic acid into large molecular weight compounds.

To achieve this, *S. cerevisiae* cells were grown to exponential phase on media containing lactate or oleic acid as sole carbon source. These cells were then harvested and resuspended in equivalent media containing radiolabelled lactic or oleic acid. Glucose (2%) was added to test samples, and no glucose was added to control samples. The assimilation of ^{14}C-lactic acid or ^{3}H-oleic acid by *S. cerevisiae* cells into large molecular weight TCA-precipitable material was then measured. In *S. cerevisiae*, both lactate and oleic acid assimilation were rapidly repressed by glucose. Therefore the *S. cerevisiae* cells stopped the assimilation of these secondary carbon sources and apparently switched quickly to glucose assimilation. This confirmed the generally held view that *S. cerevisiae* does not assimilate both glucose and secondary carbon sources at the same time.

The next step is to investigate the effects of glucose on carbon assimilation in *C. albicans*. Once again, the approach was to test the assimilation of radiolabelled carbon sources by the cell. The same procedures were followed as for *S. cerevisiae*, with *C. albicans* cells being grown on lactate or oleic acid and then the assimilation of ^{14}C-lactic acid or ^{3}H-oleic acid into TCA-precipitable material was measured after glucose addition [63].

Unlike *S. cerevisiae*, *C. albicans* was still able to assimilate both lactate and oleic acid for some hours after addition of glucose. Lactate metabolism appeared to continue relatively normal because only minor effects were observed in the lactate uptake following glucose addition. Tests with the other secondary carbon source (oleic acid) showed similar results. Therefore, *C. albicans* is able to assimilate lactate and glucose at the same time. Similarly, both oleic acid and glucose can be assimilated by *C. albicans* at the same time. This suggests that glucose has a minimal immediate impact on the ability of *C. albicans* to assimilate secondary carbon sources at least over the timescales examined [63].

Therefore, there are significant differences between *C. albicans* and *S. cerevisiae* with respect to the regulation of their assimilation of alternative carbon sources. Apparently in *S. cerevisiae*, glucose and secondary carbon sources are not assimilated at the same time. In contrast, in *C. albicans*, the continued stability of gluconeogenic and glyoxylate cycle enzymes after glucose exposure correlates with the ability of *C. albicans* cells to continue to assimilate alternative carbon sources, even after glucose addition. Hence, the hypothesis that significant metabolic differences exist between *C. albicans* and *S. cerevisiae* was confirmed [63].

3. Glucose-accelerated protein degradation in *Candida albicans*

The previous section examined the impact of glucose on Pck1 and Icl1 expression and the assimilation of alternative carbon sources such as lactic and oleic acid in *C. albicans*. So far, the author's data confirmed that transcript profiling results were described by Yin *et al*. [54] and Rodaki *et al*. [55]. Numerous *S. cerevisiae* transcripts, including those encoding gluconeogenic enzymes (*FBP1* and *PCK1*), are repressed by glucose [54]. Similarly, 180 genes in *C. albicans*, including gluconeogenic and glyoxylate cycle enzymes were, down-regulated, even in response to very low concentrations of glucose (0.01%) [55]. The results presented in the previous section confirmed that the *ScICL1* and *ScPCK1* genes in *S. cerevisiae* and the *CaICL1* and *CaPCK1* genes in *C. albicans* are exquisitely sensitive to glucose.

While *S. cerevisiae* and *C. albicans* displayed similar responses at the transcriptional level, they diverged significantly at the post-transcriptional and metabolic levels. The *C. albicans* Icl1 and Pck1 enzymes were expressed during growth on lactate and oleic acid and were not destabilised by the addition of 2% glucose. In contrast, their orthologues in *S. cerevisiae* were rapidly destabilised by glucose. Consequently, this appeared to affect carbon assimilation, allowing *C. albicans* to continue to assimilate alternative carbon sources even after exposure to glucose. In contrast, following glucose addition to *S. cerevisiae* cells, Icl1 and Pck1 were degraded and the cells stopped assimilating lactic acid or oleic acid. These new findings showed that there are fundamental differences in the regulation of carbon assimilation in *C. albicans* compared to *S. cerevisiae* [63]. The next step is to examine the basis for these differences and in particular, possible differences in glucose-accelerated protein degradation between *C. albicans* and *S. cerevisiae*. The focus of these studies was on Icl1.

Entian and Schüller [46] reported the genetic characterisation of *C. albicans* gluconeogenic and glyoxylate cycle genes. The *C. albicans FBP1, PCK1, MLS1* and *ICL1* genes were all isolated by functional complementation of the corresponding *S. cerevisiae* deletion mutants. Remarkably, the regulation of the heterologously expressed *C. albicans* gluconeogenic and glyoxylate cycle genes in *S. cerevisiae* was similar to that of their *S. cerevisiae* orthologues. Therefore, in this project we expressed *C. albicans ICL1* in *S. cerevisiae* and tested whether CaIcl1 is destabilised by glucose in *S. cerevisiae*. The other aims of this section are to test whether *C. albicans* has retained the ability to destabilise target proteins in response to glucose and to examine the signals and mechanisms that trigger glucose-mediated destabilisation of target proteins in *C. albicans*.

To test whether *C. albicans* is able to degrade proteins in response to glucose, the *S. cerevisiae ICL1* gene was expressed in *C. albicans*. To achieve this, one *C. albicans ICL1* allele was replaced with a tagged *S. cerevisiae ICL1* ORF. The *ScICL1* locus in *S. cerevisiae* was first tagged using primers with Myc$_3$-URA3, and the genomic DNA from this tagged was PCR amplified using primers to create the *CaICL1p-ScICL1-MYC$_3$-URA3* cassette [63]. This cassette was transformed into the *CaICL1* locus in *C. albicans ICL1/ICL1*. Before going further, it was necessary to test whether the *ScICL1-MYC$_3$-URA3* sequence was integrated accurately into the *CaICL1* genomic locus. Three primer pairs were designed to amplify overlapping fragments of the *CaICL1p-ScICL1-MYC$_3$-URA3* locus based on the *in silico* sequence [63]. PCR amplification using these primers yielded the desired bands, establishing that the newly created strain *ScICL1-MYC$_3$-URA3* sequence had integrated correctly into the *CaICL1* locus in the *C. albicans* genome [63].

Then Western blots were performed to test whether the ScIcl1-Myc$_3$ protein was detectable in these *C. albicans* transformants. The two positive clones were grown to stationary phase overnight on an alternative carbon source in the absence of glucose. Controls were included to confirm expression of the tagged ScIcl1 in *C. albicans*. In both new strains, an Icl1 band of the predicted size (62 kDa) was observed, which was the right size compared to the controls.

To further ensure the correct replacement of the *C. albicans ICL1* ORF with the tagged *S. cerevisiae ICL1* ORF, the functionality of this *ScICL1* ORF was tested in *C. albicans*. The *ScICL1-MYC$_3$-URA3* cassette was amplified from genomic DNA and transformed into *C. albicans ICL1/icl1* cells selecting heterozygote for uridine prototrophs. Once again, correct insertion of the *ScICL1-MYC$_3$-URA3* sequence was confirmed by diagnostic PCR using the three primer pairs as before and also tested by another three primer pairs to confirm the construction of the *C. albicans ScICL1-MYC$_3$-URA3/icl1* strain [63].

Western blots were performed to confirm the expression of the Myc-tagged *ScICL1* ORF *S. cerevisiae* in *C. albicans ScICL1 MYC$_3$ URA3/icl1* background. Two positive clones were grown to stationary phase on lactate-containing medium and protein subjected to Western blotting. This showed the expression of the tagged ScIcl1 of about 62 kDa in *C. albicans*. As expected the ScIcl1 protein was not expressed during growth on glucose because it was expressed from the endogenous *CaICL1* promoter that is glucose repressed [63].

The phenotype of this *C. albicans ScICL1-MYC$_3$-URA3/icl1* mutant was then tested by growing in different carbon sources: glucose, fructose, lactate, oleic acid, pyruvate and acetate. The mutants were compared with control *C. albicans ICL1/ICL1, ICl1/icl1* and *icl1/icl1* strains. The presence of the *ScICL1* gene in a *C. albicans icl1* background was sufficient to restore growth on lactate, oleic acid, pyruvate and acetate. This growth was comparable to the positive *ICL1/ICL1* control strain and contrasted with the negative *icl1/icl1* control, which was only able to grow on glucose and fructose. This indicated that the tagged *ScICL1* was functional in *C. albicans* [63].

Having confirmed the genotype, expression and functionality of the *ScICL1* ORF in *C. albicans*, the next step was to test the effects of glucose on the levels of the ScIcl1 protein when expressed in *C. albicans*. The *C. albicans ScICL1-MYC$_3$-URA3*//icl1 strain was first grown on alternative carbon sources (lactate or oleic acid), and then glucose was added to a final concentration of 2%. Samples were then taken at regular intervals, proteins extracted, and ScIcl1-Myc$_3$ levels examined by Western blotting. Control cultures to which no glucose was added, were also examined. This showed that ScIcl1 levels remained high in *C. albicans* cells grown on the alternative carbon sources. However, following the addition of 2% glucose to *C. albicans* cells, ScIcl1 was degraded. This indicates that *C. albicans* has retained the capacity to destabilise target proteins in response to glucose [63].

C. albicans is clearly capable of degrading target proteins following exposure to glucose. Therefore, why is CaIcl1 not degraded following glucose addition? Has CaIcl1 lost the specific signal that would target it for glucose-accelerated degradation? To test this, the CaIcl1 protein was expressed in *S. cerevisiae.*

To achieve this, the *S. cerevisiae ICL1* ORF was replaced with a Myc$_3$-tagged *C. albicans ICL1* ORF. The *C. albicans ICL1-MYC$_3$-URA3* was PCR amplified using the primers and transformed into *S. cerevisiae* strain (Ura$^-$, Leu$^-$) selecting for uracil prototrophs. Correct integration of the *CaICL1-MYC$_3$-URA3* cassette into the *ScICL1* locus was confirmed by diagnostic PCR using three primer pairs. In this way, a new *S. cerevisiae* strain was constructed containing a *ScICL1p-CaICL1-MYC$_3$-URA3* mutation [63].

Western blots were performed to test whether the CaIcl1-Myc$_3$ protein of the predicted 61 kDa size was expressed in *S. cerevisiae*. Cells were grown on alternative carbon sources in the absence of glucose and compared to positive and negative controls. These Western blots confirmed that CaIcl1 61 kDa was expressed in *S. cerevisiae* during growth on lactate or oleic acid and that CaIcl1-Myc$_3$ was in the correct size compared to the positive control in which CaIcl1-Myc$_3$ was expressed in *C. albicans*. Interestingly, CaIcl1-Myc$_3$ was expressed in *S.*

cerevisiae cells grown on lactate or oleic acid, but not in cells grown on glucose. This was to be expected when the *CaICL1-MYC*$_3$ ORF was expressed from the *ScICL1* promoter [63].

Having confirmed the genotype of the *S. cerevisiae* mutant expressing the *C. albicans ICL1* ORF, the next step was to test the effects of glucose on the CaIcl1-Myc$_3$ protein levels in *S. cerevisiae*. The *S. cerevisiae* strain was grown on lactate or oleic acid, and then glucose was added to a final concentration of 2%. Cells were harvested at various time periods thereafter, protein extracts prepared, and CaIcl1-Myc$_3$ protein levels measured by Western blotting. The results showed that CaIcl1-Myc$_3$ remained at high levels in *S. cerevisiae* during growth on the alternative carbon sources. Even upon the addition of 2% glucose, the levels of CaIcl1-Myc$_3$ remained high in *S. cerevisiae*. Minimal decay of the CaIcl1-Myc$_3$ protein was observed even 4 hours after glucose addition. These data suggest that the *C. albicans* Icl1 protein has lost the signals that trigger destabilisation in response to glucose [63].

The above work suggested that *C. albicans* has retained the ability to degrade target proteins in response to glucose, but that CaIcl1 has lost the specific signal(s) that trigger this glucose-accelerated protein degradation. What is the nature of this degradation signal that has been lost by CaIcl1?

Ubiquitination is known to play a role in the glucose-accelerated degradation of gluconeogenic enzymes in *S. cerevisiae* [57]. Previously, Entian and Barnett [45] demonstrated that Ubc8 functions in the catabolite degradation of fructose-1,6-bisphosphatase in *S. cerevisiae*. Earlier, Johnson *et al.* [69] showed that ubiquitin acts as a degradation signal in *S. cerevisiae*. Therefore, consensus ubiquitination target sites were examined in CaIcl1 and ScIcl1 using Ubpred (Predictor of protein ubiquitination site, from htt/www.ubpred.org/index.html) [70 - 73].

Based on this bioinformatic comparison, the ScIcl1 sequence contains strong consensus ubiquitination sites at amino acids 158 and 551, but there is a lack of high confidence ubiquitination targets in CaIcl1. This prediction was based on high level of confidence which is described in Ubpred system containing score range $0.84 \leq s \leq 1.00$, 0.197 for sensitivity and 0.989 for specificity. These included the hydrophobic nature of the ubiquitination target site for the high confidence prediction (TEDQFKENGVKK), which is contrast to the low- and medium- confidence sites that contain acidic and basic residues in the putative ubiquitination site (NGVKK; FNWPKAMSVD) [70 - 73]. Therefore, the presence of consensus ubiquitination sites in these proteins correlated with glucose-accelerated degradation.

Hence, the next step is to test whether ScIcl1 decay rates in *C. albicans* are affected by inactivation of polyubiquitin (*UBI4*).

To achieve this, the experimental goal was to introduce the Myc$_3$-tagged *S. cerevisiae ICL1* ORF into a *C. albicans ubi4/ubi4* mutant [74]. The *ScICL1-MYC*$_3$*-URA3* cassette was PCR amplified using primers and transformed into *C. albicans ubi4/ubi4* cells selecting for uridine prototrophs. The correct insertion of the *ScICL1-MYC*$_3$*-URA3* into the *CaICL1* locus was confirmed by diagnostic PCR with the same primer pairs as before. These amplified the conjoined sequence of the *CaICL1* promoter and the *ScICL1* ORF. The successful and accurate insertion of the *ScICL1-MYC*$_3$*-URA3* cassette into *C. albicans ubi4/ubi4* mutant was confirmed in this way.

Western blotting was then performed to test whether a ScIcl1-Myc$_3$ protein of the predicted size was expected in the *ubi4/ubi4* cells. Cells were grown overnight on the alternative carbon sources (lactate and oleic acid) in the absence of glucose. A new Myc$_3$-containing protein of 62 kD was observed indicating that the ScIcl1-Myc$_3$ protein was expressed on YPL and was the right size [63].

Having confirmed the genotype and the expression of the *ScICL1* ORF in *C. albicans ubi4/ubi4* cells, the next step was to test the effects of glucose on ScIcl1-Myc$_3$ protein levels. The *ubi4/ubi4* cells were grown on lactate or oleic acid and then glucose was added to a final concentration of 2%. Interestingly, ScIcl1-Myc$_3$ cells were more stable in *C. albicans ubi4/ubi4* cells than in wild type *C. albicans* cells after addition of 2% glucose. However, the inactivation of the *UBI4* (polyubiquitination) locus did not completely inhibit the degradation of the ScIcl1-Myc$_3$ protein such that it became as stable as ScIcl1-Myc$_3$ in wild type *C. albicans* cells in the absence of glucose. This might be because residual ubiquitination remains in *ubi4/ubi4* cells thanks to the presence of a second ubiquitin-encoding locus in *C. albicans* (*UBI3*) [74]. Nevertheless, it was concluded that the inactivation of *UBI4* (polyubiquitin) inhibits the glucose-accelerated degradation of ScIcl1 in *C. albicans*. Ubiquitination plays a role in glucose-accelerated protein decay in this fungus.

As stated above, ScIcl1 contains two high confidence putative ubiquitination sites located at residues 551 and 158, whereas CaIcl1 contains no such sites. Therefore, we reasoned that if ubiquitination plays a role in glucose-accelerated protein decay in *C. albicans*, then the addition of a ubiquitination site to CaIcl1 would confer glucose-accelerated degradation upon this protein. Therefore, the next experimental objective is to introduce the carboxyl-terminal ubiquitin site from ScIcl1 (TEDQFKENGVKK) into CaIcl1, together with the Myc$_3$ tag into wild type polyubiquitin containing *C. albicans* cells [63].

To achieve this, a *ScUBI*-site-*MYC$_3$-URA3* cassette was PCR amplified from *S. cerevisiae* genomic DNA and transformed into *C. albicans ICL1/ICL1* cells. To confirm the correct integration of this cassette at the 3′-end of the *CaICL1* ORF in these cells, uridine prototrophic transformants were subjected to diagnostic PCR using the same primer pairs as before and new primer pairs. This PCR amplification yielded the desired bands, establishing that the *ScUBI-MYC$_3$-URA3* was correctly integrated at the *C. albicans ICL1* locus [63].

Having established the genotype of the new strain (*C. albicans ICL1-ScUBI*-site-*MYC$_3$-URA3*), the next step is to confirm the expression of the CaIcl1 protein carrying the carboxyl-terminal ubiquitination site and the Myc$_3$ tag. Therefore, Western blots were performed to test the presence and size of the tagged protein. Five positive *C. albicans* clones were grown on an alternative carbon source (lactate) in the absence of glucose, protein extracts were made, and Western blots were performed, probing for the Myc epitope. A new Icl1-Myc$_3$ band of about 61 kD was observed, confirming that the Icl1 protein was expressed on YPL and that it had a similar size to the positive control ScIcl1-Myc$_3$ [63].

Having confirmed the genotype of the new strain and the expression of the CaIcl1 protein with the carboxyl-terminal ubiquitination site in *C. albicans* cells, the next step is to test the effects of glucose on the stability of this protein. The new strain was grown on lactic or oleic acid and glucose was added to a final concentration of 2%. Cells were harvested at various time periods thereafter; protein was extracted and these were subjected to Western blotting. Interestingly the CaIcl1-Ubi-Myc_3 protein was rapidly degraded following glucose addition to cells grown on lactate or oleic acid. In conclusion, the addition of a ubiquitination site to CaIcl1 accelerates its degradation in response to glucose in *C. albicans* [63].

The above observations strongly suggest that specific proteins can be targeted for degradation in *C. albicans* following exposure to glucose, and these proteins are degraded via ubiquitination. If this is the case, it should be theoretically possible to detect ubiquitinated forms of these proteins. Hence immuno-precipitation experiments were then performed in an attempt to demonstrate ubiquitinated forms of the CaIcl1-Myc_3 protein in *C. albicans.* Proteins were extracted from *C. albicans ICL1-UBI*-site-*MYC_3-URA3* cells 20, 40 and 120 minutes after glucose addition. Analogous control extracts were also prepared from *S. cerevisiae* and *C. albicans* cells expressing ScIcl1+Myc_3, CaIcl1+Myc_3 and untagged parental strains grown on lactate plus glucose and lactate alone. These extracts were immunoprecipitated with an anti-Myc antibody that was predicted to precipitate Icl1 proteins having carboxyl-terminal Myc_3 tags. These immunoprecipitates were then subjected to Western blotting with an anti-ubiquitin antibody to test whether any of these Myc_3-tagged Icl1 proteins carry ubiquitin sequences. The Western blots were also probed with the anti-Myc antibody to confirm that Myc-tagged Icl1 proteins had been immunoprecipitated. This was the case. Interestingly, a weak ubiquitin-containing band of a length consistent with Icl1-Myc_3 proteins was detected. Such bands were observed in three replicate experiments. These weak bands were observed for the ScIcl1-Myc_3 CaIcl1-Ubi-Myc_3 proteins following glucose addition (both proteins carry ubiquitination sites). However, no ubiquitination of these proteins was observed in the absence of glucose, or for the CaIcl1-Myc_3 protein (which lacks a strong ubiquitination site) or for the untagged control cells [63].

These data suggest that when *S.cerevisiae* Icl1 or an artificial *C. albicans* Icl1 carrying a ubiquitination signal is expressed in *C. albicans*, it becomes ubiquitinated and destabilised in response to glucose. However, the native *C. albicans* Icl1 protein is not destabilised by glucose. Therefore, in response to glucose, target proteins became ubiquitinated and then degraded in *C. albicans* [63].

What natural *C. albicans* proteins might be subjected to ubiquitin-mediated, glucose-accelerated protein degradation? To address this, bioinformatic tools were used to predict possible ubiquitination sites in glycolytic, gluconeogenic and glyoxylate cycle enzymes in *S. cerevisiae* and *C. albicans.* Five enzymes were selected for analysis: Fbp1, Pck1, Mdh1, Eno1 and Mls1. Based on this analysis, *S. cerevisiae* Fbp1, Pck1 and Eno1 appear to carry strong ubiquitination sites, while only Eno1 *C. albicans* appears to have a high confidence ubiquitination site. In conclusion, while these central metabolic pathways are highly conserved between *S. cerevisiae* and *C. albicans,* these organisms appear to display significant differences in the presence of ubiquitination sites in the orthologous enzymes [63]

4. Overview of Metabolic Adaptation in *Candida albicans*

A previous study suggested that *C. albicans* might be capable of using more than one carbon source at the same time during growth in specific niches in the host [34]. This study was based on the analysis of specific promoter-green fluorescent protein (GFP) fusions during systemic candidiasis. Almost all *C. albicans* cells infecting the kidney expressed GFP fusions with glycolytic promoters (*PYK1, PFK2*). Meanwhile one third to one-half of cells infecting the kidney also expressed *ICL1*- and *PCK1*-GFP fusions, suggesting that anabolic and catabolic pathways might be expressed at the same time. If this is the case, in principle, this would allow this pathogenic yeast to better utilise the complex mixture of available carbon sources in host niches. This working hypothesis would be consistent with earlier studies, suggesting that *C. albicans* is a glucose Crabtree-negative yeast. In other words, this pathogen retains respiratory activity even following exposure to glucose [44]. During growth on glucose, *ADH1* mRNA levels rise to maximum levels during late exponential growth phase and then decline to low levels in stationary phase [75]. The *ADH1* mRNA is relatively abundant during growth on galactose, glycerol, pyruvate, lactate or succinate, and less abundant during growth on glucose or ethanol. However, alcohol dehydrogenase levels do not correlate closely with *ADH1* mRNA levels. This locus may be controlled at both transcriptional and post-transcriptional levels, or other differentially regulated *ADH* loci may exist in *C. albicans* [75].

Interestingly, a significantly smaller proportion of glucose is fermented to ethanol by *C. albicans* than by *S. cerevisiae* [75]. This is consistent with the low amounts of ethanol produced by *C. albicans* observed in this study.

S. cerevisiae is not able to assimilate both non-fermentable carbon sources and glucose at the same time because of glucose repression. Hence, we predicted that these yeasts have evolved different responses to glucose. Therefore, in this study, I analysed the regulation of carbon assimilation in *C. albicans* focussing on genes/enzymes involved in gluconeogenesis and the glyoxylate cycle. I tested *ICL1* and *PCK1* gene expression, Icl1 and Pck1 protein stability and the impact of glucose on the assimilation of non-fermentable carbon sources. The author compared their *C. albicans* responses to those of *S. cerevisiae* under equivalent conditions. The following conclusions can be drawn from these findings.

First, gluconeogenic and glyoxylate cycle mRNAs are sensitive to glucose in both *C. albicans* and *S. cerevisiae*. This reconfirmed previous findings from Aberdeen Fungal Group Laboratory [54, 55] and other laboratories [76]. Dramatic decreases in *ICL1* and *PCK1* mRNA levels were observed in *C. albicans* cells after exposure to 2% glucose. This glucose concentration is higher than the levels of glucose homeostatically maintained in human blood (about 0.1%). However, it is already known that *C. albicans* responds to lower glucose concentrations within the physiological range of blood glucose [54, 55]. Therefore, *C. albicans* is able to respond to blood glucose levels during disseminated haematological infections. Interestingly, patients with diabetes who often have elevated blood glucose levels, have a higher risk of systemic *Candida* infections [14], and dietary glucose enhances *C. albicans* colonisation and invasion [77].

The second main observation was that the Icl1 and Pck1 proteins are stable in *C. albicans* following glucose exposure. The addition of 2% glucose to *C. albicans* cells growing on lactate or oleic acid did not trigger the degradation of the Icl1 and Pck1 proteins, at least within the 4 hours examined. This is in contrast to the situation in *S. cerevisiae*, where the addition of 2% glucose triggered the rapid degradation of the Icl1 and Pck1 proteins. The estimated half-lives for these proteins in *S. cerevisiae* are more than 20 hours [78] indicating that these proteins are very stable. This probably represents a significant difference in the physiological responses of these pathogenic and benign yeasts to glucose. *C. albicans* is able to establish infections in complex niches, many of which contain a rich mixture of alternative carbon sources [34]. The stability of the Icl1 and Pck1 proteins in *C. albicans*, even in the presence of glucose, provided the first clue that this pathogen might be able to assimilate alternative carbon sources at the same time as glucose in these carbon-rich niches.

The third conclusion was that *C. albicans* is able to assimilate both glucose and alternative carbon sources at the same time. It was shown that glucose addition has no major impact on the assimilation of the alternative carbon sources (lactate and oleic acid). The maintenance of gluconeogenic and glyoxylate cycle enzymes, therefore, appears to allow *C. albicans* to continue to assimilate alternative carbon sources, even following glucose addition. Therefore, during a transient exposure to glucose in the bloodstream, for example, *C. albicans* would be able to maintain anabolic metabolism. Also, after phagocytosis, when the genes of glyoxylate cycle and gluconeogenesis have been induced [34], these pathways probably remain active some time afterwards because of the stability of their enzymes. It was reported that the glyoxylate cycle helps to protect *C. albicans* against host anti-microbial defences by facilitating anabolic metabolism in the absence of fermentable carbon sources [79]. Barelle *et al.* [34] indicated that the pathogen *C. albicans* regulates central carbon metabolism in a niche-specific manner during disease establishment and progression. These authors reported two stages *C. albicans* activate the glyoxylate cycle and gluconeogenesis in response to phagocytosis during the early stage of infection and this is followed by glycolytic metabolism when the fungus colonises tissue. This metabolic flexibility is thought to increase the biological fitness of this pathogen within its host. It is conceivable that the prolonged activity of the anabolic pathways might further increase the fitness of this pathogen.

In conclusion, the regulation of central carbon metabolism in *S. cerevisiae* and *C. albicans* seems to have evolved in ways that reflect their different biological niches. *S. cerevisiae* has adapted to grow rapidly when high concentrations of sugars become available from fruit (*from feasts to famine*) [10], whereas *C. albicans* appears to have adapted to utilise the complex mixtures of carbon sources that are available in the GI tract or the bloodstream for example. The next step in this study is to test whether *C. albicans* has retained the ability to target accelerated protein degradation in response to glucose.

Next, the reverse cloning was done by replacing the *S. cerevisiae ICL1* ORF in *S. cerevisiae* with a Myc_3-tagged *C. albicans ICL1* ORF. The aim was to test whether the CaIcl1 protein was destabilised by glucose when expressed in *S. cerevisiae.* This revealed that the CaIcl1 protein was not destabilised in response to glucose when expressed in *S. cerevisiae.* This indicated that the *C. albicans* Icl1 protein has lost the signal that triggers destabilisation in response to glucose.

The *S. cerevisiae* Fbp1 protein is destabilised by glucose via ubiquitination [64]. Therefore, we reasoned that the CaIcl1 protein might have lost ubiquitination signals, which could account for the stability of the CaIcl1 protein in *S. cerevisiae* following glucose addition. Indeed, a bioinformatic analysis revealed that while ScIcl1 carries ubiquitination sites, CaIcl1 does not.

To test whether ubiquitination might play a role in glucose-accelerated protein degradation in *C. albicans*, the impact of *UBI4* inactivation upon ScIcl1 degradation was tested. Interestingly,

http://dx.doi.org/10.5772/62406

inactivation of the polyubiquitin gene slowed ScIcl1 degradation in *C. albicans* in response to glucose. This was consistent with the idea that ubiquitination contributes to glucose-accelerated protein degradation in *C. albicans.*

If this was the case, the addition of a ubiquitination signal should confer glucose-accelerated degradation upon the stable CaIcl1 protein. This was tested, showing that a carboxyl-terminal ScIcl1 ubiquitination signal was sufficient to trigger the rapid degradation of CaIcl1 following glucose addition to *C. albicans* cells [63].

Finally, direct biochemical evidence for the involvement of ubiquitination in glucose-accelerated protein degradation in *C. albicans* was obtained by showing that ubiquitin co-immunoprecipitated with the ScIcl1 and CaIcl1-Ubi proteins in *C. albicans*, but only when cells were exposed to glucose [63].

In conclusion, *C. albicans* is capable of destabilising target proteins in response to glucose, and this destabilisation is mediated by ubiquitination. The lack of ubiquitination sites on the *C. albicans* Icl1 and Pck1 proteins probably accounts for the observation that these glyoxylate cycle and gluconeogenic enzymes are not destabilised by glucose in *C. albicans.*

5. Conclusion and Future Perspectives

Overall, the topic was to explore the impact of glucose on the assimilation of alternative carbon sources and catabolite inactivation in *C. albicans.* To achieve this, the effects of glucose on the transcriptional and post-transcriptional regulation of key genes and enzymes were studied, and the molecular mechanisms that trigger protein destabilisation in response to glucose were examined. These effects were then compared with glucose responses in *S. cerevisiae.*

Gene expression in both *C. albicans* and *S. cerevisiae* is sensitive to glucose. In both yeasts, *ICL1* and *PCK1* mRNA expression levels were down-regulated in response to glucose. This confirmed the previous microarray studies in *S. cerevisiae* [54] and in *C. albicans* [55].

ICL1 and *PCK1* are involved in the utilisation of alternative carbon sources such as organic and fatty acids, and these genes are repressed by glucose in *S. cerevisiae*. Indeed gluconeogenic and glyoxylate cycle genes have been shown to be repressed by glucose concentrations as low as 0.01% in *S. cerevisiae* [54]. Similarly, *C. albicans* genes involved in central carbon metabolism respond rapidly to the addition of glucose. Indeed the *PCK1* and *ICL1* genes have been shown to be repressed by glucose at levels as low as 0.1% [55]. These observations imply that the utilisation of alternative carbon sources could be repressed by glucose in *C. albicans*. Given that if *C. albicans* genes involved in the utilisation of alternative carbon sources are glucose- regulated in a similar fashion to those in *S. cerevisiae*, then it might be expected that these genes would be repressed during systemic infections. However, during phagocytosis by macrophages, *C. albicans* cells appear to up-regulate the glyoxylate cycle, as the expression of the isocitrate lyase (*ICL1*) and malate synthase (*MLS1*) genes is induced [80]. The same applies to the gluconeogenic gene, *PCK1* [34]. Furthermore both *ICL1* and *PCK1* appear to be expressed in some *C. albicans* cells during systemic kidney infections [34]. Various studies have shown that genes involved in gluconeogenic and glyoxylate cycle contribute to fungal virulence [34, 62, 79].

C. albicans often occupies niches that contain complex mixtures of carbon sources. Our initial working hypothesis, therefore, was that *C. albicans* might exploit many of these diverse carbon sources rather than focussing on glucose alone. Therefore, the tight glucose repression of the *PCK1* and *ICL1* genes seemed somewhat surprising [54, 55, 76] because this was inconsistent with our working hypothesis. Our subsequent discovery that the Pck1 and Icl1 enzymes were not destabilised by glucose was more consistent with this working hypothesis. Catabolite inactivation – the rapid degradation of specific enzymes following glucose exposure – is a well-defined phenomenon in *S. cerevisiae.* In the yeast, the gluconeogenic enzyme Fbp1 is rapidly degraded when cells are shifted from media with poor carbon sources to rich media containing glucose [59]. Consistent with this, in this project it was found that both the Icl1 and Pck1 proteins were rapidly degraded in *S. cerevisiae* in response to glucose. This was the case when cells were pre-grown on lactic acid or oleic acid. In contrast, the *C. albicans* Icl1 and Pck1 proteins were not destabilised in response to glucose when cells were exposed to glucose. The stability of the CaIcl1 and CaPck1 enzymes in the presence of glucose suggested that *C. albicans* might be capable of continuing to utilise alternative carbon sources even when glucose became available. This suggestion was more consistent with our working hypothesis that *C. albicans* has evolved to utilise carbon sources simultaneously in complex niches.

To examine this, the impact of glucose on the ability of *C. albicans* to assimilate radiolabelled lactic acid or oleic acid was tested and compared with that of *S. cerevisiae.* These incorporation studies confirmed the divergent behaviour of these yeasts with respect to their patterns of carbon assimilation. In *S. cerevisiae*, the assimilation of lactic and oleic acid was repressed by glucose and subsequent growth was reliant on glucose. In contrast, in *C. albicans*, the utilisation of lactic and oleic acid was not repressed by glucose. Hence, the utilisation of alternative carbon sources by *C. albicans* was not repressed by glucose, and thus the subsequent growth of this pathogen was supported by assimilating both glucose and alternative carbon sources [63].

In summary, both *C. albicans* and *S. cerevisiae* displayed similar responses to glucose at the transcriptional level, but their responses at post-transcriptional and metabolic levels differed significantly. Therefore, *C. albicans* can assimilate both glucose and alternative carbon sources at the same time, whereas *S. cerevisiae* is not able to do so (Fig. 1). This is predicted to play a significant role in the growth of this fungus during infection in the human host [41]. This could be tested by reprogramming the Icl1 and Pck1 enzymes to be glucose- sensitive in *C. albicans.* The prediction is that this engineered *C. albicans* strain would grow less well on mixed carbon sources containing glucose, and hence would display attenuated virulence. Additional experiments that could be carried should test the impact of carbon sources other than glucose, (such as lactose, galactose or fructose) [Ting and Sandai, unpublished] on the stability of gluconeogenic and glyoxylate cycle enzymes in *C. albicans.* Fructose, lactose and galactose are commonly found in the diet, and significant differences are thought to exist between *C. albicans* and *S. cerevisiae* with regard to the regulation of galactose utilisation [81, 82].

Another additional experiment could involve the broad screening of central metabolic enzymes in *C. albicans* for consensus ubiquitination target sites, beyond the preliminary screen performed here. This would help to extend the predicted impact of glucose on central metabolic pathways. This preliminary bioinformatic screen of gluconeogenic and glyoxylate cycle enzymes has indicated that the *S. cerevisiae* Icl1, Fbp1, Eno1 and Pck1 proteins carry high confidence ubiquitination sites (Fig. 2). Previous studies have shown that ScFbp1 is catabolite inactivated in a glucose-dependent manner via ubiqutination and proteasomal degradation [59]. In contrast, in *C. albicans*, only Eno1 carries a high confidence ubiquitination site. This bioinformatic analysis is consistent with the suggestion that gluconeogenesis and the glyoxylate cycle are insensitive to glucose or at least glucose stimulated, ubiquitin-mediated protein degradation in *C. albicans* [63].

The next main step in this project involved testing whether *C. albicans* has retained the molecular capability of destabilising target proteins in response to glucose. Examinations of Icl1 protein levels in both *S. cerevisiae* and *C. albicans* revealed that while Icl1 is rapidly degraded in response to glucose in *S. cerevisiae*, Icl1 remains stable in *C. albicans*. To test whether the *C. albicans* Icl1 protein has lost the signal that triggers destabilisation in response to glucose, the *C. albicans ICL1* ORF was expressed in *S. cerevisiae*. Interestingly, the *C. albicans* Icl1 protein was not destabilised in response to glucose when it was expressed in *S. cerevisiae*. This was consistent with the idea that the *C. albicans* Icl1 protein has lost the signal required to trigger glucose-accelerated degradation [66].

The next step is to test whether *C. albicans* has retained the ability to degrade target proteins in response to glucose. To investigate this, the tagged *S. cerevisiae* Icl1 protein was expressed in *C. albicans*. This tagged *S. cerevisiae* Icl1 protein was rapidly degraded when the *C. albicans* cells were exposed to glucose. This indicated that *C. albicans* has retained the molecular apparatus that mediates glucose-accelerated protein decay (or "catabolite inactivation").

What apparatus mediates this glucose-accelerated degradation? In *S. cerevisiae*, ubiquitination plays an important role in the rapid proteasome-mediated degradation of Fbp1 in response to glucose [57]. Therefore, the amino acid sequences of ScIcl1 and CaIcl1 were screened for consensus ubiquitination sites. This revealed that while the ScIcl1 sequence has strong ubiquitination sites, the CaIcl1 sequence does not (Fig. 3). Therefore, to examine whether ubiquitination plays a role in glucose-accelerated protein degradation in *C. albicans*, the impact of a polyubiquitin (*ubi4/ubi4*) null mutation [74] on the degradation of ScIcl1 in *C. albicans* was tested. The tagged *ScICL1* ORF was expressed in this *C. albicans ubi4/ubi4* mutant and its decay rate was measured in the presence and absence of glucose. Compared to the controls, the degradation of ScIcl1 was relatively slow in the *C. albicans ubi4/ubi4* mutant. This suggested that ubiquitination plays a role in glucose-accelerated protein degradation in *C. albicans*.

To test this further, we investigated the effects of introducing a *S. cerevisiae* ubiquitination site on to the carboxyl-terminus of the stable CaIcl1 protein. This CaIcl1-Ubi protein was destabilised in response to glucose in *C. albicans* (Fig. 3). This confirmed that ubiquitination plays a key role in glucose-accelerated protein degradation in *C. albicans*. It is also confirmed that *C. albicans* has retained the molecular apparatus that destabilises target proteins in response to glucose. In summary, *C. albicans* cells have retained the molecular apparatus that degrades target proteins in response to glucose, but CaIcl1 has lost the signal that triggers this destabilisation. As a result, the stability of CaIcl1 enzyme in the presence of glucose allows *C.*

albicans cells to continue to use alternative carbon sources such as lactic and oleic acid rather than switching to glycolysis.

What is the apparatus required to trigger glucose accelerated decay? Ubiquitin- mediated protein degradation occurs via the proteasome [83]. This is a conserved molecular machine comprised of numerous protein subunits. Proteins are targeted to the proteasome via ubiquitination, which involves several steps (Fig. 4). Ubiquitin is activated in a two-step process involving the E1 and E2 enzymes and the hydrolysis of ATP. The primed ubiquitin molecule, once attached to an E2 enzyme via a thioester linkage, is then ligated to the target protein via an E3 ligase which provides the substrate specificity. A previous PhD student in the Aberdeen Fungal Group Laboratory [84] has already shown that proteasomal subunits are highly conserved across the fungal kingdom and are conserved in *C. albicans* (Fig. 4). Furthermore, E1, E2 and E3 enzymes are conserved in *C. albicans* (Fig 4) [85], which are consistent with the ubiquitination apparatus being retained in this pathogen. Presumably, the inactivation of components of this system could block glucose-accelerated protein degradation in *C. albicans.*

In *S. cerevisiae,* Ubc8 appears to be the ubiquitin-conjugating enzyme involved in glucose-accelerated protein degradation. Ubc8 has been described as a ubiquitin-conjugating enzyme that negatively regulates gluconeogenesis by mediating the glucose-induced ubiquitination of Fbp1 [57, 64, 85, 86]. Interestingly the Ubc8 protein appears to be conserved in *C. albicans* [87]. Additional ubiquitin-conjugating enzymes exist in *C. albicans,* such as Ubc4 and Ubc6, and these might also be involved. However, all these *UBC* genes remain uncharacterised in *C. albicans,* and therefore it is not yet known whether these genes play a role in glucose-accelerated protein degradation. Interestingly however, *UBC8* is the only ubiquitin-related gene that is up-regulated at the transcriptional level following glucose exposure in *C. albicans* (Table 1). Therefore, Ubc8 is an excellent candidate for the ubiquitin-conjugating enzyme that mediates glucose-accelerated protein degradation in *C. albicans.* Clearly, a future experiment that could be carried out would be to create a *C. albicans ubc8/ubc8* mutant and to test whether this mutation blocks glucose-accelerated protein degradation in *C. albicans*. Other *UBC* genes might also be inactivated to test the possibility that they are not involved in glucose-accelerated protein degradation [63].

These findings are relevant to our understanding of *C. albicans* growth and survival in the host, and hence to *C. albicans* pathogenicity. *C. albicans* persists as commensal during colonisation in the healthy human GI tract where monosaccharides (such as glucose, fructose and galactose) and disaccharides (such as sucrose and lactose) can be abundant [88]. These sugars probably help to sustain the fungus, for example, during the first 6 months of a host's life when new born infants consume milk and hence lactose [89]. Both disaccharides and monosaccharides may supply a carbon-rich environment for microbes such as *C. albicans,* and they are also absorbed into the bloodstream [82]. However, during systemic infections *C. albicans* cells invade the bloodstream and often internal organs such as kidney. Glucose is present in the bloodstream but appears to become limited in systemic microenvironments that are colonised during infection of organs. At this point, the fungal cells probably switch to gluconeogenesis and glyoxylate cycle metabolism to utilise the available alternative carbon sources [34]. Also, during phagocytosis, by macrophages and neutrophils, *C. albicans* cells switch to the assimilation of alternative carbon sources, activating genes such as *ICL1* [34, 62, 79, 89] that are required for full pathogenicity [34, 79]. It would appear from the findings in this chapter, that

http://dx.doi.org/10.5772/62406

C. albicans has evolved in such a manner that this fungus can continue to assimilate these alternative carbon sources, even after exposure to glucose. The presumption is that this ability to use several of carbon sources in these complex and carbon-rich microenvironments contributes to the growth and pathogenicity of *C. albicans* in these microenvironments. Possibly the greatest challenge for the future is to elucidate exactly what carbon sources individual *C. albicans* cells assimilate *in vivo* during commensalism, mucosal infection and systemic candidiasis and to elucidate the contribution of transcriptional and post-transcriptional control mechanisms to this regulation.

This carbon metabolism of *C. albicans* might be investigated further by examining the ability of mutant *C. albicans* cells that carry the *ICL1-ubi* allele to grow and assimilate carbon *in vivo*. These *C. albicans* cells express Icl1 that is destabilised by glucose because of the addition of the carboxyl-terminal ubiquitination site. In principle, Icl1 would be degraded and cells no longer able to metabolise via the glyoxylate cycle following glucose addition. As a result, those cells would presumably be less able to course infections and would be less able to compete for available nutrients against other microorganisms such as endogenous bacteria in the GI tract compared to their wild type. It is likely to show less successful colonisation, virulence and fitness due to this defect in its ability to assimilate both glucose and alternative carbon sources at the same time [63].

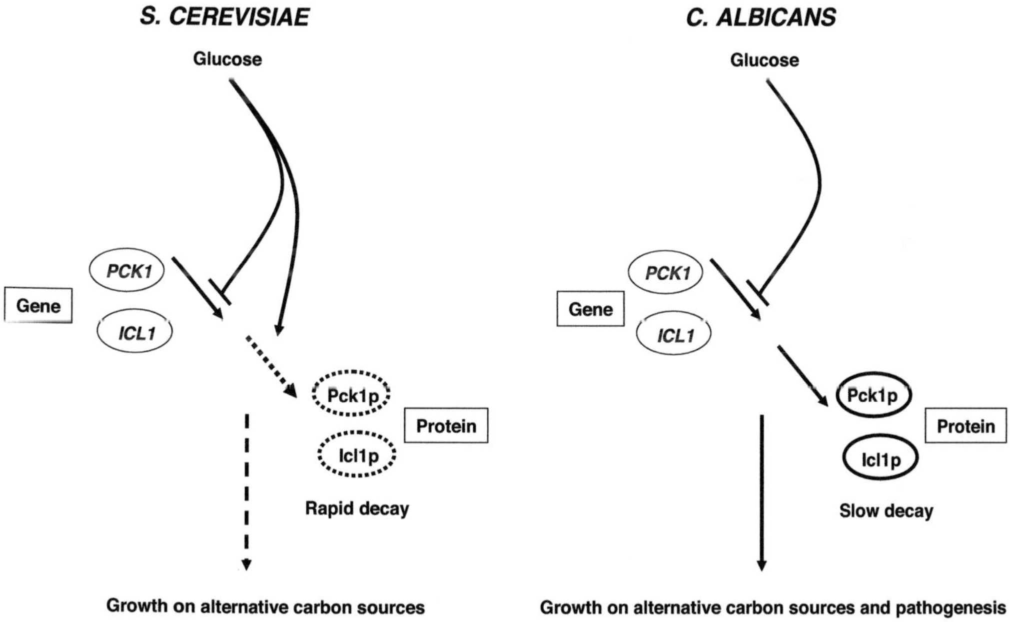

Figure 1. Proposed model of the impact of glucose on the assimilation of alternative carbon sources by *S. cerevisiae* and *C. albicans*. In *C. albicans* and *S. cerevisiae* transcription of both *ICL1* and *PCK1* are repressed by glucose. However, their regulation at post-transcriptional levels and metabolism diverge significantly. The *S. cerevisiae* Icl1 and Pck1 proteins are rapidly destabilised in response to glucose and the assimilation of alternative carbon sources is repressed by glucose. In contrast, in *C. albicans* the Icl1 and Pck1 proteins decay slowly in response to glucose and continue to assimilate both glucose and alternative carbon sources at the same time.

In addition, it would be interesting to conduct further investigations of the impact of other carbon sources such as galactose, fructose, sucrose, fatty acid and amino acid on carbon assimilation in *C. albicans*. For example galactose might also trigger glucose-like repression in *C. albicans* [82]. The behaviour of *C. albicans* towards other carbon sources differs from *S. cerevisiae*. It would be interesting to define the effects of these carbon sources on the levels and activities of glycolytic, gluconeogenic, glyoxylate cycle and fatty acid β-oxidation enzymes. Which other carbon sources trigger the ubiquitination-mediated degradation of these proteins in *C. albicans*? How do these mechanisms affect the ability of *C. albicans* to assimilate lipid, carbohydrate, protein and other organic acids in their human host during commensalism and infection? Such studies will provide a more complete physiological understanding of *C. albicans* for the future research.

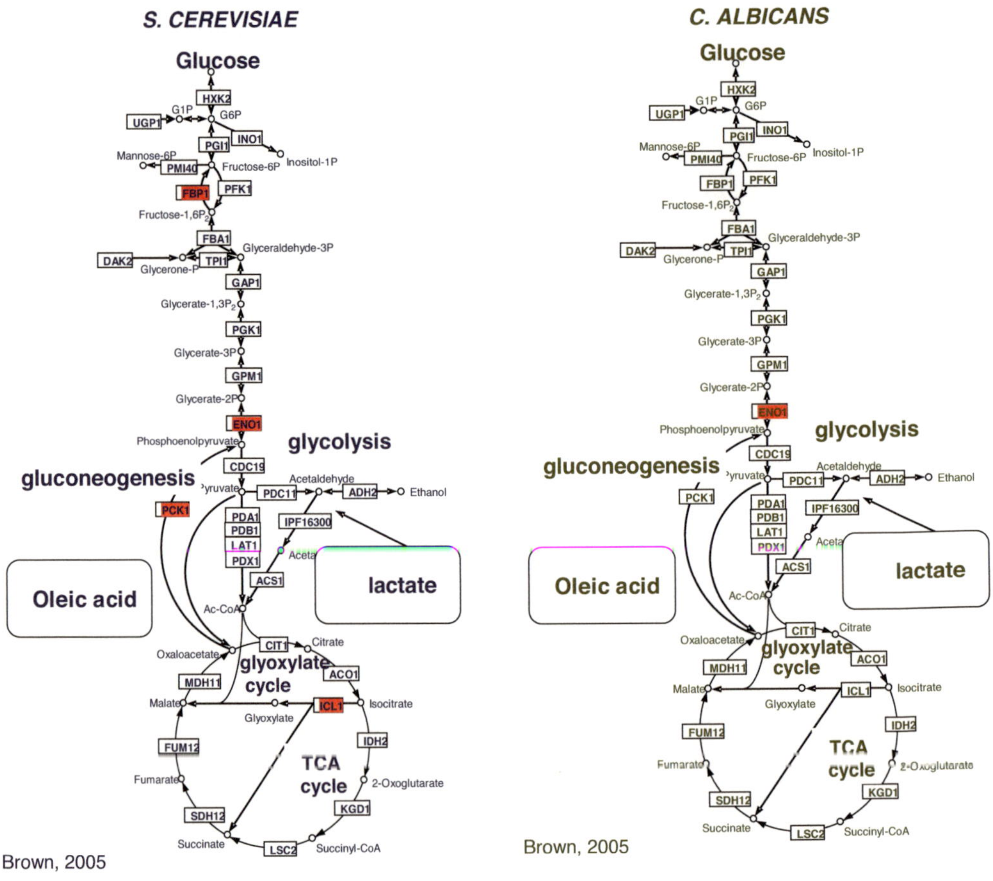

Figure 2. Bioinformatic prediction of ubiquitination sites in glycolytic, gluconeogenic and glyoxylate cycle enzymes from *S. cerevisiae* and *C. albicans*. Icl1, Pck1, Eno1 and Fbp1 were examined. Those carrying high confidence ubiquitination sites are highlighted in red.

http://dx.doi.org/10.5772/62406

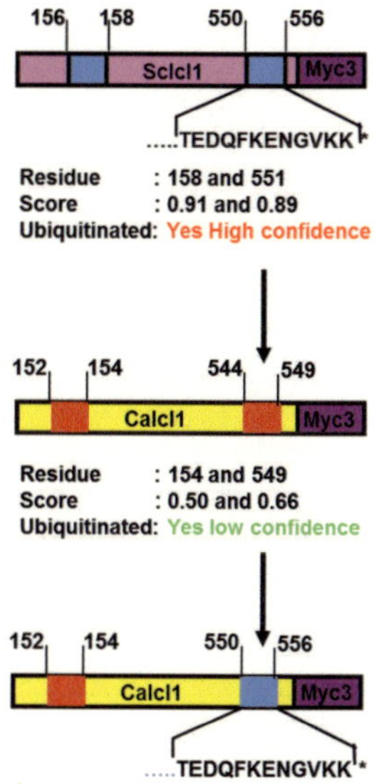

Figure 3. Role of ubiquitin-mediated protein degradation in enzyme destabilisation in C. albicans in response to glucose. Bioinformatics comparison of CaIcl1 and ScIcl1 reveals a lack of putative ubiquitination target in CaIcl1. Introduction of carboxyl-terminal ScUbi-site in CaIcl1 plus Myc-tagging protein and testing the impact of glucose on the turnover of CaIcl1 with C-terminal ScUbi-site. Adding back a Ubi-site accelerates degradation in response to glucose.

Candida dataset *Candida* gene Systematic orf19Number common			Expression Ratio glucose Concentration (%) 0.0 0.01 0.1 1.0	*Saccharomyces dataset* S. cerevisiae gene homology Systematic common		Expression Ratio glucose Concentration (%) 0.0 0.01 0.1 1.0	Description
CA5729	orf19.7438	*UBA1*	-1.2 1.0 -1.2 -1.1	YKL210W	*UBA1*	1.0 -1.4 -1.1 -1.2	Ubiquitin-activating enzyme (by homology)
CA3898	orf19.5074	*UBA2*	-1.3 -1.0 -1.2 -1.2	YDR390C	*UBA2*	1.0 -1.2 1.1 1.0	Ubiquitin-activating -like enzyme (by homology)
CA2926	orf19.4209	*UBA3*	1.1 -1.0 1.0 -1.1	YPR066W	*UBA3*	1.0 -1.1 1.3 1.4	Ubiquitin-like protein activating enzyme
CA0531	orf19.8686	*UBC1*	1.2 1.0 1.4 1.2	YDR177W	*UBC1*	1.0 -1.2 1.1 1.1	Ubiquitin-conjugating enzyme (by homology)
CA5977	orf19.7571	*UBC4.3*	1.3 1.1 1.1 1.1	YBR082C	*UBC4*	1.0 1.1 1.7 1.7	E2 ubiquitin-conjugating

Candida dataset *Candida* gene Systematic orf19Number common			Expression Ratio glucose Concentration (%) 0.0 0.01 0.1 1.0	*Saccharomyces dataset* S. cerevisiae gene homology Systematic common		Expression Ratio glucose Concentration (%) 0.0 0.01 0.1 1.0	Description
							enzyme, 3-prime end
CA5648	orf19.7347	*UBC6*	-1.0 1.0 1.1 -1.0	YER100W	*UBC6*	1.0 1.0 1.2 1.6	E2 ubiquitin-conjugating enzyme (by homology)
CA4199	orf19.4540	***UBC8***	**1.3 2.1 3.6 2.5**	YEL012W	*UBC8*	1.0 1.1 -1.0 -1.1	Ubiquitin-conjugating enzyme (by homology)
CA5109	orf19.6424	*UBC9*	1.0 1.2 1.1 1.0	YDL064W	*UBC9*	1.1 1.3 1.2 -1.1	E2 ubiquitin-conjugating enzyme (by homology)
CA5769	orf19.5411	*UBC12*	-1.1 1.0 -1.1 1.1	YLR306W	*UBC12*	1.0 -1.6 -1.3 -1.5	E2 ubiquitin-conjugating enzyme (by homology)
CA0417	orf19.2225	*UBC13*	1.2 1.1 1.1 1.1	YDR092W	*UBC13*	1.1 -1.4 -1.3 -1.2	E2 ubiquitin-conjugating enzyme (by homology)
CA3263	orf19.2697	*UBR12*	-1.2 1.0 -1.1 -1.1	YLR024C	*UBR2*	1.0 -1.6 -1.7 -1.6	Ubiquitin-protein ligase (by homology)
CA3262	orf19.2695	*UBR11.3*	-1.1 1.0 -1.1 -1.1	YGR184C	*UBR1*	1.0 -1.4 -1.4 -1.3	Ubiquitin-protein ligase, 3′ end (by homology)
CA1279	orf19.3628	*RSP5*	-1.0 1.1 1.2 1.2	YER125W	*RSP5*	1.0 1.1 1.0 -1.1	Ubiquitin-protein ligase (by homology)
CA5435	orf19.3237	*UFD4*	-1.1 1.3 1.3 1.4	YKL010C	*UFD4*	1.0 -1.4 -1.4 -1.3	Ubiquitin fusion degradation protein (by homology)

http://dx.doi.org/10.5772/62406

Candida dataset *Candida* gene Systematic orf19Number common			Expression Ratio glucose Concentration (%) 0.0 0.01 0.1 1.0	*Saccharomyces dataset* S. cerevisiae gene homology Systematic common		Expression Ratio glucose Concentration (%) 0.0 0.01 0.1 1.0	Description
CA2803	orf19.5776	*IPF11711*	-1.1 1.3 1.3 1.3	YDR457W	*TOM1*	1.0 1.2 1.1 1.1	Ubiquitin-protein ligase (by homology)
CA6150	orf19.5892	*IPF1857*	-1.3 1.4 -1.1 1.1	YJR036C	*HUL4*	1.0 -1.8 -1.9 -2.9	similar to Saccharomyces cerevisiae Hul4p hect domain E3 ubiquitin-protein ligase (by homology)

Table 1. Expression of *C. albicans* and *S. cerevisiae* homologues involved in protein ubiquitination [55].

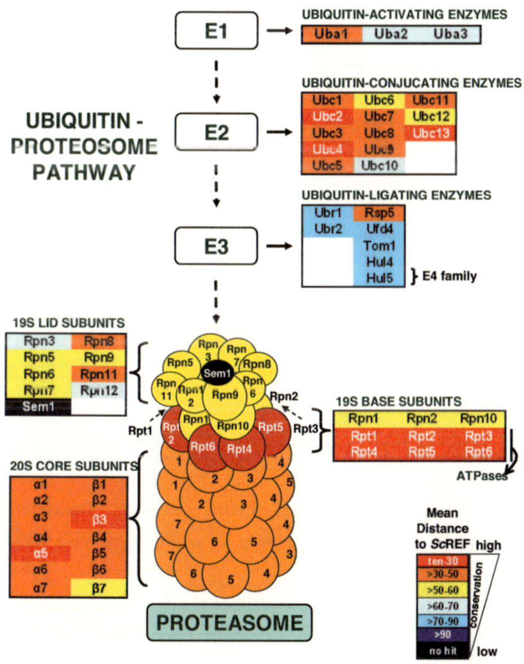

Figure 4. Protein conservation in the proteasome. Each protein is colour-coded according to its mean distance to *Sc*REF scores (scale bottom right: high *Sc*REF scores represent low sequence conservation). Each subunit of the actual machine (20S core particle and 19S cap) has been colour -coded based on the mean of the mean distance to *Sc*REF values for the proteins that form it in all species. Rpn13 (*Sc*REF distance = 82) is not included in the picture. Ubiquitin-related enzymes have been reviewed by Hochstrasser (1996), and protein component of the machine was identified based on the review by Sharon and co-workers (2006). In the ubiquitin-ligating enzymes, except for the Ubr1 and Ubr2 enzymes, all the others are hect-domain proteins [84].

Acknowledgements

I would like to thank Professor Alistair JP Brown for his advice and support throughout this project. I would also like to thank the Malaysian Ministry of Higher Education and Universiti Sains Malaysia for providing financial support. I am grateful to the members of Aberdeen Fungal Group, Institute of Medical Sciences, University of Aberdeen, UK and the staff of Advanced Medical and Dental Institute, Universiti Sains Malaysia for all their support and friendship. Thanks to my family and friends for their love and support.

Author details

Doblin Sandai*

Address all correspondence to: doblin@usm.my

Infectomics Cluster, Advanced Medical and Dental Institute, Universiti Sains Malaysia, Bertam Penang, Malaysia

References

[1] Calderone RA and Gow NAR. Host recognition by *Candida* species In: *Candida* and Candidiasis Calderone 1st edn. ASM Press, Washington DC: 2002; 67- 86.

[2] Cutler JE. Putative virulence factors of *Candida albicans*. Annual Reviews Microbiology. 1991; 45: 187- 218.

[3] Sudbery P, Gow NAR, and Berman J. The distinct morphogenic states of *Candida albicans* Trends in Microbiology. 2004; 12: 317- 324.

[4] Mathews HL and Witek-Janusek L. Host defence against oral, esophageal, and gastrointestinal candidiasis. *Candida* and Candidiasis. EMBO Journal. 2004; 13: 179- 192.

[5] Odds FC, Gow NA, and Brown AJP. Fungal virulence studies come of age. Genome Biology. 2001; 2(3): REVIEWS1009.

[6] Berman J and Sudbery PE. *Candida albicans*: a molecular revolution built on lessons from budding yeast. Nature Review Genetic. 2002; 3: 918- 930.

[7] Copping VMS, Barrelle CJ, Hube B, Gow NAR, Brown AJP, and Odds FC. Exposure of *Candida albicans* to antifungal agents affects expression of *SAP2* secreted proteinase genes. Journal of Antimicrobial Chemotherapy. 2005; 55: 645- 654.

[8] Sanglard D and Odds FC. Resistance of *Candida albicans* spcecies to antifungal agents: molecular mechanisms and clinical. Journal of Antimicrobial Agent Chemotheraphy. 2006; 50: 1383- 1392.

[9] Pappas PG, Kauffman CA, Andes D, Benjamin DK, Calandra TF, Edward JE, Filler SG, Fisher JF, Kullberg BJ, Ostrosky-Zeichner L, Reboli AC, Rex JH, Walsh TJ, and Sobel JD. Clinical practice guidelines for the management of candidiasis: 2009 update by the Infectious Diseases Society of America. Clinical Infectious Disease.2009; 48: 503- 535.

[10] Carlson M. Glucose repression in yeast. Current Opinion of Microbiology. 1999; 2: 202- 207.

[11] Johnston M. Feasting, fasting and fermenting glucose sensing in yeast and other cells. Trends in Genetic. 1999; 15: 29- 33.

[12] Gancedo JM. Yeast repression catabolite repression. Microbiology Molecular Biology Review. 1998; 62: 334- 361.

[13] Santangelo GM. Glucose signalling in *Saccharomyces cerevisiae*. Microbiology and Molecular Biology. 2006; 70: 253- 282.

[14] Odds FC. *Candida* and Candidiosis 2nd edn. Bailliere Tindall, London; 1998.

[15] Ruhnke M. Skin and mucous membrane infections. In: *Candida* and candidiasis (Ed. Caldrone RA) ASM Press, Washington DC: 2002; 307- 325.

[16] Kullberg BJ and Filler SG. Candidemia. In: *Candida* and Candidiasis (Ed. Calderone, R.A.) ASM Press, Washington DC: 2002; 327- 340.

[17] Soll DR. Phenotype switching. In: *Candida* and Candidiasis (Ed. Calderone, R.A) ASM Press, Washington DC: 2002; 123- 142.

[18] Piispanen AE and Hogan DA. PEPped up: induction of *Candida albicans* virulence by bacteria cell wall fragments. Cell Host Microbes. 2008; 4: 1- 2.

[19] Soll DR. *Candida* commensalism and virulence: the evolution ofphenotypic plasticity. Acta Tropica. 2001; 81: 101- 110.

[20] Senet JM. *Candida* adherence phenomena from commensalism to pathogenicity. International Microbiology. 1998; 1: 117- 122.

[21] Nair RG and Samaranayake LP. The effect of oral commensal bacteria on *Candida* adhesion to human buccal epithelial cells *in vitro*. Journal of Medical Microbiology. 1996; 45: 179- 185.

[22] Hostetter M. Adhesins and ligands involved in the interaction of *Candida spp.* with epithelial and endothelial surfaces. Clinical Microbiology Reviews.1994; 7: 29- 42.

[23] Pfaller MA. Nosocomial candidiasis: emerging species, reservoirs, and modes of transmission. Clinical Infection. 1996; 22: S89- S94.

[24] Bendel CM, Hess DJ, Garni RM, Henry-Stanley M, and Wells CL. Comparative virulence of *Candida albicans* yeast and filamentous forms in orally and intravenously inoculated mice. Critical Care Medicine. 2003; 31: 501- 507.

[25] Cole GT, Halawa AA, and Anaissie EJ. The role of the gastrointestinal tract in hematogenous candidiasis: from the laboratory to the bedside. Clinical Infection. 1996; 22: S73- S88.

[26] Sims CR, Ostrosky-Zeichner L, and Rex JH. Invasive candidiasis in immunocompromised hospitalised patients. Archives of Medical Research. 2005; 36: 660- 671.

[27] Sobel JD. Treatment of vaginal *Candida* infections. Expert Opinion on Pharmacotherapy. 2002; 3: 1059- 1065.

[28] Munro CA and Hube B. Anti-fungal therapy at the HAART of viral therapy, Article. Trends in Microbiology. 2002; 10: 173- 177.

[29] Odds FC, Brown AJP, and Gow NAR. Antifungal agents: mechanism of action. Trends in Microbiology. 2003; 11: 272- 279.

[30] Ghannoum MA and Kuhn DM. Voriconazole – better chances for patients with invasive mycoses. European Journal of Medical Research. 2003; 7: 242- 256.

[31] Gonzalez GM, Tijerina R, Najvar LK, Baconegra R, Rinaldi M, Loebenberg, and Graybill JR. *In vitro* and *in vivo* activities of posaconazole against Coccidioides immitis. Journal of Antimicrobial Agents Chemotheraphy. 2002; 46: 1352- 1356.

[32] Olsen SJ, Mummaneni V, Rolan P, Norton J, and Grasela DM. Ravuconazole single ascending oral dose study in healthy subjects. Presented at: 40th Interscience Conference on Antimicrobial Agents and Chemotherapy; September 17- 20, 2000; Toronto, Ontario, Canada. Abstract 838.

[33] Walker LA, Munro CA, de Bruijn I, Lenardon MD, McKinnon A, and Gow NA. Stimulation of chitin synthesis rescues *Candida albicans* from echinocandins. PLoS Pathogens. 2008; 4: e1000040.

[34] Barelle CJ, Priest CL, MacCallum DM, Gow NA, Odds FC, and Brown AJP. Niche-specific regulation of central metabolic pathways in a fungal pathogen. Cellular Microbiology. 2006; 8: 961- 971.

[35] Fradin C, De Groot P, MacCallum DM, Schaller M, Klis F, Odds FC, and Hube B. Granulocytes govern the transcriptional response, morphology and proliferation of *Candida albicans* in human blood. Molecular Microbiology. 2005; 56: 397- 415.

[36] Garcia-Sanchez S, Mavor A, Russell CL, Argimon S, Dennison P, Enjalbert B, Brown AJP. Global roles of Ssn6 in Tup1- and Nrg1-dependent gene regulation in the fungal pathogen, *Candida albicans*. Molecular Biology of the Cell. 2005; 16: 2913- 2925.

[37] Rubin-Bejerano I, Fraser I, Grisafil P, and Fink GR. Phagocytosis by neutrophills induces an amino acid deprivation response in *Saccharomyces cerevisiae* and *Candida albicans*. Proceedings of the National Academy Science USA. 2003; 100: 11007- 11012.

[38] Lorenz MC, Bender JA, and Fink GR. Transcription response of *Candida albicans* upon internalisation by macrophages. Eukaryotic Cell. 2004; 3: 1076- 1087.

[39] Dickinson JR, Dawes IW, Boyd ASF, and Baxter RL. CNMR studies of acetate metabolism during sporulation of *Saccharomyces cerevisiae*. Proceeding of the National Academy of Sciences USA. 1983; 80: 5847- 5851.

[40] Lorenz MC and Fink GR. Life and death macrophage: role of the glycoxylate cycle in virulence. Eukaryotic Cell. 2002; 1: 657- 662.

[41] Brown AJP. Integration of metabolism with virulence in *Candida albicans*. In: *Fungal Genomics*. (Ed. Brown AJP). Mycota XIII, Springer-Verlag, Heidelberg: 2005; 185- 203.

[42] Jones T, Federspiel NA, Chibana H, Dungan J, Kalman S, Magee BB, Newport G, Thorstenson YR, Agabian N, Magee PT, Davis RW, and Scherer S. The diploid genome sequence of *Candida albicans*. Proceedings of the National Academy of Sciences USA, 2004; 101: 7329- 7334.

[43] Piskur J, Rozpedowska E, Polakova S, Merico A, and Compagno C. How did *Saccharomyces* evolve to become a good brewer? Trends in Genetics. 2006; 4: 183- 6.

[44] Niimi M, Kamiyama A, and Tokunaga, M. Respiration of medically important *Candida* species and *Saccharomyces cerevisiae* in relation to glucose effect. Medical and Veterinary Mycology. 1988; 26: 195- 198.

[45] Entian KD and Barnett JA. Regulation of sugar utilization by *Saccharomyces cerevisiae*. Trends in Biochemistry Science. 1992; 17: 506- 510.

[46] Entian KD and Schüller HJ. Glucose repression (carbon catabolite repression) in yeast. In: Yeast Sugar Metabolism: Biochemistry, Genetics, Biotechnology and Applications (Eds. Zimmermann FK, Entian KD) Technomic, Basel: 1997; pp. 409- 434.

[47] Ronne H. Glucose repression in fungi. Trends in Genetics. 1995; 11: 12- 17.

[48] Bojunga N, Kötter P, and Entian KD. The succinate/fumarate transporter Arc1p of *Saccharomyces cerevisiae* is part of the gluconeogenic pathway and its regulated by Cat8. Molecular and General Genetics.1988; 260: 453- 461.

[49] Scholer A and Schüller HJ. A carbon source-responsive promoter element necessary for activation of the isocitrate lyase gene *ICL1* is common to genes of the gluconeogenic pathway in the yeast *Saccharomyces cerevisiae*. Molecular of Cell Biology. 1994; 14: 3613- 3622.

[50] Caspary F, Hartig A, and Schüller HJ. Constitutive and carbon source-responsive promoter elements are involved in the regulation expression of the *Saccharomyces cer-*

evisiae malate synthase gene *MLS1*. Molecular of General Genetics. 1997; 255: 619-627.

[51] Proft M, Grzesitza D, and Entian KD. Identification and characterization of regulatory elements in the phosphoenolpyruvate carboxykinase gene *PCK1 of Saccharomyces cerevisiae*. Molecular of Genomic Genetics. 1995; 246: 367- 373.

[52] Niederacher D, Schüller HJ, Grzesita D, Gutlish H, Hauser HP, Wagner T, and Entian KD. Idenfication of UAS elements and binding proteins necessary for derepression of *Saccharomyces cerevisiae* fructose-1, 6-bisphosphatase.Current Genetics. 1992; 22: 363-370.

[53] Lutfiyya LL, Iyer VR, Derisi J, Devit MJ, Brown PO, and Johnston M. Characterization of three related glucose repressors and genes they regulate in *Saccharomyces cerevisiae*. Genetics. 1998; 150: 1377- 1391.

[54] Yin Z, Wilson S, Hauser NC, Tournu H, Hoheisel JD, and Brown AJP. Glucose triggers different global responses in yeast depending on the strength of the signal, and transiently stabilizes ribosomal protein mRNAs. Molecular Microbiology, 2003; 48: 713- 724.

[55] Rodaki A, Enjalbert B, Young T, Odds FC, Gow NAR, and Brown AJP. (2009) Glucose promotes stress resistances in the fungal pathogen, *Candida albicans*. Molecular Biology of the Cel. 2009; 22: 4845- 55.

[56] Mager WH and Planta J. Coordinate expression of ribosomal protein genes in yeast as a function of cellular growth rate. Molecular Cell Biochemistry. 1991; 104: 181- 187.

[57] Schüle T, Rose M, Entian KD, Thumm M, Wolf, DH. Ubc8p function in catabolite degradation of fructose-1, 6-bisphosphatase in yeast. EMBO Journal. 2000; 19: 2161-2167.

[58] Horak J, Regelmann J, and Wolf DH. Two distinct proteolytic systems responsible for glucose-induced degradation of fructose-1,6-bisphosphatase and the Gal2p transporter in the yeast *Saccharomyces cerevisiae* share the same protein components of the glucose signaling pathway. Journal of Biochemistry. 2002; 277: 8248- 8254.

[59] Hammerle M, Bauer J, Rose M, Szallies A, Thumm M, Dusterhus S, Mecke D, Entian KH, and Wolf DH. Protein of newly isolated mutants and the amino-terminal proline are essential for ubiquitin-proteasome-catalysed catabolite degradation of fructose-1,6-bisphosphatase of *Saccharomyces cerevisiae*. The American Society for Biochemistry and Molecular Biology. 1998; 25: 25000- 25005.

[60] Sosinska GJ, de Groot PWJ, de Mattos T, Dekker HL, de Koster CG, Hellingwerf KJ, and Klis FM. Hypoxic conditions and iron restriction affect the cell-wall proteome of *Candida albicans* grown under vagina-simulative condition. Microbiology. 2008; 154: 510- 520.

[61] Hube B, Stehr F, Bossenz M, Mazur A, Kretschmer M, and Schafer W. Secreted lipase of *Candida albicans*: cloning, characterisation and expression analysis of a new gene family with at least ten members. Archives of Microbiology. 2000; 174: 362- 374.

[62] Lorenz MC, Bender JA, and Fink GR. Transcriptional response of *Candida albicans* upon internationalization by macrophages. Eukaryotic Cell. 2004; 3: 1076- 1087.

[63] Sandai D, Yin Z, Selway L, Stead D, Walker J, Leach MD, Bohovych I, Ene IV, Kastora S, Budge S, Munro CA, Odds FC, Gow NA, and Brown AJP. The evolutionary rewiring of ubiquitination targets has reprogrammed the regulation of carbon assimilation in the pathogenic yeast *Candida albicans*. Microbiology. 2012; 11(3): e00495-e00512.

[64] Regelmann J, Schule T, Josupeit FS, Horak J, Rose M, Entian KD, Thumm M, and Wolf, DH. Catabolite degradation of fructose-1,6-bisphosphate in the yeast *Saccharomyces cerevisiae*: a genome-wide screen identifies eight novel GID genes and indicates the existence of two degradation pathways. Molecular Biology of the Cell. 2003; 14: 1652- 1663.

[65] Wickerham LJ. Taxonomy of yeast. Department Agriculture of Technical Bulletin. 1952; 1929: 1- 19.

[66] Williamson MI, Samaranayake LP, and Mac Farlane TW. Biotypes of *Candida albicans* using the AP1 20C System. FEMS Microbiology. 1986; 37: 27- 29.

[67] Rokas A and Hittinger CT. Transcription rewiring: the proof is in the eating. Current Biology. 2007; 17: 1007- 1013.

[68] Lorenz MC and Zhou H. Carnitine acetyltransferases are required for growth on non-fermentable carbon sources but not for pathogenesis in *Candida albicans*. Microbiology. 2003; 154: 500- 509.

[69] Johnson ES, Bartel B, Seufert W, and Varshavsky A. Ubiquitin as a degradation signal. EMBO Journal. 1992; 11: 497- 505.

[70] Hastie T, Tibshirani R, and Friedman JH. The elements of statistical learning: data mining, inference, and prediction. Vol. 58. New York, NY, Springer Verlag; 2001; 236-244.

[71] Hitchcock AL, Auld K, Gygi SP, and Silver PA. A subset of membrane-associated proteins is ubiquitinated in response to mutations in the endoplasmic reticulum degradation machinery. Proceedings of the National Academy Science USA. 2003; 100: 12735- 12740.

[72] Peng J, Schwartz D, Elias JE, Thoreen CC, Cheng D, Marsischky G, Roelofs J, Finley D, and Gygi SP. A proteomics approach to understanding protein ubiquitination. Nature Biotechnology. 2003; 21: 921- 926.

[73] Rost B, Liu J, Nair R, Wrzeszczynski K O, and Ofran Y. Automatic prediction of protein function. Cell Molecular of Life Science. 2003; 60: 2637- 2650.

[74] Leach MD, Stead DA, Argo E, MacCallum DM, and Brown AJP. Molecular and proteomic analyses highlight the importance of ubiquitination for the stress resistance, metabolic adaptation, morphogenetic regulation and virulence of *Candida albicans.* Molecular Microbiology. 2011; 10: 1365- 2958.

[75] Bertram G, Swoboda RK, Gow NAR, Gooday GW, and Brown AJP. Structure and regulation of the *Candida albicans ADH1* gene encoding an immunogenic alcohol dehydrogenase. Yeast. 1996; 12: 115- 128.

[76] Lorenz DR, Cantor CR, and Collins JJ. A network biology approach to aging in yeast. Proceedings of the National Academy Science USA. 2009; 106: 1145- 1150.

[77] Vargas SL, Patrick CC, Ayer GD, and Hughes WT. Modulating the effects of dieting carbohydrate supplementation on *Candida albicans* and invasion in neutropenic mouse. Infection and Immunity. 1993; 61: 619- 626.

[78] Rost B. Review: protein secondary structure predictions continue to rise. Journal of Structure Biology. 2001; 134: 204- 218.

[79] Lorenz MC and Fink GR. Life and death macrophage: role of the glycoxylate cycle in virulence. Eukaryotic Cell. 2002; 1: 657- 662.

[80] Lorenz MC, and Fink GR. The glyoxylate cycle is required for fungal virulence. Nature. 2001; 412: 83-86.

[81] Askew C, Sellam A, Epp E, Hogues H, Mullick A, Nantel A, and Whiteway M. Transcription regulation of carbohydrate metabolism in the human pathogen *Candida albicans.* PloS Pathogens. 2009; 5: e1000612.

[82] Sabina J and Brown V. Glucose sensing network in *Candida albicans*: a sweet spot for fungal morphogenesis. Eukaryotic Cells. 2009; 8: 1314- 1320.

[83] Horak J. Down-regulation of model yeast proteins by ubiquitin-dependent proteolysis. Physiology Research. 2004; 53: 99- 102.

[84] Nikolaou E. Phylogenetic diversity of fungal stress signalling pathways. PhD Thesis, University of Aberdeen Scotland. UK: 2009.

[85] Qin S, Nakajima B, Nomura M, and Arfin SM. Cloning and characterisation of a *Saccharomycess cerevisiae* gene encoding a new member of the ubiquitin-conjugating protein family. Journal of Biological Chemistry. 1991; 266: 15549- 15554.

[86] Hochstrasser M. Ubiquitin-dependent protein degradation. Annual Reviews Genetics. 1996; 30: 405- 439.

[87] Oh J, Fung E, Schlecht U, Davis RW, Giaever G, Onge R P, Deutschbauer A, and Nislow C. Gene annotation and drug target discovery in *Candida albicans* with a tagged transposon mutant collection. PLoS Pathogens. 2010; 6(10): 1001140.

[88] Khatib R, Riederer KM, Ramanathan J, and Baran Jr. J. Facel fungal flora in healthy volunteers and inpatients. Mycoses. 2001; 44: 151- 156.

[89] Leibovitz E. Neonatal consensus: clinical picture, management controversies and consensus, and new therapeutic options. Journal of Antimicrobial Chemotheraphy. 2002; 49 (Suppl. 1): 69-73.

Chapter 13

Infection and Infertility

Wei Wu, Qiuqin Tang, Hao Gu, Yiqiu Chen, Yankai Xia, Jiahao Sha and Xinru Wang

Additional information is available at the end of the chapter

http://dx.doi.org/10.5772/62500

Abstract

Infection is a multifactorial process, which can be induced by a virus, bacterium, or parasite. It may cause many diseases, including obesity, cancer, and infertility. In this chapter, we focus our attention on the association of infection and fertility alteration. Numerous studies have suggested that genetic polymorphisms influencing infection are associated with infertility. So we also review the genetic influence on infection and risk of infertility.

Keywords: infection, infertility, virus, bacterium, parasite, polymorphism, genetics

1. Introduction

The search for source of infection and infertility has been an active area of study for many years. Because the source of infection is complex, we divided the source of infection into three groups: virus, such as mumps virus, hepatitis B virus, human papillomavirus, herpes simplex virus, and human immunodeficiency virus; bacteria, such as *Chlamydia trachomatis* and *Helicobacter pylori*; and parasite, such as *Toxoplasma gondii*. First, we review the association of these infections and infertility. Because genetic influence may play important roles in regulating the infection in fertility, we also discuss the genetic effects on infertility, mainly the gene polymorphisms influencing infection and infertility in the following sections.

2. Infection and fertility alteration

2.1. Mumps virus infection and fertility

Even though Hippocrates described mumps many years ago and its vaccine has been available for long time, the disease continues to spread in the world. Mumps, a disease of droplet contact, is transmitted to the population via the respiratory tract. The viruses multiply in upper respiratory tract mucosa and are carried to the affinity organs, such as the inner ear, pancreas and mammary glands, testis, and ovaries. [1]

Mumps virus is an RNA virus, which causes inflammatory reactions. Infections of mumps virus cause a variable clinical symptom. At the very beginning of infection, the virus attacks the testes, destroying the testicular parenchyma and reducing androgen production. [2] Most commonly they lead to fever and parotitis, and about 30% of male adolescents with mumps will develop orchitis. [3] Because orchitis is the most common complication in men, the disease sometimes develops in adult patients.

Previous studies consisting of about 300 patients with mumps orchitis were carried out between 1951 and 1970. Following mumps orchitis, cytogenic deterioration, with regard to sperm morphology, is a long-lasting effect. Spermiogenesis was greatly disrupted in half of the patients. In many patients whose testes were not atrophied, poor fertility was found persistently. According to the observations, sperm morphology was the most influenced, of the characteristics that were studied, and sperm count might be the least affected. [4] In conclusion, mumps virus infection is a risk factor for male infertility.

2.2. Hepatitis B virus infection and infertility

Hepatitis B virus (HBV) is a double-stranded DNA virus, which is one of the most common viruses threatening health of human beings. [5] HBV infection has been a very serious public health problem worldwide, especially in Asia. HBV infection was found to be related to decreased instability of sperm chromosome, sperm function, [5] and impaired sperm viability and normal morphology. [6] Recent work has confirmed that sperm is possibly a vector for vertical transmission of HBV. [7] However, little is known about the influence of HBV infection on sperm functions, which is vital for the fertility of those HBV carriers.

In 1985, it was discovered that HBV DNA was in spermatozoa and proposed that HBV may be a cause of male infertility by damaging spermatozoa. [8] But the mechanisms of the HBV impacting on human sperm remain unclear. Therefore, the studies of the influences of viral proteins on sperm function and the explanation of the pathways involved are critically important for male reproduction. HBs is the main component of HBV envelope proteins, so its effects on sperm functions, such as motility, fertilizing ability of sperm, and the according pathways require full studies. [5] Other studies indicate that HBV infection induces adverse influence on sperm chromosomes. Fluorescence in situ hybridization technique can visualize HBV DNA sequences that integrate into sperm chromosomes. Consequently, HBV enters germ line of male and integrates into the genome. [8]

Results of some studies indicated that HBs were able to reduce the human sperm fertilizing ability by inducing loss of sperm mitochondrial membrane, which potentially leads to the decrease of sperm fertilizing ability. [9] With increased concentrations of HBs, sperm were found to lose mitochondrial membrane potential and have decreased sperm motility and sperm fertilizing ability was affected. However, the molecular mechanism of HB-induced reproduction dysfunction needs to be explored in the future.

HBV can be transmitted vertically to the offspring through the male germ line because HBV may do harm to sperm function. [8] Some observations concerning the viral infection indicate that woman carriers of HBV may have reduced fertility potential, but further work is needed to explore the field and understand the effect of chronic viral infection on the reproduction. [10] So more attention should be immediately paid to the patients with HBV infection in the aspect of reproductive health.

2.3. *Chlamydia trachomatis* infection and infertility

Chlamydia trachomatis is an intracellular bacterium and needs living cells to multiply. Its chromosome includes about 1 million base pairs. Identified serotypes of *C. trachomatis* are eighteen. This kind of bacterium's cell cycle is quite different from that of others. [11]

C. trachomatis infections are considered to be the most common sexually transmitted bacterial infections all over the world. [12] The infection cycle starts with the entry of an infectious particle into an epithelial cell. *Chlamydia* infections cause great medical, economic, and even social problems. To diagnose *C. trachomatis* infection, nucleic acid amplification tests are done. [13]

Many studies have studied the link between chlamydial infection and semen quality. Some *in vitro* and *in vivo* studies tried to study the relationship between chlamydial infection and markers in spermatozoa. The establishment of a causal relationship between chlamydia and male infertility would have important effects on public health. [12] However, *C. trachomatis* infections are more harmful to the reproductive health of women than to men.

C. trachomatis is one of the major causes of mucopurulent cervicitis, which leads to about three kinds of complications and pelvic inflammatory disease in female. [14] Chlamydial pelvic inflammatory disease (PID) is a significant preventable cause of infertility and bad pregnancy outcome. According to a study about chlamydial infection and women, significantly higher prevalences of IgA and IgG antibodies were found among individuals suffering from infertility. The results of polymerase chain reaction (PCR) testing indicated that the women with positive IgA and IgG antibodies might possibly have been infected with *C. trachomatis* before. However, this study had some limitations, such as many bias and small sample size. [15]

Consequently, additional studies are necessary to get more epidemiologic data about *C. trachomatis* infection and to formulate useful prevention and intervention actions such as health education among adolescents. When talking about the treatment of this infection, the use of azithromycin should be considered during pregnancy. Treatment of sex partners is vital for reducing the risk of re-test after treatment.

2.4. *Toxoplasma gondii* infection and infertility

Toxoplasma gondii is a very common protozoan parasite infecting warm-blooded animals, including both mice and humans. About one-third of the human population has been exposed to it. [16] Approximately 50% of the humans are infected and developed a disease named toxoplasmosis, which is one of the most common parasitic zoonoses throughout the world. In different regions within any country and among different population groups based on various social, cultural lifestyle, and environmental factors, the prevalence of *T. gondii* always varies. [17]

Some studies indicate that low socioeconomic status has contributed to *T. gondii* exposure. [18] Another risk factor of the exposure might be the consumption of raw fruits and vegetables that were contaminated with *T. gondii* oocysts. Globally, very limited amount of studies of the agricultural population about the prevalence of *T. gondii* infection are conducted by researchers. The goal of a study was to investigate the prevalence and possible risk factors of toxoplasmosis among female farmworkers in a region of Turkey. [17]

In adults, *T. gondii* does not cause serious diseases, but in women infected with *T.gondii*, life-threatening complications such as congenital disease or even abortion occurs in the developing fetus. [19] However, there were some relations between infection of *Toxoplasma* and the sperm quality in human population. Zhou et al. [20] found that *Toxoplasma* infection in infertile human couples was higher than that in fertile ones. It may be related to the antisperm antibodies that were higher in infected human couples. A recent research of *T. gondii* infection in men with sterility indicated that among the cases of man's sterility, some of them were serologically *Toxoplasma*-IgG, IgM, and CAg positive. It was concluded that *T. gondii* infection may influence men's fertility. [21] Lu et al. concluded that acute infection of *T. gondii* can cause male infertility, and Sun et al. [22] concluded that acute *T. gondii* infection can devastate the reproductive function of infected male mice experimentally. Researchers used rats to study the effect of toxoplasmosis on male reproduction and found that in the *Toxoplasma*-infected group, sperm motility was decreased significantly. However, in median sperm concentration, they did not find any significant difference in infected animals and controls. Results indicate that there is possibly a correlation between toxoplasmosis and disturbed reproduction in male rats. [23]

Furthermore, a large-scale experiment with greater amount of animals and generations will be required to study the significant effect statistically. [24] Based on current researches, control programs of *Toxoplasma* infection in many countries should be implemented. Faster and reliable diagnostic tests should also be developed for male and female. [17]

2.5. Human papillomavirus infection and infertility

It was estimated that the prevalence of human papillomavirus was at about 12% globally in 2012, [25, 26] despite licensure of HPV vaccines in over 50% of the countries. Recent data indicate that in the United States more than 10 million people are newly infected every year and 79 million people are currently affected. [27] Inconsistent vaccination rates may contribute to continuing prevalence of this virus. [28, 29] Furthermore, in 2010, the whole cost of preventing and treating HPV-associated disease was said to be $8.0 billion. [30] Consequently, more attention has to be paid to the HPV infection.

Over 100 HPV types could spread by skin-to-skin contact, including sex, oral sex, sexual intercourse, and other contacts, involving the skin surfaces and genitals. People are commonly susceptible to this virus distributing in the skin and mucous membranes. It has been estimated that more than 50% sexually active populations will acquire the HPV infection during their whole lifetime, [31] and the risk of infection increases with the lack of condom use, the number of sexual partners, and smoking. [32, 33] Majority of sexually active adults may possibly acquire HPV during their lifetime. Generally, with the increasing amount of lifetime sexual partners, the risk of developing illness caused by HPV increases. [30] The human papillomavirus is considered to be one of the most common sexually transmitted viruses affecting fertility.

HPV is a kind of pathogen that induces chronic infections without any specific symptoms. It is generally accepted that sexually transmitted viruses can cause some changes in infertility. According to a summary of findings, there are some effects of HPV on sperm parameters. For example, HPV infections can alter sperm motility. On the other hand, HPV may increase sperm DNA fragmentation and change semen pH. In general, studies indicate that HPV infection is a factor adversely affecting male fertility or even resulting in infertility.

The studies that report on the differences in sperm quality between uninfected and infected men are discordant. *In vitro* studies have demonstrated that after incubation with specific HR-HPV DNA, higher motility of normal spermatozoa was found. [34] Additionally, there have been quite different influences of seminal HPV infection on some sperm parameters; a few studies have demonstrated that in HPV-infected men, sperm motility decreased, but they do not provide significant information on which sperm parameter could indicate HPV infection.

However, there was no significant difference in sperm quality between HPV-infected men and the uninfected. A study suggests that the presence of HPV may not affect sperm quality. In another recent study, about 300 semen samples of male partners of couples treated by IVF were screened for the HR-HPV DNA infection. [34] Between infected and uninfected men, the HPV DNA infection did not differ significantly. That is to say, sperm quality does not be impaired by the presence of HPV.

It was interesting that HPV-infected couples with the help of assisted reproduction technique might have an increased risk of pregnancy loss compared with the controls, according to a study. [35] However, additional larger studies are necessary to demonstrate the findings before clinical application and support the possibility of reducing the risk of the infection by assisted reproductive technology (ART). [36] Surely, including HPV infection, there are a great amount of other factors that cause infertility. [37] Small sample sizes and limited range of HPV types tested may possibly explain the discrepancies. In conclusion, studies of diverse results will promote more discussions about the influences of HPV infection on infertility.

2.6. Herpes simplex virus (HSV) infection and infertility

The Herpesviridae family consists of over 200 species infecting birds, mammals, fish, and so on. [38] In accordance with the World Health Organization (WHO), about 90% of the Earth's population is infected by viruses of the Herpesviridae family. HSV can be categorized into two types: HSV-1 and HSV-2. Through direct contact with sites of viral shedding or with mucocutaneous fluids carrying the virus, individuals can contract HSV-1. HSV-1, the most prevalent virus among herpes viruses, is transmitted through oral secretions or sores, causing ocular and oral manifestations. Diseases caused by the virus are pharyngitis, tonsillitis, and gingivostomatitis, causing inflammation of the pharynx and tonsils and swelling of the gums. [39] During sexual contact with people having a genital HSV-2 infection, someone can get HSV-2 infection. Additionally, HSV-2 may possibly enhance the risk of acquiring HIV. Generally, someone infected with it does not know the infection is present in his/her body. When it induces symptoms, it is extremely painful.

Some studies have established the association between HSV infection and male infertility. By semen analysis, researchers compare mean sperm count and morphology of samples. Using real-time PCR method, researchers find a prevalence of HSV DNA in semen. [40] According to a study of 279 infertile women attending an *in vitro* fertilization and embryo transfer program, the positivity rate for HSV was about 6.30%. [41] In order to investigate the prevalence of HSV in the infertile men, a study used serologic testing and PCR to test semen and blood samples. The PCR results indicated that the prevalence of HSV in semen was about 12%. [39] However, more researches should be conducted to correctly compare infertile individuals with and without HSV.

HSV targets the reproductive system, and the infection among males and females leads to infertility problems, but the mechanism seems different in the two populations. As shown in transgenic mice and in some experiments, it seems to affect the semen in males. [42] Interestingly, there have been no specific semen parameter associated with the HSV infection so far. [43] In women, HSV infection is a risk factor for infertility. The causal relationship between the infection and infertility in males and females would be established through further researches.

2.7. *Helicobacter pylori* infection and infertility

Helicobacter pylori is a spiral-shaped, microaerophilic organism, a member of the genus *Helicobacter*, and infects humans, especially at the gastroduodenal tract level. [44] Its genome is as small as 1667 kb, its niche is restricted, and the genome expresses a small amount of metabolic events. However, due to specific virulence determinants, *H. pylori* has been able to establish an adaptive evolutionary machinery. [45]

H. pylori infection is not limited in the gastroduodenal tract; *H.pylori* infection causes other digestive illness too. In the 1990s, some epidemiological studies indicated that *H. pylori* infection might be related to extra-digestive diseases affecting the heart and the blood vessels; then further studies showed that the disorders associated with this infection also affect the oropharynx, skin, and various other systems, such as the respiratory, endocrine, immune, hemopoietic, and central nervous systems. [46, 47]

Recently, more and more evidence in the literature indicates that *H. pylori* infection seems to negatively influence the reproductive function. Moretti et al. first investigated the association of *H. pylori* infection and female infertility. They reported an increased prevalence of *H. pylori* infection in female patients with fertility disorders compared to controls. [48] Several years later, a Japanese retrospective survey including almost 200 female patients supported the observation. [49] Figura et al. reported that the anti–*H. pylori* antibody levels in serum samples were higher in individuals with reproductive disorders than in controls and suggested that the risk of infertility may be increased by *H. pylori* infection. [48] Furthermore, Moretti et al. [50] found that the prevalence of *H. pylori* infection was higher in male patients with fertility problems than in controls.

Through various mechanisms, such as the release of molecular mimicry, inflammatory mediators, and systemic immune response, *H. pylori* infection can directly or indirectly impair reproductive functions. [51] Before considering reproductive disorders as another manifestation of extra-digestive diseases related to *H. pylori* infection, it is significant to carry out further studies about the prevalence of *H. pylori* infection in patients and controls, and particularly to perform study evaluating reproductive potential after *H. pylori* infection. [50] Furthermore, biologic researches to explain the relationship between *H. pylori* infection and infertility are required.

2.8. Bacterial semen infection and infertility

Almost 15% of cases of male infertility can be explained by infections about genitourinary tract. [52] Both infections and inflammation in the male reproductive system may impair the sperm cell, function, and the overall spermatogenetic process, [53 – 55] altering qualitative and quantitative sperm.

The bacteria, viruses, and fungi that contribute to semen infection may be sexually transmitted or come from the urinary tract; their effect on impairing male fertility has already been discussed. [56]

The sperm bacterial contamination is very normal and might contribute to the impairment of semen quality in infertile patients. Some studies have investigated the effect of bacterial semen infection in male fertility, but the putative influence of bacteria on semen quality is still inconsistent. [57]

Bacteria can affect the male reproductive function directly, by reducing the acrosome reaction, causing the agglutination of motile sperm, and changing cell morphology, and indirectly, by producing reactive oxygen species caused by the inflammatory response to bacterial infection. [58] The negative effect of bacteria on sperm motility is known to all. [55, 59] The findings of Moretti et al. [60] show that in all groups except for in two, sperm motility was reduced significantly. Moretti et al. suggested that the existence of bacteria would possibly alter the sperm quality. In the positive group, the mean sperm concentration for bacteria was significantly less than that in controls, whereas the value was always considered normal for WHO. Findings reported by other researchers [53, 57] indicate that *Escherichia coli, Enterococcus faecalis,* and *Ureaplasma* urealyticum have negative influence on semen quality of infertile patients. Alterations frequently observed in spermatozoa attributed to bacteria in both *in vitro* and *in vivo* conditions are reduced sperm concentration, sperm morphological alterations, loss of motility, and impaired acrosome reactions.

However, there is no absolute agreement on the detrimental effect of bacteria in the semen. A research reported that the bacteria isolated from the genitourinary tracts of men do not have any influence on semen quality; however, bacteria always impaired the antioxidant ability of sperm in infertile patients with pathological semen parameters. [55]

The exact molecular mechanism that the male fertility is affected by bacteria infection is not only multifactorial but also complex, and it is still a puzzle. [60] More studies based on the molecular approach should be applied to this problem to provide new explanation to the microorganisms contacting with sperm and eventually monitoring the health of male genitourinary organs. In fact, re-evaluating sperm characteristics of patients treated would help to confirm the role of bacterial presence of the observed sperm abnormalities.

2.9. Human immunodeficiency virus infection and infertility

Initially, in the 1980s, human immunodeficiency virus (HIV) was found in the mononuclear cell fraction of the semen of one HIV-1-seropositive man and two men developing acquired immunodeficiency syndrome. [61] In the early period of the epidemic, those individuals diagnosed as HIV positive were not estimated to live a long life. [62] Since the HIV and AIDS were identified, in the management and long-term prognosis for infected people, vital advances have been made.

According to the WHO, about 75 million people have been infected with the HIV and more than 30 million humans have died of it. During the past 20 years, it has been extensively researched on the field of HIV infection, which invades the human immune system. In Sub-Saharan Africa remaining severely influenced, about 1 in 20 adults is infected by HIV and the number accounts for 71% of the infected people globally. [63]

With the appearance and especially the development of the immunodeficiency syndrome pandemic, attention of the sexual transmission of viruses in human population and its health effects has peaked accordingly. [61] HIV that causes AIDS is the most enormously studied virus among the sexually transmitted viruses. Some studies assessed the influence of HIV infection on sperm parameters in HIV-positive men. Researchers analyzed the association between markers of HIV infection and characteristics of semen. For example, a significant correlation between sperm count and CD4 cell count was demonstrated. Compared with fertile men, HIV-positive men's semen volume, sperm motility, and total sperm count were impaired. Dulioust et al. [64] investigated almost 200 HIV-infected men free from AIDS symptoms on the semen characteristics. Standardized methodology was used to analyze the semen samples collected. However, they did not observe any relation between HIV infection and semen characteristics. In the study of HIV-infected men, the semen changes may be not remarkable enough to affect fecundity greatly. The perfect study design of larger patient size is a longitudinal cohort study, which describes semen parameters during the development of an HIV infection. [65]

Studies showed that fertility was lower in HIV-1–infected women than the controls in Sub-Saharan Africa. It was the first time to suggest that HIV/AIDS was related to the fertility defects. [66] Recently, more studies indicate that fertility rates in HIV-infected women have decreased in the United States. [67] Among HIV-1–infected women, subfertility may be explained by biological alterations in reproductive physiology. Based on a reproductive endocrinology, HIV-infected women are more likely to have amenorrhea and protracted anovulation compared to the uninfected women. [68, 69] Many studies have linked HIV infection with premature ovarian failure. Additionally, pregnancy-related problems will continue after conception. In several clinical studies, it is more common that HIV-infected women may have pregnancy loss. [66] The correlation between HIV infection and infertility is a significant area for further research and investigation. The observations of those studies demonstrate that access to investigating infertility and treating HIV-positive individuals is very limited in many countries. Healthcare professionals who care for these patients must pay more attention to conduct effective strategies to change the situation. [62] Researchers should design more treatments to minimize the risk of HIV transmission and to better understand the influences HIV and its treatments have on reproductive competence and fertility. [66]

3. Genetics influence on infection and risk of infertility

About 7% of men from the general population are infertile and 11.3% of married women suffering from infertility. [70, 71] Genetic inheritance could influence risk of many diseases like infertility. Over the last two decades, the genes responsible for many rare reproductive disorders have been identified by genetic linkage mapping with multiple affected individuals. [72] In male infertility, a cause for infertility cannot be identified in almost half cases. Severe spermatogenesis impairment is likely a genetic condition in many male infertility cases. [73] In female infertility, genetic factors also contribute to risk of many diseases, such as uterine fibroids, endometriosis, and tubal damage. Common genetic variants in complex diseases are simpler to detect by population studies (case–control study). Genome-wide association study (GWAS) is a developed method to study the genetic variants in population-based studies. GWAS methods could provide a powerful approach for mapping disease gene. [74] Single nucleotide polymorphisms (SNP) array and next-generation sequencing (NGS) could provide critical new date on rare variants. More than 30 million SNPs that segregate in human population have been identified. Gene discoveries from GWAS may not provide results that translated immediately into the clinic. They are the starting point to understand disease biology and already provided novel insights into biological pathways and novel biomarkers. [74]

In previous part, we have reviewed the association of infection and infertility, since gene polymorphism could influence infertility and infection status could also been influenced by gene polymorphism; therefore, we summarize the literatures reporting genetics influence on infection and risk of infertility below, because male and female infertility have different causes and subgroups; here we discussed them in two aspects.

3.1. Gene polymorphism influence infection and risk of male infertility

Even though many articles have been reported the association of gene polymorphism with male infertility, the association between gene polymorphism influencing infection and male infertility is limited to only two reports. [75, 76] As we know, unique immune environment of the testis is very important for spermatogenesis. Cytokines play critical roles in the maintenance of immune environment of the testis. Members of the interleukin-1 (IL-1) family are pleiotropic cytokines involved in the regulation of junction dynamics during spermatogenesis and further increase on infection. Recently, the polymorphism of the human IL-1B gene (C + 3953T) has been reported to associate with male infertility in asthenozoospermic patients from an Indian population. [75] In that study, the author found that the genotype frequencies of the IL 1B Taq C/T polymorphism were significantly higher in asthenozoospermic patients

(OR=10.4; CI, 2.50–43.96). Meanwhile, the author also found the association of variable number tandem repeat (VNTR) polymorphism of the interleukin (IL)-1 receptor antagonist gene (ILRN) with male infertility before. [76] The study indicated that risk of IL1RN2 polymorphism with male infertility (OR=1.43; CI, 1.1546–1.7804). In these two articles, we can find that the polymorphisms of IL-1 were both studied in these articles. One reason might be that these two studies carried by one research group and another reason might be that IL-1 plays important roles in testicular microenvironment. However, the total numbers of male subjects recruited in these two studies were limited to 452–689. So, it may lack sufficient statistical data to show the real association. Besides, the males in these studies were all Indians; therefore, further confirmation of the association in other ethnic population are needed. In addition, interactions of gene–gene and gene–environment factors were not considered. Environmental exposure of some chemicals or habits and customs of subjects such as smoking or drinking could influence the association of gene polymorphism and infertility. [77, 78] So we have reason to believe that the infection status could also impact the association of polymorphism and risk of infertility. Subjects with the same polymorphisms but different infection status may have different risk of infertility. Similarly, subjects with the same infection status but different polymorphisms may also have different risks. Thus, more complete researches are needed to determine the association of genetic polymorphism influencing infection and risk of male infertility in different subgroups and different infection status.

The associations between gene polymorphism and male infertility have been relatively widely investigated. However, the associations of gene polymorphism influencing infection and risk of male infertility were rarely confirmed. This may be the reason that researchers often focus on the polymorphism of genes playing roles in spermatogenesis. Since infection could increase the risk of infertility, more gene polymorphisms influencing infection are needed to be confirmed to be associated with male infertility in the future.

3.2. Gene polymorphisms influence infection and risk of female infertility

Tubal factor infertility (TFI) is one of the most common female infertility, and chronic inflammation induced by *C. trachomatis* can lead to TFI. The immune response is linked to cytokine secretion pattern, which is influenced by the host genetic background. So the associations between polymorphism of cytokine and TFI have caused researchers' concern. The HLA systems control immune responses by representing antigenic epitopes to immune T cells. By analyzing HLA class II alleles (DQA1 and DQB1) and CHSP60-specific lymphoproliferative responses in TFI patients and healthy controls, Kinnunen et al. [79] found that DAQ1*0102 and DQB1*0602 alleles together with IL-10-1082AA genotype were more significantly frequently in the TFI patients. Cohen et al. [80] also found that HLA-DR1*1503 and DRB5*0101 alleles were more commonly in *C. trachomatis* microimmunofluorescence seronegative women with infertility, and these alleles may lead to an immunologically mediated mechanism of protection against *C. trachomatis* infection–induced TFI. In 2015, Jansen et al. [81] analyzed the association of HLA-A rs1655900: G>A and susceptibility of *C. trachomatis* infection in a STD cohort and found that the carriage of HLA-A rs1655900 has no effect on susceptibility but might be

http://dx.doi.org/10.5772/62500

protective to the development of late complications, especially tubal pathology could be relevant.

As one of the most important cytokines, the associations between IL polymorphisms and *C. trachomatis*–related female infertility also have been widely studied. To investigate the genetic basis of Chlamydia-associated infertility and various manifestations of tubal damage, Ohman et al. [82] studied polymorphisms in cytokine genes, including IL-10, interferon (IFN)-gamma, tumor necrosis factor (TNF)-alpha, transforming growth factor (TGF)-beta1, and IL-6, by a case–control study. The results suggested that IL-10 AA genotype and the TNF-alpha A-allele could increase the risk of severe tubal damage in women with *C. trachomatis* –related TFI. Meanwhile, in an *in vitro* study, to study the relationship between IL-10 promoter polymorphism and cell-mediated immune response, the researcher analyzed lymphocyte proliferation and cytokine, including IL-10, IFN-gamma, TNF-alpha, IL-2, IL-4, and IL-5, in subjects with different IL-10 genotypes. Results indicated that impaired cell-mediated response to *C. trachomatis* is associated with IL-10 genotype in subjects with high IL-10–producing capacity. [83] Unlike mentioned in male infertility, IL-B and IL-1RN gene polymorphisms are not associated with *C. trachomatis* –related TFI. [84] A polymorphism of NALP3 (gene symbol CIAS1) has been associated with decreased IL-1 levels and increased occurrence of vaginal Candida infection. Witkin et al. [85] selected women undergoing *in vitro* fertilization and tested polymorphism in intron 2 of the gene coding for NALP3 from their DNA. Researcher concluded that the CIAS1 7 unit repeat polymorphism could increase the likelihood of mycoplasma infection–associated female infertility.

Mannose-binding lectin (MBL) could activate the complement, modifies inflammation, and is involved in apoptotic cell clearance. [86] To study the role of MBL in tubal damage and female fertility, in 2010, Laisk et al. [87] performed a case–control study and found that MBL2 low-producing genotypes were associated with an increased incidence of pathogens associated with genital tract infections, hyper-producing MBL2 genotype HYA/HYA and low-producing MBL2 genotypes were associated with susceptibility to TFI, high-producing genotype HYA/LYA has a protective effect. In 2011, Laisk et al. [88] also compared four polymorphisms in MBL2 by a case–control study and found that the low-producing MBL2 genotypes were associated with susceptibility to TFI. Besides, the low-producing genotypes showed association of early pregnancy loss in IVF treatment.

Besides the most studied genetic polymorphisms, major histocompatibility complex class I chain–related A (MICA) gene is a potential host genetic candidate for *C. trachomatis* infections. To study the effect of MICA on the susceptibility to *C. trachomatis* infection and its association with tubal pathology, researcher selected 214 infertile women and found that women with tubal infertility more often had antibodies to *C. trachomatis*. Results suggested that the MICA locus might modify host susceptibility to *C. trachomatis* infection. [89]

From the literatures mentioned above, we can see that most of them are mainly in the study of TFI induced by *C. trachomatis*, the reason may be that *C. trachomatis* is the most common bacterial cause of sexually transmitted infections. [90] The numbers of subjects recruited in above studies are also limited (from 113 [79] to 811 [81]), and most of them were below 300 subjects. The mechanism of the genetic polymorphism is also limited. Besides, the interactions of these genetic polymorphisms were not carried in these studies. Thus, further study, including more detail mechanism and more subjects from different countries or race, is needed.

In conclusion, genetic inheritance influences the risk of many reproductive disorders; genetic polymorphism could also increase the risk of infertility. The studies demonstrating the polymorphisms influencing infection and infertility were relatively rare. To date, studies on reproductive and genetic inheritance have used relatively small samples. More and more cohorts have been established or in preparation, so further genetic maker studies in larger samples with detail phenotypes and clinical information should be considered into disease risk classification. Along with detail environment and gene information, gene–gene and gene–environment interactions also shall be added in further studies. Since GWAS method has been widely improved to study other diseases, we can carry out infection and infertility researches by GWAS, so more and more genetic polymorphisms influencing infection and risk of infertility can be found out in the future. The system researches can provide theoretical and experimental support for clinical diagnosis and treatment guide.

Author details

Wei Wu[1*], Qiuqin Tang[2], Hao Gu[1], Yiqiu Chen[1], Yankai Xia[1], Jiahao Sha[3] and Xinru Wang[1*]

*Address all correspondence to: wwu@njmu.edu.cn; xrwang@njmu.edu.cn

1 State Key Laboratory of Reproductive Medicine, Department of Toxicology, School of Public Health, Nanjing Medical University, Nanjing, China

2 State Key Laboratory of Reproductive Medicine, Department of Obstetrics, Nanjing Maternity and Child Health Care Hospital Affiliated to Nanjing Medical University, Nanjing, China

3 State Key Laboratory of Reproductive Medicine, Nanjing Medical University, Nanjing, China

References

[1] Kanda, T. *et al.* Case of mumps orchitis after vaccination. *International Journal of Urology* 21, 426–428 (2014). doi:10.1111/iju.12305.

[2] Whyte, D. *et al.* Mumps epidemiology in the mid-west of Ireland 2004–2008: increasing disease burden in the university/college setting. *Euro surveillance : bulletin Europeen sur les maladies transmissibles = European communicable disease bulletin* 14, 11–15, (2009). pii:19182.

[3] Otto, W. *et al.* Ongoing outbreak of mumps affecting adolescents and young adults in Bavaria, Germany, August to October 2010. *Euro surveillance : bulletin Europeen sur les maladies transmissibles = European communicable disease bulletin* 15, 21–24, (2010).pii: 19748.

[4] Bartak, V. Sperm count, morphology and motility after unilateral mumps orchitis. *Journal of Reproduction and Fertility* 32, 491–494 (1973).

[5] Zhou, X. L. *et al.* Effects of hepatitis B virus S protein on human sperm function. *Human Reproduction* 24, 1575–1583 (2009). doi:10.1093/humrep/dep050.

[6] Huang, J. M. *et al.* Effects of hepatitis B virus infection on human sperm chromosomes. *World Journal of Gastroenterology* 9, 736–740 (2003).

[7] Huang, J. M. *et al.* Studies on the integration of hepatitis B virus DNA sequence in human sperm chromosomes. *Asian Journal of Andrology* 4, 209–212 (2002).

[8] Bu, Z. *et al.* Effect of male hepatitis B virus infection on outcomes of in vitro fertilization and embryo transfer treatment: insights from couples undergoing oocyte donation. *International Journal of Clinical and experimental Medicine* 7, 1860–1866 (2014).

[9] Hadchouel, M. *et al.* Presence of HBV DNA in spermatozoa: a possible vertical transmission of HBV via the germ line. *Journal of Medical Virology* 16, 61–66 (1985).

[10] Englert, Y. *et al.* Medically assisted reproduction in the presence of chronic viral diseases. *Human Reproduction Update* 10, 149–162 (2004). doi:10.1093/humupd/dmh013.

[11] Paavonen, J. & Eggert-Kruse, W. Chlamydia trachomatis: impact on human reproduction. *Human Reproduction Update* 5, 433–447 (1999).

[12] Joki-Korpela, P. *et al.* The role of Chlamydia trachomatis infection in male infertility. *Fertility and sterility* 91, 1448–1450 (2009). doi:10.1016/j.fertnstert.2008.06.051.

[13] Black, C. M. Current methods of laboratory diagnosis of Chlamydia trachomatis infections. *Clinical Microbiology Reviews* 10, 160–184 (1997).

[14] Mardh, P. A., Ripa, T., Svensson, L. & Westrom, L. Chilamydia trachomatis infection in patients with acute salpingitis. *The New England Journal of Medicine* 296, 1377–1379 (1977). doi:10.1056/NEJM197706162962403.

[15] Siemer, J. *et al.* Chlamydia trachomatis infection as a risk factor for infertility among women in Ghana, West Africa. *The American Journal of Tropical Medicine and Hygiene* 78, 323–327 (2008).

[16] Hill, D. & Dubey, J. P. Toxoplasma gondii: transmission, diagnosis and prevention. *Clinical Microbiology and Infection* 8, 634–640 (2002). pii: S1198-743X(14)62509-X.

[17] Yentur Doni, N., Simsek, Z., Gurses, G., Yildiz Zeyrek, F. & Demir, C. Prevalence and associated risk factors of Toxoplasma gondii in female farmworkers of southeastern

Turkey. *Journal of Infection in Developing Countries* 9, 87–93 (2015). doi:10.3855/jidc.5824.

[18] Alvarado-Esquivel, C., Campillo-Ruiz, F. & Liesenfeld, O. Seroepidemiology of infection with Toxoplasma gondii in migrant agricultural workers living in poverty in Durango, Mexico. *Parasites & Vectors* 6, 113 (2013). doi:10.1186/1756-3305-6-113.

[19] Montoya, J. G. & Remington, J. S. Management of Toxoplasma gondii infection during pregnancy. *Clinical Infectious Diseases* 47, 554–566 (2008). doi:10.1086/590149.

[20] Zhou, Y. H. *et al.* [Survey of infection of Toxoplasma gondii in infertile couples in Suzhou countryside]. *Zhonghua nan ke xue = National Journal of Andrology* 8, 350–352 (2002).

[21] Qi, R., Su, X. P., Gao, X. L. & Liang, X. L. [Toxoplasma infection in males with sterility in Shenyang, China]. *Zhonghua nan ke xue = National Journal of Andrology* 11, 503–504 (2005).

[22] Sun, L. H., Fan, F., Wang, J. J. & Gong, J. [Acute Toxoplasma gondii infection affects the reproductive function of male mice]. *Zhonghua nan ke xue = National journal of andrology* 14, 55–57 (2008).

[23] Terpsidis, K. I. *et al.* Toxoplasma gondii: reproductive parameters in experimentally infected male rats. *Experimental Parasitology* 121, 238–241 (2009). doi:10.1016/j.exppara.2008.11.006.

[24] Dvorakova-Hortova, K. *et al.* Toxoplasma gondii decreases the reproductive fitness in mice. *PloS One* 9, e96770 (2014). doi:10.1371/journal.pone.0096770.

[25] Markowitz, L. E. *et al.* Human papillomavirus vaccine introduction--the first five years. *Vaccine* 30 Suppl 5, F139–148 (2012). doi:10.1016/j.vaccine.2012.05.039.

[26] Noronha, A. S., Markowitz, L. E. & Dunne, E. F. Systematic review of human papillomavirus vaccine coadministration. *Vaccine* 32, 2670–2674 (2014). doi:10.1016/j.vaccine.2013.12.037.

[27] Dunne, E. F. *et al.* CDC grand rounds: Reducing the burden of HPV-associated cancer and disease. *Morbidity and Mortality Weekly Report* 63, 69–72 (2014). pii: mm6304a1.

[28] Brisson, M., Drolet, M. & Malagon, T. Inequalities in Human Papillomavirus (HPV)-associated cancers: implications for the success of HPV vaccination. *Journal of the National Cancer Institute* 105, 158–161 (2013). doi:10.1093/jnci/djs638.

[29] Jeudin, P., Liveright, E., Del Carmen, M. G. & Perkins, R. B. Race, ethnicity, and income factors impacting human papillomavirus vaccination rates. *Clinical Therapeutics* 36, 24–37 (2014). doi:10.1016/j.clinthera.2013.11.001.

[30] Pereira, N. *et al.* Human Papillomavirus infection, infertility, and assisted reproductive outcomes. *Journal of Pathogens* 2015, 578423 (2015). doi:10.1155/2015/578423.

[31] Stanley, M. Pathology and epidemiology of HPV infection in females. *Gynecol Oncol* 117, S5–10 (2010). doi:10.1016/j.ygyno.2010.01.024.

[32] Goldstone, S. *et al.* Prevalence of and risk factors for human papillomavirus (HPV) infection among HIV-seronegative men who have sex with men. *The Journal of Infectious Diseases* 203, 66–74 (2011). doi:10.1093/infdis/jiq016.

[33] Nyitray, A. G. *et al.* Age-specific prevalence of and risk factors for anal human papillomavirus (HPV) among men who have sex with women and men who have sex with men: the HPV in men (HIM) study. *The Journal of Infectious Diseases* 203, 49–57 (2011). doi:10.1093/infdis/jiq021.

[34] Golob, B. *et al.* High HPV infection prevalence in men from infertile couples and lack of relationship between seminal HPV infection and sperm quality. *BioMed Research International* 2014, 956901 (2014). doi:10.1155/2014/956901.

[35] Perino, A. *et al.* Human papillomavirus infection in couples undergoing in vitro fertilization procedures: impact on reproductive outcomes. *Fertility and Sterility* 95, 1845–1848 (2011). doi:10.1016/j.fertnstert.2010.11.047.

[36] Garolla, A. *et al.* Human papillomavirus sperm infection and assisted reproduction: a dangerous hazard with a possible safe solution. *Human Reproduction* 27, 967–973 (2012). doi:10.1093/humrep/des009.

[37] Yang, Y., Jia, C. W., Ma, Y. M., Zhou, L. Y. & Wang, S. Y. Correlation between HPV sperm infection and male infertility. *Asian Journal of Andrology* 15, 529–532 (2013). doi:10.1038/aja.2013.36.

[38] Cardone, G., Heymann, J. B., Cheng, N., Trus, B. L. & Steven, A. C. Procapsid assembly, maturation, nuclear exit: dynamic steps in the production of infectious herpesvirions. *Advances in Experimental Medicine and Biology* 726, 423–439 (2012). doi:10.1007/978-1-4614-0980-9_19.

[39] Kapranos, N., Petrakou, E., Anastasiadou, C. & Kotronias, D. Detection of herpes simplex virus, cytomegalovirus, and Epstein-Barr virus in the semen of men attending an infertility clinic. *Fertility and Sterility* 79 Suppl 3, 1566–1570 (2003). doi:S0015028203003704.

[40] Amirjannati, N. *et al.* Molecular and serologic diagnostic approaches; the prevalence of herpes simplex in idiopathic men infertile. *Iranian Journal of Reproductive Medicine* 12, 327–334 (2014).

[41] Dereli, D. *et al.* Screening for herpes simplex virus in infertile women. *Genitourinary Medicine* 71, 131–132 (1995).

[42] Huttner, K. M., Pudney, J., Milstone, D. S., Ladd, D. & Seidman, J. G. Flagellar and acrosomal abnormalities associated with testicular HSV-tk expression in the mouse. *Biology of Reproduction* 49, 251–261 (1993).

[43] el Borai, N. *et al.* Detection of herpes simplex DNA in semen and menstrual blood of individuals attending an infertility clinic. *Journal of Obstetrics and Gynaecology Research* 23, 17–24 (1997).

[44] Goodwin, C. S. & Worsley, B. W. Microbiology of Helicobacter pylori. *Gastroenterology Clinics of North America* 22, 5–19 (1993).

[45] Fraser, C. M. *et al.* Genomic sequence of a Lyme disease spirochaete, Borrelia burgdorferi. *Nature* 390, 580–586 (1997). doi:10.1038/37551.

[46] Figura, N. *et al.* Extragastric manifestations of Helicobacter pylori infection. *Helicobacter* 15 Suppl 1, 60–68 (2010). doi:10.1111/j.1523-5378.2010.00778.x.

[47] Franceschi, F., Gasbarrini, A., Polyzos, S. A. & Kountouras, J. Extragastric Diseases and Helicobacter pylori. *Helicobacter* 20 Suppl 1, 40–46 (2015). doi:10.1111/hel.12256.

[48] Figura, N. *et al.* Helicobacter pylori infection and infertility. *European Journal of Gastroenterology & Hepatology* 14, 663–669 (2002).

[49] Kurotsuchi, S. *et al.* The plausibility of Helicobacter pylori-related infertility in Japan. *Fertility and Sterility* 90, 866–868 (2008).doi:10.1016/j.fertnstert.2007.06.097.

[50] Moretti, E., Figura, N., Collodel, G. & Ponzetto, A. Can Helicobacter pylori infection influence human reproduction? *World Journal of Gastroenterology* 20, 5567–5574 (2014). doi:10.3748/wjg.v20.i19.5567.

[51] de Korwin, J. D. [Does Helicobacter pylori infection play a role in extragastric diseases?]. *La Presse medicale* 37, 525–534 (2008). doi:10.1016/j.lpm.2007.07.029.

[52] Pellati, D. *et al.* Genital tract infections and infertility. *European journal of obstetrics, gynecology, and reproductive biology* 140, 3–11 (2008). doi:10.1016/j.ejogrb.2008.03.009.

[53] Henkel, R. & Schill, W. B. Sperm separation in patients with urogenital infections. *Andrologia* 30 Suppl 1, 91–97 (1998).

[54] Urata, K. *et al.* Effect of endotoxin-induced reactive oxygen species on sperm motility. *Fertility and Sterility* 76, 163–166 (2001). pii:S0015-0282(01)01850-7.

[55] Sanocka-Maciejewska, D., Ciupinska, M. & Kurpisz, M. Bacterial infection and semen quality. *Journal of Reproductive Immunology* 67, 51–56 (2005). doi:10.1016/j.jri.2005.06.003.

[56] Haidl, G. Macrophages in semen are indicative of chronic epididymal infection. *Archives of andrology* 25, 5–11 (1990).

[57] Fraczek, M. & Kurpisz, M. Mechanisms of the harmful effects of bacterial semen infection on ejaculated human spermatozoa: potential inflammatory markers in semen. *Folia histochemica et cytobiological/Polish Academy of Sciences, Polish Histochemical and Cytochemical Society* 53, 201–217 (2015). doi:10.5603/fhc.a2015.0019.

[58] Tremellen, K. Oxidative stress and male infertility--a clinical perspective. *Human reproduction update* 14, 243–258 (2008). doi:10.1093/humupd/dmn004.

[59] Fraczek, M., Szumala-Kakol, A., Jedrzejczak, P., Kamieniczna, M. & Kurpisz, M. Bacteria trigger oxygen radical release and sperm lipid peroxidation in in vitro model of semen inflammation. *Fertility and Sterility* 88, 1076–1085 (2007). doi:10.1016/j.fertnstert.2006.12.025.

[60] Moretti, E. *et al.* The presence of bacteria species in semen and sperm quality. *Journal of Assisted Reproduction and Genetics* 26, 47–56 (2009). doi:10.1007/s10815-008-9283-5.

[61] Dejucq, N. & Jegou, B. Viruses in the mammalian male genital tract and their effects on the reproductive system. *Microbiology and Molecular Biology Reviews* 65, 208–231 (2001); first and second pages, table of contents. doi:10.1128/MMBR.65.2.208-231.2001.

[62] Yudin, M. H., Shapiro, H. M. & Loutfy, M. R. Access to infertility services in Canada for HIV-positive individuals and couples: a cross-sectional study. *Reproductive Health* 7, 7 (2010). doi:10.1186/1742-4755-7-7.

[63] Chatterjee, A. N., Saha, S. & Roy, P. K. Human immunodeficiency virus/acquired immune deficiency syndrome: Using drug from mathematical perceptive. *World Journal of Virology* 4, 356–364 (2015). doi:10.5501/wjv.v4.i4.356.

[64] Dulioust, E. *et al.* Semen alterations in HIV-1 infected men. *Human Reproduction* 17, 2112–2118 (2002).

[65] van Leeuwen, E., van Weert, J. M., van der Veen, F. & Repping, S. The effects of the human immunodeficiency virus on semen parameters and intrauterine insemination outcome. *Human Reproduction* 20, 2033–2034; author reply 2034–2035 (2005). 10.1093/humrep/deh875.

[66] Kushnir, V. A. & Lewis, W. Human immunodeficiency virus/acquired immunodeficiency syndrome and infertility: emerging problems in the era of highly active antiretrovirals. *Fertility and sterility* 96, 546–553 (2011). doi:10.1016/j.fertnstert.2011.05.094.

[67] Massad, L. S. *et al.* Pregnancy rates and predictors of conception, miscarriage and abortion in US women with HIV. *AIDS* 18, 281–286 (2004). pii: 00002030-200401230-00018.

[68] Chirgwin, K. D., Feldman, J., Muneyyirci-Delale, O., Landesman, S. & Minkoff, H. Menstrual function in human immunodeficiency virus-infected women without acquired immunodeficiency syndrome. *J Acquired Immune Deficiency Syndromes and Human Retrovirology* 12, 489–494 (1996).

[69] Cejtin, H. E. *et al.* Effects of human immunodeficiency virus on protracted amenorrhea and ovarian dysfunction. *Obstetrics & Gynecology*108, 1423–1431 (2006). 10.1097/01.AOG.0000245442.29969.5c.

[70] Krausz, C., Escamilla, A. R. & Chianese, C. Genetics of male infertility: from research to clinic. *Reproduction* 150, R159–174 (2015). doi:10.1530/REP-15-0261.

[71] Briceag, I. *et al.* Fallopian tubes--literature review of anatomy and etiology in female infertility. *Journal of Medicine and Life* 8, 129–131 (2015).

[72] Botstein, D. & Risch, N. Discovering genotypes underlying human phenotypes: past successes for mendelian disease, future approaches for complex disease. *Nature Genetics* 33 Suppl, 228–237 (2003). doi:10.1038/ng1090.

[73] Aston, K. I. Genetic susceptibility to male infertility: news from genome-wide association studies. *Andrology* 2, 315–321 (2003). doi:10.1111/j.2047-2927.2014.00188.x.

[74] Montgomery, G. W., Zondervan, K. T. & Nyholt, D. R. The future for genetic studies in reproduction. *Molecular Human Reproduction*20, 1–14 (2014). doi:10.1093/molehr/gat058

[75] Jaiswal, D., Trivedi, S., Agrawal, N. K., Singh, R. & Singh, K. Association of interleukin-1beta C + 3953T gene polymorphism with human male infertility. *Systems Biology in Reproductive Medicine* 59, 347–351 (2013). doi:10.3109/19396368.2013.830234.

[76] Jaiswal, D., Trivedi, S., Singh, R., Dada, R. & Singh, K. Association of the IL1RN gene VNTR polymorphism with human male infertility. *PLoS One* 7, e51899 (2012). doi: 10.1371/journal.pone.0051899.

[77] Huo, X. *et al.* Bisphenol-A and female infertility: a possible role of gene-environment interactions. *International Journal of Environmental Research and Public Health* 12, 11101–11116 (2015). doi:10.3390/ijerph120911101.

[78] Yarosh, S. L., Kokhtenko, E. V., Starodubova, N. I., Churnosov, M. I. & Polonikov, A. V. Smoking status modifies the relation between CYP1A1*2C gene polymorphism and idiopathic male infertility: the importance of gene-environment interaction analysis for genetic studies of the disease. *Reproductive Sciences* 20, 1302–1307 (2015). doi: 10.1177/1933719113483013.

[79] Kinnunen, A. H. *et al.* HLA DQ alleles and interleukin-10 polymorphism associated with Chlamydia trachomatis-related tubal factor infertility: a case-control study. *Human Reproduction* 17, 2073–2078 (2002).

[80] Cohen, C. R. *et al.* Immunogenetic correlates for Chlamydia trachomatis-associated tubal infertility. *Obstetrics & Gynecology* 101, 438–444 (2003). pii:S0029784402030776.

[81] Jansen, M. E., Brankovic, I., Spaargaren, J., Ouburg, S. & Morre, S. A. Potential protective effect of a G>A SNP in the 3'UTR of HLA-A for Chlamydia trachomatis symptomatology and severity of infection. *Pathogens and Disease* (2016). doi:10.1093/femspd/ftv116.

[82] Ohman, H. *et al.* Cytokine polymorphisms and severity of tubal damage in women with Chlamydia-associated infertility. *Journal of Infectious Diseases* 199, 1353–1359 (2009). doi:10.1086/597620.

[83] Ohman, H. *et al.* IL-10 polymorphism and cell-mediated immune response to Chlamydia trachomatis. *Genes & Immunity* 7, 243–249 (2006). doi:10.1038/sj.gene.6364293.

[84] Murillo, L. S. *et al.* Interleukin-1B (IL-1B) and interleukin-1 receptor antagonist (IL-1RN) gene polymorphisms are not associated with tubal pathology and Chlamydia trachomatis-related tubal factor subfertility. *Human Reproduction* 18, 2309–2314 (2003).

[85] Witkin, S. S. *et al.* Genetic polymorphism in an inflammasome component, cervical mycoplasma detection and female infertility in women undergoing in vitro fertilization. *Journal of Reproductive Immunology* 84, 171–175 (2010). doi:10.1016/j.jri.2009.11.005.

[86] Dommett, R. M., Klein, N. & Turner, M. W. Mannose-binding lectin in innate immunity: past, present and future. *Tissue Antigens* 68, 193–209 (2006). doi:10.1111/j.1399-0039.2006.00649.x.

[87] Laisk, T. *et al.* Association of CCR5, TLR2, TLR4 and MBL genetic variations with genital tract infections and tubal factor infertility. *Journal of Reproductive Immunology* 87, 74–81 (2010). doi:10.1016/j.jri.2010.06.001.

[88] Laisk, T., Peters, M. & Salumets, A. Mannose-binding lectin genotypes: potential role in tubal damage and adverse IVF outcome. *Journal of Reproductive Immunology* 92, 62–67 (2011). doi:10.1016/j.jri.2011.09.004.

[89] Mei, B. *et al.* Association of MICA gene polymorphisms with Chlamydia trachomatis infection and related tubal pathology in infertile women. *Human Reproduction* 24, 3090–3095 (2009). doi:10.1093/humrep/dep339.

[90] Paavonen, J. Chlamydia trachomatis infections of the female genital tract: state of the art. *Annals of Medicine* 44, 18–28 (2012). doi:10.3109/07853890.2010.546365.

Section 4

Veterinary Genital Tract Infections

Chapter 14

Infection and Infertility in Mares

K. Satué and J.C. Gardon

Additional information is available at the end of the chapter

http://dx.doi.org/10.5772/63741

Abstract

In cyclic mares, the uterine environment can easily disturbed due to inflammatory processes that occur secondary to microbial invasion. Different aerobic and anaerobic bacteria can enter the uterus during natural mating, artificial insemination, reproductive examination or parturition. The postpartum period is a critical phase since due to relaxation of the uterus and cervix may favor recurrent infections air intake (pneumovagina) or urine collection in mares with poor perineal conformation. Infections are mainly caused by opportunistic or commensal microorganisms, such as *Streptococcus zooepidemicus, hemolytic Escherichia coli* and *Staphylococcus aureus*. Other microorganisms like *Taylorella equigenitalis, Klebsiella pneumoniae* and *Pseudomona aeruginosa* are transmitted through venereal route. Regarding to the fungal endometritis, the most common fungi include *Candida* and *Aspergillus*. These microorganisms cause infertility as a result of repeated inseminations during the breeding season and proliferate when the natural immune system is weakened in mares with advanced age and multiparous, or after repeated use of antibiotics. Indeed, in susceptible mare to endometritis, uterine defense mechanisms involving phagocytosis and opsonization by neutrophils, local synthesis of antibodies, mucociliary activity, vascular and myoelectric activity permeability are compromised, leading to fluid accumulation in response to inflammation and infertility.

Keywords: cycling mare, infectious diseases, reproduction

1. Introduction

The ability to maintain a uterine environment compatible with embryonic and fetal life is essential for reproductive efficiency in horses. However, the uterine environment is easily disturbed by an inflammatory process following aerobic and anaerobic bacterial invasion, which can occur during natural breeding, artificial insemination (AI), reproductive examination, parturition, postnatal infection (pneumovaginal infections), and mostly during a delayed postnatal cleaning of the uterus as a result of poor conformation [1].

These bacterial uterine infections cause conception and embryo survival failures despite many repeated breeding during the season. In the horse industry, endometritis due to uterine infectious of bacterial origin brings about 25–60% economic losses, leading to infertility. In pregnant mares, these infectious diseases can appear as failure to conceive, early fetal losses, mid-gestational abortion, placentitis, birth of a septic neonate, postpartum metritis, or delays in rebreeding and can be related with other systemic pathologies of viral, bacterial, and fungal origin [2]. Besides in nonpregnant mares, these infections are most often caused by opportunistic or commensal and venereal microorganisms, with a large variety of species have been isolated.

The healthy mare has three functional genital seals forming a barrier between the external environment and the uterine lumen [3, 4].

- Lips of vulva: examination of vulvar and perineal conformation should be included in all prebreeding examinations or evaluations for infertility. The vulva should be a vertical position aligned with the anal opening. The labia should be tight, with most of length below the tuber ischii. The vulvar lips may become parted as a consequence of malformation caused by previous traumatic injuries. In older multiparous mares, there is a tendency for extreme relaxation of the vulvar lips, particularly during estrus, as well as tilting of the dorsal aspect of the vulva becomes horizontal as it is pulled cranially over the tuber ischii. These anatomic changes predispose the mare to pneumavagina (windsucking) and pneumouterus, ultimately causing urine to pool in the cranial vagina producing ascending infection and contaminate the uterus when the cervix is open. Pneumovagina may lead to an urovagina (urine pooling within the vagina) when the vestibule and urethral opening are displaced cranially. In this situation, contamination with fecal material adds to the increased risk of infection.

- Vulvovaginal constriction: immediately in front of the external urethral opening is the vulvovaginal constriction or vestibular seal. In genitally healthy mares, this forms the second line of defense against aspirated air and fecal material. In a normal mare, the vestibulovaginal area remains sealed even when the vulvar labia are parted. Compromised vestibulovaginal sphincter function is suspected when air is sucked into the vagina of compromised secondary to rectovaginal tears and other foaling injuries.

- Cervix: forms the important third (and last) protective physical barrier to protect the uterus from the external environment. The cervix must also relax during estrus to allow intrauterine ejaculation or insemination of semen and drainage of uterine fluid, late pregnancy, and the immediate postpartum period. An inflammation of the cervix is usually associated with endometritis and/or vaginitis.

If the closure of the vulva is compromised, it results in the development of a pneumovagina with consequent aspiration of bacteria and other contaminated products [5]. The initial development of vaginitis can result in cervicitis and acute endometritis and therefore can lead subfertility. Usually, in mares, contamination of the caudal reproductive tract with bacteria during pregnancy can result in embryonic death. In late pregnancy, it can result in the development of placentitis and abortion [4, 6].

http://dx.doi.org/10.5772/63741

The more severe conformational abnormalities result in failure of the vulval closing, increasing fecal contamination since the vulva forms a platform in which feces can collect. In these cases, the vulval lips are angled at 25° for even 50° to the vertical. According to Bradecamp [6], defective vulval conformation can be:

- Congenital, rare to find.
- Acquired, which is due to vulval enlarging resulting for the repeated foaling, injury to perineal tissue and poor body condition (old, thin mares). Older and pluriparous mares are frequently affected with pneumovagina. However, in cases of young mares that are in work and have little body fat and/or poor vulval conformation, it can develop these pathology.

Pneumovagina might occur during estrus when the perineal tissues are more relaxed. Some mares make a noise while walking; however, the diagnosis of other mares may be difficult by the absence of noises. The pathognomonic sign is the presence of hyperemia and a frothy exudate in the anterior vagina, on examination with a speculum. Poor cervical dilation may reduce uterine clearance, while cervical damage or incompetence may predispose to infection. Finally, susceptible mares may accumulate more fluid within their uterus than normal mares because of a greater production of glandular secretions secondary to inflammation. The consequence of decreased physical clearance is that bacteria, inflammatory by-products and fluid remain in the uterine lumen, inducing more inflammation, mucosal cell damage, and fibrosis. The persistent inflammation may result in premature luteolysis. Ultimately, chronic inflammation results in degenerative changes within the endometrium and reduced fertility [5–7].

Real-time ultrasound examination of the uterus may reveal the presence of air or urine as hyperechoic or hypoechoic foci seen at the opposed luminal surfaces, respectively. Cytological and histological examination of the endometrium may demonstrate significant numbers of neutrophils indicative of an endometritis [6]. The clinical presentation of acute or chronic reproductive tract infections in the mare is salpingitis, cervicitis, and vaginitis [2, 5].

2. Vulvitis, vaginitis, and cervicitis

Vulvitis (inflammation of the vulva), vaginitis (inflammation of the vagina), and cervicitis (inflammation of the cervix) can develop due to different reasons such as difficult labor, chronic contamination of the reproductive tract due to poor conformation, sexually transmitted diseases, or mating. Bruises and hematomas (a pool of blood under the surface of the skin) of the vagina may be found in mares following delivery of a foal. Severe inflammation of the vulva and vagina, including local tissue death, may also occur [8]. Infectious vaginitis and cervicitis may occur as part of the uterine infection process or as a result of local irritation or laceration. Vaginal injuries secondary to breeding or parturition may lead to abscess formation and adhesions [9].

The sinus and fossa clitoral (the folded lining near the clitoris) should always be considered as a location of bacterial growth. The clitoral swabs are taken from the clitoral fossa and the clitoral sinuses to rule out acquired *Pseudomonas aeruginosa*, *Klebsiella pneumoniae*, and *Taylorella equigenitalis*. The signs of severe inflammation can include an arched back, elevated tail, poor appetite, straining, swelling of the vulva, and a foul smelling, watery discharge. Signs begin 1–4 days after birth and last for 2–4 weeks. In most cases, supportive care and treatment with antibiotics are sufficient [10].

Among causes that produce infectious vulvitis and vaginitis include contamination by *P. aeruginosa* and *K. pneumoniae* or venereal transmission produced by equine coital exanthema, contagious equine metritis (CEM), and dourine. Although the primary route of transmission is venereal, outbreaks have been documented in which transmission occurred through contaminated supplies and instruments or by the use of a single glove for rectal examination of many mares [11].

P. aeruginosa and *K. pneumoniae* cervicitis can be spread between horses by venereal transmission. Bacteriological studies should be routinely performed on recently introduced mares and stallions to prevent such infections. Culture is also indicated if there is an increased incidence of endometritis on a stud farm. Pre- and post-ejaculation urethral swabs and semen obtained from stallions should be cultured. Routine washing of the stallion penis with antiseptic solution before and after breeding is contraindicated because it may disturb the normal bacterial flora of the penile surface and promote growth of these pathogenic bacteria [1, 12]. Mares infected with *P. aeruginosa* and *K. pneumoniae* discharge greenish-tinged pus with a sweet "grape-like" odor by endometritis.

Equine coital exanthema is a benign venereal disease caused by equine herpesvirus type-3 (EHV-3). EVH-3 is a member of the subfamily Alphaherpesvirinae [13]. Although the primary route of transmission is venereal, outbreaks have been documented in which transmission occurred through contaminated supplies and instruments or by the use of a single glove for rectal examination of many mares [14]. Clinical signs in mares might develop 4–8 days after sexual contact and are clearly expressed by the presence of numerous circular red nodules up to 2 mm in diameter on three different parts of the genital tract: vulvar and vaginal mucosa, the clitoral sinus, and perineal skin. These lesions primarily develop into vesicles, then into pustules and eventually rupture, leaving shallow, painful, ulcerated areas that may amalgamate into larger lesions. Edema can develop in the perineum and may extend between the thighs. Sometimes, ulcers will be found on the teats, nasal mucosa, and lips. Secondary infection of the ulcers by *Streptococcus* spp. is common, causing ulcers which exude a mucopurulent discharge, and the mare may become febrile. Without these secondary bacterial infection occurs, skin healing is complete within 3 weeks, but clitoral and vaginal ulcers heal slowly. Skin lesions persist for long periods as unpigmented scars; however, pregnancy rates are not reduced. Lesions in stallions are similar to those described in mares and are found on both the penis and prepuce. Therefore, copulation may be difficult because intromission is painful, and the stallion usually refuses to mount and copulate. If copulation does occur during the ulcerative stage, ulcers can cause bloody ejaculates, reducing sperm viability [11]. Although coitus is the major route of exposure for stallions and mares, mares can be infected by AI or thorough indirect contact with contaminated veterinary instruments or equipment, gynecological examination or testing for pregnancy [11, 14, 15].

http://dx.doi.org/10.5772/63741

Dourine also produces vulvitis, vaginitis, and cervicitis in the mare. Dourine is sexually transmitted disease caused by the protozoan parasite, *Trypanosoma equiperdum*. This pathology is spread during natural or artificial breeding, foaling, and in the milk of infected mares. Transmission from stallions to mares is more common, but mares can also transmit the disease to stallions. The incubation period is a few weeks to several years. *T. equiperdum* can be found in the vaginal secretions of infected mares and the seminal fluid, mucous exudate of the penis, and sheath of stallions. Affected animals include swelling of the vagina and vulva and mucopurulent vaginal discharge pus by their vulva (females) or urethra (males). Inflammation of vulva and vagina may extend along the perineum to the ventral abdomen and mammary gland. The genital region, perineum, and udder may become depigmented. Clinical signs of dourine can be nonspecific and include fever (temperature greater than 38.6°C), conjunctivitis, weight loss, skin plaques that may become depigmented, and neurologic signs [1, 16]. Dourine usually not causes endometritis, but abortion can occur with more virulent strains [17–19]. Approximately 50–70% of infected horses die [1, 16, 18, 20].

CEM is a transmissible, venereal disease of horses produced by the bacterium *T. equigenitalis*. Compared with other breeds, Thoroughbred horses appear to be more severely affected by the disease. Due to the animals may be asymptomatic, the disease is difficult to detect and control. CEM is a serious disease because it is highly contagious and can have a devastating effect on equine reproductive efficiency. Transmission may also occur indirectly by AI or contact with contaminated hands, instruments used for practitioners or at breeding facilities following international horse shipments. Undetected carrier mares and stallions are the source of infection of the disease during the breeding season. Normally, a carrier stallion can infect several mares before the disease is diagnosed. The sites of persistence in mares that are clitoral carriers are the clitoral sinuses (medial and lateral) and the clitoral fossa [21], for an extended period of time [18]. Mares with CEM shows edema and hyperemia of the vaginal mucosa, cervix and endometrium [18], resulting in infertility, failures to conceive (revealed by an early return to estrus after breeding), or spontaneous abort [22].

Other microorganisms that have been isolated from fossa and sinus clitoral are *Escherichia coli, Streptococcus faecalis, Corynebacterium* spp., *Staphylococcus aureus*, β-hemolytic Streptococcus, *Bacillus, Enterobacter aerogenes*, Pasteurella spp., α-hemolytic Streptococcus, Citrobacter, and Proteus [23]. When suspected carrier status level of the clitoris, the clitoris is advisable to treat/lobby before examining the uterus to prevent the risk of transmission of infection to the cervix.

3. Endometritis

Despite significant research and study, endometritis continues to be a major clinical problem in broodmare practice and a major source of subfertility. Appropriate diagnosis and treatment are imperative when attempting to get these mares in foal. Many cycling mares fail to conceive due to infections in their reproductive tracts and for this reason they are called "dirty mares." Dirty mares or mares with endometritis refer to the acute or chronic inflammatory process involving the endometrium. Reduction of fertility associated with endometritis—both acute and chronic—has been recognized for many years. This subfertility is due to an inappropriate environment within the uterus for the development of the embryo. In some cases, the endometritis may cause early regression of the corpus luteum (CL). One of the main obstacles in producing the maximum number of live, healthy foals from mares bred during the previous season is the mare, which is susceptible to persistent, acute endometritis following breeding [24–26]. A combination of a bacteriological and a cytological examination improved the diagnostic performance in subfertile mares [27].

Positive cytology to *E. coli* and β-hemolytic streptococci is highly associated with the presence of neutrophil in the stratum compactum and spongiosum on uterus. The low volume, lavage technique is a rapid and accurate method for diagnosing mares with endometritis, and the risk of false-positive samples is considered to be minimal when compared with other flushing techniques described [28].

The key to successful management of these mares is to identify them before or shortly after breeding and manage them appropriately. Treatment generally consists of a combination of uterine lavage and ecbolic administration to enhance uterine clearance and administration of intrauterine antibiotics [29–32].

Overall, endometritis is classified as follows [33]:

- Venereal infectious endometritis.
- Nonvenereal infectious endometritis.
- Persistent post-mating endometritis.
- Endometriosis (chronic degenerative endometritis).
- Chronic infectious endometritis.

The uterine lumen of the normal fertile mare is bacteriology sterile despite the fact that the reproductive tract is contaminated with bacteria from the act of breeding, foaling, and veterinary procedures. As it has been previously expressed mares with imperfect vulval conformation can input air with bacteria into the genital tract, which can develop into endometritis. The uterus responds to these bacteria with a rapid influx of neutrophils killing the bacteria rapidly (within 24 hours). Then, these inflammatory products are mechanically removed, and the endometritis resolves itself. Usually, the failure to resolve this inflammation results in what is commonly known as "susceptible" mare. This "susceptible" mares have a delay in uterine clearance, and the inflammatory products accumulate as uterine fluid. Such mares have a reduced pregnancy rate due to an inappropriate environment for the early development of the embryo [34]. However, the reproductive tract of mare possesses various mechanisms to protect itself against infection: physical barriers as vulva, vestibulovaginal sphincter, and cervix, local immune mechanisms and the physical ability to eliminate products of inflammation, as described below. The uterine infections become established when one or several of these natural defense mechanisms fail or become overwhelmed. These infections become established when normal defense fails to clear potentially pathogenic organisms that are introduced into the uterus. The most common sources of uterine contamination include coitus, parturition, AI, septic genital examination, and manipulation. Age, parity, number of barren years, and uterine biopsy grade influence likelihood of persistence of infection [2].

3.1. Mechanisms of defense of uterus in the mare

3.1.1. Physical barriers

The uterine cavity is protected from ascending infection by several anatomic structures. The first line of defense in the prevention of contamination of the vagina and eventually the uterus is provided by the seal of the normal vulvar labia. The second physical barrier is the vestibulovaginal sphincter. And the third important anatomic barrier is the cervix. However, in some mares, compromised cervical function is observed, and its entity may remain open during anestrus and even diestrus. The most common cause of cervical incompetence is a lesion consequent to dystocia [3]. A plan for treatment and prevention of uterine infection should include a plan to reestablish normal barrier function. Surgical procedures such as episioplasty, vestibulovaginoplasty, and rectovaginal tear repair should be considered if indicated and reestablish the uterine contractility in the elimination of bacteria, fluid, and inflammatory products from the uterus after breeding [35].

3.1.2. Immunity and uterine defense

An adaptive immune response in the mare's uterus has been demonstrated. The endometrium of the mare is inhabited by T lymphocytes. Genitally normal mares had greater numbers of CD4+ (TH cells) and CD8+ cells (TC cells) in the stratum compactum than in the stratum spongiosum. The density of these cells was either increased during estrus or found to be independent of cycle stage. Also it was not influenced by age and larger numbers of CD4+ and CD8+ cells that are present in the uterine body than in the uterine horns. Following insemination or mares with endometritis, the number of CD4+ and CD8+ cells is increased. Thus, the number of CD4+ cells doubled in lymphoid aggregates, and the number of CD8+ cells in the luminal and glandular epithelium increases. Therefore, an adaptive response is initiated following antigenic stimulation of the endometrium [24, 36].

As the most common etiological agent in bacterial endometritis, *Streptococcus equi* spp. *zooepidemicus* (*S. zooepidemicus*) is commonly used in most experimental models because of its relative ease of laboratory handling and identification. Antigens of *S. zooepidemicus* are processed through an endocytic pathway and are presented on the membrane surface of cells that express class II major histocompatibility complex (MHC) molecules. Presentation of class II MHC molecules to CD4+ cells is limited to "professional" antigen-presenting cells (APCs), such as dendritic cells, macrophages, and B cells. "Nonprofessional" APCs, for instance, certain epithelial cells, fibroblasts, and vascular endothelial cells, can present antigen in the context of class II MHC molecules. But APCs cells fail to deliver a co-stimulatory signal and present antigen for short-term periods during a continued inflammatory response. Cells in the equine endometrium expressing MHC class II include macrophages, monocytes, dendritic cells, lymphocytes, vascular endothelial cells, and uterine luminal epithelium. Expression of MHC

II molecules was greater in normal mares in estrus than in diestrus. The distribution of these molecules was predominantly under the luminal epithelium, with occasional foci in the stratum compactum and infrequently in the stratum spongiosum. This pattern is reliable with antigen presentation [36–38].

On the other hand, cytokines play an important role in the reproductive processes [39]. The complexity of their regulation is due to pleiotropism of cytokines, where each cytokine has multiple target cells of different organs and where responses may differ according to cell type. The response to endometritis is mediated by inflammatory mediators such as leukotriene B4 (LTB4) and prostaglandins (PG) E2. Mares susceptible to endometritis have a higher expression of pro-inflammatory cytokines (interleukin-1 β-I; L-1β), IL-6, and tumor necrosis factor-α (TNF-α) during estrus and IL-1β and TNF-α during diestrus [24, 34]. An overregulated endometrial gene expression of pro- and anti-inflammatory cytokines (IL-1β, IL-6, IL-8) and a systemic acute phase response (APR) have been described in mares with experimentally induced *E. coli* endometritis [40], as it has gene expression of cytokines in response to AI with dead spermatozoa in resistant and susceptible mares [24, 36].

In response to endometritis, endometrial mRNA transcripts of pro-inflammatory cytokines are excellently regulated in resistant mares. These resistant mares have an initial high-expression levels followed by normalization within a short period of time. By contrast, susceptible mares have an extended expression of pro-inflammatory cytokines, leading to the hypothesis that an unbalanced endometrial gene expression of inflammatory cytokines might play an important role in the pathogenesis of persistent endometritis [36, 38]. In addition, endometritis gives rise to a systemic APR and an up-regulated endometrial gene expression of serum pro- and anti-inflammatory cytokines and serum amyloid type A (SAA) [28, 36].

The contact of endometrium with infectious agents results in altered synthesis and secretion of inflammatory mediators (cytokines and arachidonic acid metabolites) and disturbs endometrial functional balance of PGE2, PGI, PGF2α, and leucotrienes [41]. The events leading to endometritis are initiated by a local reaction to the primary antigen, with production of inflammatory mediators, especially PGE2, and neutrophil influx. Increased vascular permeability resulting from proinflammatory mediators exacerbates the neutrophil influx and leakage of serum proteins into the uterus [2, 42]. PGF2α is considered as the most accurate markers of inflammation during endometritis for use in practice [42]. Furthermore, in sustained endometritis in mares, PG may not only cause early luteolysis or early pregnancy loss but may also be related to endometrial fibrosis pathogenesis by stimulating collagen deposition [43].

3.1.3. Immunoglobulins

The predominant immunoglobulins (Igs) in the uterine secretions are IgG, IgM, and IgA produced within the endometrium. Uterine Ig concentration does not differ between mares susceptible and resistant to endometritis, suggesting that this is not a major factor in susceptibility to infection. Susceptible mares tend to have slightly higher concentrations of intrauterine Ig than do resistant mares, but susceptible mares are less efficient at opsonizing streptococci during acute infection [44, 45]. The inoculation with *T. equigenitalis* results in both local and systemic titer increases in antibody [1]. Following intrauterine inoculation with *S. zooepidemi-*

http://dx.doi.org/10.5772/63741

cus, this activity is not only strain specific but also comprises heat-stable and heat-labile components. In general, mares susceptible to endometritis have similar or higher levels of free Ig in the uterus. The common inference is a dysfunction in the humoral response to intrauterine infection, which does not contribute significantly to enlarge susceptibility to endometritis. Investigation of bacterial Ig-binding proteins, would lead to a better understanding of the humoral response to intrauterine infection and its role in susceptibility to endometritis. Certainly, Ig-binding proteins have been identified in uterine secretions and deplete hemolytic complement activity in vitro [44].

3.1.4. Neutrophils

In addition to the traditional functions, neutrophils are able to release DNA in response to infectious stimuli, forming neutrophil extracellular traps and killing pathogens [46]. Neutrophil chemotaxis is induced by bacteria, endotoxin, spermatozoa, semen extenders, and sterile water and saline solutions. A massive entry of neutrophils into the uterine lumen occurs in both susceptible and resistant mares after local exposure to foreign proteins. In some mares, this stimulation causes a persistent-induced endometritis. Therefore, neutrophils play an important role in this phenomenon, and their effects are exacerbated if bacteria are present.

Susceptible mares have higher nitric oxide (NO), which is a bactericidal agent produced by macrophages and neutrophils following incorporation of microorganisms than can cause myometrial relaxation in their uterine secretions and greater inducible NO expression compared with resistant mares. The NO facilitates smooth muscle relaxation, but its role in persistent endometritis is a possible role of NO, either directly or in a NO-associated pathway, in delayed uterine clearance [47]. The activated neutrophils also are an important source of reactive oxygen species (ROS), which can play a role in the pathogenesis of endometritis in mares [42, 48].

Resistant mares are able to eliminate most fluid in response to the effects of oxytocin and PG on the myometrium. Susceptible mares fail to eliminate fluid often because of intrinsic endometrial or myometrial pathology that reduces uterine contractions less efficient in uterine clearance. The phagocytic activity of neutrophils is higher on entry into the uterine cavity [44]. Phagocytic activity may be highest during estrus since in ovariectomized mares treated with estrogens neutrophil phagocytic activity was greater. Phagocytic activity of circulating neutrophils is no different between susceptible and resistant mares; however, phagocytic activity and life span of uterine neutrophils are significantly reduced in susceptible mares. Susceptible mares also have additional uterine clearance problems and accumulate more fluid, which may contribute to a reduction in the viability of neutrophils [24, 44].

Young mares experimentally inoculated with *S. zooepidemicus* clear infection within a few hours, whereas barren mares inoculated with *S. zooepidemicus* and *P. aeruginosa* have a delayed elimination of bacteria [37].

Opsonizing activity in the uterus has a peak of 8 hours after inoculation with *Streptococcus*. Studies using heat-treated uterine fluid suggest that complement is not a primary opsonizing factor in the uterus. In this way, the uterine environment of endometritis susceptible mares seems to be hostile to complement. In contrast, the opsonizing capacity to serum and degree of serum complement activity does not differ between susceptible and resistant mares [44, 49].

3.1.5. Physical clearance of infection

The prevention of persistent infection is due to physical clearance of pathogens and inflammatory debris from the uterus and is most effective during estrus [50]. However, mares susceptible to infectious endometritis are unable to eliminate bacteria from the uterus in the immediate post-ovulatory period [51]. Younger mares are able to eliminate both *S. zooepidemicus* and nonantigenic particles more quickly than older mares.

Some anatomic changes, such as pendulous uteri or broad ligaments, defective myometrial activity and degenerative changes to the vascular and lymphatic drainage of the uterus, are also involved in delayed uterine clearance and the pathogenesis of the endometritis. Ulceration, degeneration, or lack of cilia of the endometrium may be involved in failure of mucociliary clearance [52, 53].

In susceptible mares, myometrial contractions are less frequent and of shorter duration and intensity, perhaps because of increased fibrosis or another biochemical factors affecting uterine contractibility. Alghamdi et al. [47] informed that uterine contractions are reduced in the presence of NO, which is found in high concentration in susceptible mares.

3.1.6. Antibacterial activity of uterine secretion

Strzemienski et al. [54] reported that cell-free uterine flushes from mares in mid-diestrus possess antibacterial activity. However, Johnson et al. [55] have failed to demonstrate inherent antibacterial activity of uterine fluid from noncycling mares or from E2- or P4-supplemented ovariectomized mares. The discrepancy in the results from these studies may be based on any qualitative and quantitative differences between the uterine secretions from cycling and noncycling mares. Recently, it has been identified in the equine endometrium an antimicrobial and immunomodulator member of the transferring gene family that is expressed by epithelial cells and neutrophils. Lactoferrin's antibacterial property lies in its ability to sequester-free iron, thereby inhibiting bacterial growth. Although lactoferrin expression was overregulated during early estrus, protein staining was uninfluenced by cycle and was most intense in the glandular epithelium. According with Kolm et al. [56], expression of lactoferrin was increased in mares with delayed physical clearance during early estrus, which might represent a response to inflammation. From the point of view of host–pathogen interactions, unless a diminished response in lactoferrin expression and production were observed, it is unlikely to explain how this could be a factor in susceptibility to endometritis.

3.1.7. Mucociliary clearance in the mare

It has been suggested that mucociliary clearance may play an important role in the clearance of infections and that disruption of mucociliary currents in the susceptible mare leads to persistence of infection [33]. Mucus production and secretion and optical density are increased during estrus in mares with delayed clearance. The biological implication of these alterations in the mucus is unknown. The effects of fluid accumulation and uterine pathogens on mucociliary clearance are basis for future research [57]. Bacterial pathogens of the uterus affect the elasticity and stickiness of the uterine mucus. It was identified that *K. pneumoniae* and other gram-negative bacteria lead to the viscosity of the mucus causing a decrease in mucociliary activity, while β-hemolytic streptococci decrease the viscosity of the mucus. Additionally, it has been reported that an increase in PGE_2, LTB4, arachidonic acid metabolites and an increase in vascular permeability causes the entrance of *S. zooepidemicus* into the uterus. Therefore, if uterus cleaning delays, subclinical endometritis occurs [33].

3.2. Opportunistic infection endometritis

Infection produced by opportunistic microbes is a major cause of infertility in the mare and inflicts major losses on the equine breeding industry due to early embryonic loss, placentitis, birth of septic foals, and postpartum metritis. Early pregnancy loss is estimated to affect 25–40% of the broodmares and uterine infections reported in 25–60% of barren mares [2].

3.2.1. Bacterial endometritis

The organisms most frequently isolated from mares with acute endometritis are *S. zooepidemicus* (β-hemolytic), *E. coli* (*haemolytica*), *P. aeruginosa*, and *K. pneumoniae* [2, 58–60].

At a rate of up to 50% of the endometritis cases, *S. zooepidemicus* is globally the most considerable bacterial endometritis agent in mares [50, 58]. This most commonly isolated pathogens from the uterus of mares, suffering from infectious endometritis associated with increased age, parity, and poor vulvar conformation [28, 50, 61]. Endometritis produced by *S. zooepidemicus* can origin from a reservoir of dormant bacteria residing within the endometrium, and not only as an ascending infection [37, 62]. However, these bacteria can be introduced into the uterus by breeding because bacteria often are introduced into the uterus during coitus or AI [2].

Other commensal bacteria isolated from reproductive tract of mare include *Actinomyces pyogenes, Proteus* spp., *Staphylococcus* spp., and *Citrobacter* spp. These bacteria are occasionally supported by cytologic of histopathologic evidence of concurrent inflammation. α-Hemolytic *Streptococcus*, *Enterobacter* spp., and *Staphylococcus epidermidis* are rarely causes of endometritis and should be considered simple contaminants [2, 24]. *Corynebacterium* spp. and anaerobic bacteria such *Bacteroides fragilis* may occasionally cause endometritis in mares [26, 63]. Anaerobic bacteria and mycoplasmas have been suggested as possible causes of endometritis from postpartum and foal heat in the mare samples when the evidence of inflammation is present without aerobic bacteria [2]. The resulting disease is characterized by endometritis, vaginal discharge, and a devastating effect on fertility.

The pathogenicity of bacteria depends on their ability to adhere to the endometrium, preventing their removal by normal uterine clearance mechanisms. Adhesive proprieties of *S. zooepidemicus* are probably mediated by fibronectin-binding proteins and hyaluronic acid capsule [62]. Resistance to phagocytosis is often observed with *S. zooepidemicus* and *K. pneumoniae.* This resistance is probably mediated by antigenic variation, antiphagocytic M-protein like, hyaluronic acid capsule or polysaccharide, and Fc receptors on phagocytic cells.

M-protein-like surface proteins capable of depriving the bacterium of unspecific and specific immune reactions caused by attaching to the Fc region of IgG and IgA. The M-like proteins also bind fibrinogen [64]. Streptococci-binding fibrinogen to the M-like protein attaches to phagocytes too, yet they are not internalized. *S. zooepidemicus* is able to resist complement-mediated cell lysis, which might be mediated by the M-protein-like. The antigenicity of the M-protein-like is mainly responsible for the mounting of a protective immune response. Bacterial toxins promote deterioration of complement and exacerbate uterine inflammation [64–66].

In contrast to a true sexually transmitted diseases, persistent infectious endometritis is often the result of contamination of the uterus by the mare's fecal flora combined with compromised uterine defenses [24, 67]. Different bacteria such as *P. aeruginosa, K. pneumoniae, S. zooepidemicus,* and *E. coli* can be sexually transmitted in horses, but the magnitudes of exposure to these microorganisms are determined by the particular strain involved and active participation of the mare's uterine defense mechanisms [24]. Once the bacterium attaches and colonizes mucous membranes produces endometritis. This process is promoted by extracellular enzymes and toxins. Many strains of *P. aeruginosa* produce exotoxin A, which causes tissue necrosis due to blocking protein synthesis of host cells. Pseudomonas and other bacteria survive in nature by forming biofilms on surfaces. A biofilm is a structured consortium of bacteria embedded in a self-produced polymer matrix consisting of polysaccharide, protein, and extracellular DNA. A bacterial biofilm is a complex aggregation of microorganisms growing on a solid substrate. Biofilms are characterized by structural heterogeneity, genetic diversity, complex community interactions, and an extracellular matrix of polymeric substances, which greatly increase in the resistance to antibiotic therapy. It has been proposed that endometrial biofilms are responsible for the cases of chronic endometritis that appears to be nonresponse to conventional treatment [68].

3.2.2. Fungal endometritis

Candida spp. and *Aspergillus* spp. are the most common fungal organisms isolated from the uterus of mares with endometritis. The incidence of fungal infection in mares with endometritis is estimated to vary from 0.1% to 5%. Fungal organisms isolated from the equine uterus include *Aspergillus* spp., several *Candida* spp., *Cryptococcus neoformans, Fusarium* spp., *Hansenula anomala, Hansenula polymorpha,* several *Rhodotorula* spp., *Scedosporidium apiospermum, Saccharomyces cerevisiae, Trichosporon beigelii, Torulopsis candida, Acremonium* spp., *Actinomyces* spp., *Fusarium* spp., *Aspergillus fumigatus, Aspergillus glaucus, Aspergillus niger, Monosporium apiospermum, Monosporium* spp., *Aureobasidium pullulans, Mucor* spp., *Candida albicans, Nocardia* spp., *Candida ciferii, Paecilomyces* spp., *Candida famata, Penicillium* spp., *Candida guillermondii, Pseudallescheria boydii, Candida krusei, Rhodotorula glutinis, Candida lusitaniae, Rhodotorula minuta, Candida parapsilosis, Rhodotorula rubra, Candida pseudotropicalis, Rhodotorula* spp., *Candida rugosa, Candida stellatoides, Candida tropicalis, Torulopsis glabrata, Candida zeylanoides, Circinella* spp., *Trichosporon cutaneum, Coccidiodes immitis, Trichosporon* spp., *Cryptococcus humicolus,* and *Yarrowia lipolytica* [69].

Most mares presented with fungal endometritis have a history of previous bacterial endometritis. These mares usually undergo intense therapy that includes frequent uterine lavages and intrauterine infusion of antibiotics. The frequent uterine manipulation, associated with anatomical problems leading to pneumovagina, results in chronic contamination of the uterus. In addition, antibiotics drained from the uterus alter the normal bacterial flora in the vagina, predisposing to an excessive growth of opportunistic fungal organisms, making the vagina and external genitalia the primary reservoir for pathogens. Affected mares tend to be old and pluriparous with poor perineal conformation or maiden mares with cervical incompetence. Mares may have been treated repeatedly with intrauterine antibiotics, have normal or abnormal estrous cycles, may be presented with a history of anovulatory follicles, or have endocrine dysfunction such as equine pituitary disorders or insulin resistance. Prolonged progesterone therapy may predispose mares to fungal endometritis because cervical drainage is decreased and uterine muscular activity and neutrophil function are altered [4]. Other factors contributing to fungal infections include the presence of a moist environment, exposure to a large number of fungi and the presence of necrotic focus as occurring with trauma, abortion, and retained placenta [4, 70].

Diagnosis is based on the presence of fungal elements and inflammatory cells in endometrial smears. Yeast appears as small, round, single cell, brown to black spores on cytological smears obtained from infected mares, whereas molds have long filamentous hyphae [4, 71]. It has suggested that the hyphae are more invasive than yeast and, consequently, more difficult to treat and eliminate. *Candida albicans* can be present in both yeast and hyphal forms and therefore can penetrate deeper into the endometrium and/or growth intracellularly. However, in endometrial cytology and histology used to diagnose fungal endometritis, fungal elements only are visualized in the lumen of the uterus and not penetrate deeper in the endometrium [71].

Another important observation about the difficulty in treating fungal infections is the ability of certain species to produce biofilms, both *Candida* spp. and *Aspergillus* spp. Biofilms also give microorganisms the ability to adhere strongly to virtually and surface; therefore, proper sterilization of uterine catheters and other equipment is paramount to prevent dissemination of pathogens [69, 72].

Prolonged antibiotic therapy may be a predisposing factor for yeast overgrowth [69]. The use of antibiotic-containing semen extenders for AI may be partially responsible for the apparent increase in the number of mares with fungal endometritis. Transmission of fungal organisms from stallions has not been demonstrated, although fungi have been cultured from the urethra (*Mucor* spp.), fresh semen (*Absidia* spp.), and extended semen (*Candida* spp.) of stallions [33, 69].

Cladophialophora bantiana conducted to endometritis with infertility and uterine fluid accumulation with numerous black, hairy granules. Microscopically, the fluid presents in numerous partitions, dark fungal hyphae, and conidia in chains [73].

In terms of impairment of fertility, the significance of these organisms in the mare and the stallion is not yet well established [1]. *Mycoplasma* spp. has been isolated most frequently from the external genitalia and semen of clinically normal and infertile stallions, but their exact role in uterine infection is not well established [18]. In vitro, *Mycoplasma equigenitalium* produces a consistent cytopathic effect on the ciliated epithelium of the oviduct. *M. equigenitalium, M.*

subdolum, and *Acholeplasma* spp. are associated with infertility, endometritis, vulvitis, and abortion in mares. *M. equigenitalium* and *M. subdolum* were isolated from the genital tract of mares (5–34%) and aborted equine fetuses (7%). Also, in some situations, these organisms have been associated with endometritis, infertility, and balanopostitis in stallions [1], whereas, in other situations, they have been found in the absence of any evidence of reproductive dysfunction [18].

Chlamydia spp. has been demonstrated in the genital tract of both the stallion and the mare. While their presence is not always associated with evident clinical disease, certain species such as *Chlamidia abortus* and *Chlamidia psittaci* have detected in cases of abortion, salpingitis, and reduced semen quality in the stallion [74].

3.3. Pyometra

Pyometra may be produced by accumulation of a pus accumulation in the uterus in addition to the persistence of the CL beyond its normal lifespan [75].

Pyometra can be caused by different causes. Including interference cleaning liquid is described from the uterus, obstruction of flow caused by the cervix closed by hormonal influence or cervical pathology such as fibrosis and adhesions, or secondary to trauma, such as experienced during dystocia. Progesterone from a persistent CL can close the cervix. Similarly, exogenous progesterone administered continuously cleaning the uterine avoided. Endometrial cups have been observed as a cause of pyometra where no fetuses or fetal membranes were found within the uterine lumen [76].

Intrauterine accumulation of purulent material was observed in mares with open cervix [77]. These mares may have an innate resistance to a reduced endometrial infection, which can progress to a pyometra [4]. The most common organism associated with pyometra in the mare is *S. zooepidemicus, E. coli, Actinomyces* spp., *Pasteurella* spp., *Pseudomonas* spp., *Propionibacterium* spp., and *Candida rugosa* [78, 79].

Mares with pyometra have vulvar discharge when the cervix is relaxed or open. The pus is often creamy, it may be variable, with higher volumes associated with, watery, thin gray appearance. Smaller volumes are associated with pus cheesy exudate thickened. Rarely are clinical signs of systemic disease [79].

3.4. Venereal infectious endometritis

The bacterial diseases with potential capacity of be transmissible through fresh cooled or cryopreservated semen are *S. zooepidemicus, P. aeruginosa, K. pneumoniae, T. equigenitalis*, and *T. asinigenitalis*. Among viral diseases that can be transmitted venereal are equine arteritis (EAV) and equine herpesvirus 3 or equine coital exanthema virus, and one is a protozoan infection (*T. equiperdum*) [18, 80].

Exist other diseases that may be transmitted very infrequently by this route or that potentially could be disseminated through contamination of semen. These diseases are as follows:

http://dx.doi.org/10.5772/63741

- Internal genital infections of the testes, epididymis, and accessory sex glands, the major of which are bacterial in nature, such as *S. zooepidemicus, Salmonella abortus equi;*
- Acute to chronic systemic diseases characterized by circulation of the respective causal agents in the bloodstream, as equine infectious anemia (EIA), equine piroplasmosis;
- Infections of the urinary system with the potential for contamination of the urogenital tract, such as leptospirosis, equine rhinitis A virus infection;
- A miscellany of infective agents, including viruses, bacteria, mycoplasmas, chlamydiae, fungi, and yeast that may shed in semen [18].

Infections caused by *P. aeruginosa* and *K. pneumoniae* are often considered venereal diseases because the organisms are often introduced during coitus, AI with infected semen, or genital manipulations. *K. pneumoniae* identify as capsule types 1, 2, and 5 are highly pathogenic [1]. *K. pneumoniae* capsule types 7 and 39 have been incriminated in causing endometritis in the mare by AI, presumably with infective fresh-cooled semen [81].

Although *K. pneumoniae, P. aeruginosa,* and *S. zooepidemicus* are commensal organisms of penis and prepuce in the stallion, in cases of disturbance as a result of indiscriminate washing of the penis or too frequent washing with a surgical scrub or detergent soap. Under such circumstances, there is the potential for colonization of the penis and prepuce with the mentioned bacteria. These organisms, which rarely produce clinical disease in the stallion, can give rise to endometritis with reduced fertility in susceptible mares, especially in mares with a preexisting defect in uterine clearance [15]. Transmission of these bacteria occurs venereally, either natural breeding or AI with infective semen [18, 82].

3.4.1. Contagious equine metritis (CEM)

CEM is a transmissible, exotic, venereal disease caused by *T. equigenitalis.* This bacterium is closely adapted to the specific environmental conditions of the equine genital tract, whereby it is the only venereal transmissible bacterial agent in horses [18].

Thoroughbred horses appear to be more severely affected by the disease than other breeds. Because animals may be asymptomatic, the disease is difficult to detect and control. Due to its high contagiousness, CEM is a serious disease and can have detrimental consequences on equine reproductive efficiency. When CEM becomes established in the United States, the horse industry suffered great economic losses [1].

Initial exposure to the disease usually results in infertility. An infected mare may fail to conceive or abort. The disease frequently is associated with an endometritis [18, 83]. Abortion due to *T. equigenitalis* infection is very rare [84].

The exposure of the mare to *T. equigenitalis* can result in clinical or asymptomatic infection. After an incubation period of 2–12 days, affected mares developed odorless, grayish-white mucopurulent vulvar discharge of variable consistency and volume, which can last for up to 2 weeks or slightly longer [85]. The discharge is associated with endometritis, cervicitis, vaginitis, vulvar discharge, and return to estrus after a shortened diestrous period [86].

The infertility is temporary (only a few weeks), with adverse effect on a mare's fertility. Persistence of *T. equigenitalis* in the reproductive tract of a chronically infected mare not interfere with the maintenance of the birth of a healthy foal [18, 21]. The mare, though asymptomatic, is still infectious and can remain a carrier for several months [18, 21, 22].

In contrast to the mare, exposure of the stallion to *T. equigenitalis* does not result in infection, much less the development of any clinical signs in the vast majority of cases [87]. The stallion becomes an unapparent carrier of the bacterium, which persists as a commensal on its external genitalia without causing any adverse local or systemic effects. On very rare occasions, exposure may result in an ascending infection of the reproductive tract in the stallion [88]. In addition, *T. asinigenitalis* is transmitted through venereal for breeding or AI and causes endometritis, cervicitis, and vaginitis in experimentally infected mare [89].

3.4.2. Equine viral arteritis (EVA)

Equine viral arteritis (EVA) is a contagious viral infection affecting both mares and stallions. Prevalence of EVA ranges from 1–3% in Quarter Horses to 7% in Arabians and Thoroughbreds and to 80% in Standardbreds. Mares clinically affected with EVA may show fever, limb edema, anorexia, depression, inflammation around the eyes, nasal discharge, skin rash, and abortion. The significance of EVA infection in stallions is that certain strains can develop carrier status in 30–60% of infected stallions. Carrier stallions can transmit the virus by natural breeding or AI with fresh, cooled, or frozen semen. Mares bred with EVA-infected semen may lead to outbreaks of abortion and deaths in foals [90]. Due to these reasons, EVA is responsible for major restrictions in the international movement of horses and semen. Serologic or blood testing is used for screening both mares and stallions. Detectable antibody titers develop 2–4 weeks following exposure and are maximal at 2–4 months and remain stable for several years. If a stallion is serologically positive, the presence or absence of virus in his semen should be determined to confirm if he is a chronic carrier or shedder of the virus. The carrier state has only been documented in adult stallions. It should be emphasized that not all seropositive stallions are shedders and carriers of the virus [91].

3.5. Internal genital infections

In the stallion infection of the testes, epididymis and accessory glands may be a localized or part of a systemic disease. Though rare in occurrence, orchitis caused by a range of bacteria including *S. abortusequi, S. zooepidemicus, Burkholderia mallei, Brucella abortus, Actinobacillus equuli, P. aeruginosa, K. pneumoniae, Staphylococcus* spp., *Proteus vulgaris,* and *E. coli* can have detrimental effect for the stallion's fertility and have opportunity for venereal transmission by coitus or AI with contaminated semen to the mare [18].

3.6. Systemic diseases

Due to their potential to be transmitted by the venereal route acute and chronic systemic infectious diseases, they have come under consideration. These diseases included Eastern equine encephalomyelitis and Western equine encephalomyelitis, West Nile encephalitis, vesicular stomatitis, African horse sickness, EIA, and equine piroplasmosis. They can also pose a risk of venereal transmission if at the time of breeding or semen collection there is trauma of the stallion's genitalia, bleeding, and contamination of the ejaculate with blood containing the respective etiological agent [18].

To date, there is no evidence of occurrence of venereal transmission of any of the aforementioned diseases, with the exception of piroplasmosis, in which mare showed *Babesia* because of venereal transmission when blood from an infected stallion contaminated semen [92].

3.7. Chronic infectious endometritis

Usually, an underlying condition, such as pneumovagina, predisposes the horse to chronic infectious endometritis. The definitive diagnosis is by biopsy should show endometrial infiltration with lymphocytes and plasma cells. Chronic infectious endometritis is more common in older mares and primiparous mares with poor perineal conformation. The predisposing factors for chronic infections in mares include self-repeated contaminations, cervix fibrosis, cervical tears or adhesions, and/or "mare older maiden" syndrome and mares in which holes uterus well below the edge of the pelvis. The organisms most frequently isolated in cases of chronic infectious endometritis include the same of acute (*S. zooepidemicus, E. coli, K. pneumoniae, P. aeruginosa,* and *Candida* or *Aspergillus*). Long-term chronic, refractory infections typically involve yeast and/or gram-negative bacteria [93]. *S. zooepidemicus* is one of the most frequently pathogens isolated from uterus of mares suffering infectious endometritis. As described previously, it has the capacity to cause chronic infection latent deeply reside within the endometrial tissue [28]. Chronic inflammation may lead to fibrosis and periglandular mucus production by inadequate uterine epithelial or endometrial glands. If the elasticity, viscosity, or changes in the amount of mucus or if the cilia are damaged or denuded endometrial epithelial cell, uterine drainage will be diminished, which contributes to the accumulation of fluid and infertility [93].

A close examination of the reproductive system by rectal ultrasound can provide evidence of chronic inflammation or infection. The accumulation of fluid within the uterine lumen, endometrial edema, the presence of hyperechoic spots within the uterine lumen, and an even greater thickness of the uterine wall can all be signs of chronic infection. Culturing of endometrial biopsies or uterine fluids is more sensitive for the identification of *E. coli* when compared with culture-swab methods. Endometrial cytology identifies twice mares with acute inflammation in the culture when compared with cervical swab. A vaginal speculum examination shows evidence of inflammation and also allows to evaluate the competition lobby-vaginal sphincter. The culture of material obtained from the uterus, not always allows the diagnosis for the presence or absence of bacteria in cases of clinical endometritis [94, 95]. Obtaining a sample of endometrial cytology and further culture was used to increase the diagnostic accuracy, providing clear evidence of inflammation in conjunction with a positive culture. Mares with chronic infections often have long-standing inflammatory changes. In these cases, the prognosis is guarded because of the chronic nature of the infection and predisposing anatomical defects. Surgical correction of conformational abnormalities may try to use the Caslick procedure [93].

3.8. Chronic degenerative endometritis

Chronic degenerative endometritis or endometriosis is degenerative change that occurs in older mares or following repeated inflammation of the uterus. Degenerative fibrosis can be the result of normal aging processes or may be the end-product of a life of continuous reinfection: anyway, healing uterine mucosa causes infertility in older mares [34]. Problems related to weaken reproductive structures can cause urinary retention, a condition in which the mares do not empty completely urine, especially during estrus. Thus, the retained liquid can cause inflammation and prevent conception. The use of antibiotics is not always good. One of the disadvantages of using antibiotics is the fact that kills good and bad bacteria, leaving the animal with no natural protection against future bacterial or fungal invasions. The definitive diagnosis can only be achieved by biopsy, which shows degenerative histological changes in the uterus [93].

3.9. Persistent post-mating endometritis

Inflammation of the endometrium is caused by a response to exogenous materials introduced directly into the uterus at breeding, as components of the semen, extender in the case of AI, bacteria, and other debris [24, 96]. Two hormones, PGF2α and oxytocin, regulate myometrial contractions after the influx of neutrophils into the uterine lumen and their phagocytic activity after opsonization of the target [67]. This uterine defense mechanism reaches a pick at around 6–12 hours post-mating or AI [97]. In normal mares, most of the inflammatory products are cleared by physical uterine mechanisms within 48 hours after breeding, and the infection is cleared before the embryo leaves the fallopian tube and enters to the uterus on about days 5–6 post-ovulation [98], the uterine inflammation has to be under control by 96 hours post-ovulation to maximize survival of the embryo [67]. A susceptible mare with persistent post-mating endometritis is unable to clear such fluid by 96 hours, and the resulting prolonged inflammation generates an embryo-toxic environment. In addition, premature lysis of the CL is caused by PGF2α and subsequent progesterone deficiency, all contribute to embryo mortality and infertility [99]. This is more common in older and multiparous mares. They present with a history of short cycling and often and vaginal discharge approximately 2 weeks post-breeding [100].

4. Oophoritis and salpingitis

After abdominal surgery or peritonitis, infectious inflammation of the ovaries (oophoritis) with abscessation and peritoneal adhesions may occur. Oophoritis could be a consequence of repeated transvaginal ultrasound-guided follicular aspiration [101, 102]. Affected mares present abdominal pain, anorexia, fever of unknown origin, and weight loss. Transrectal ultrasonography can help in the diagnosis of these infections. For the extend evaluation of the lesions and confirmation of the diagnosis, laparoscopy may be achieved. Ovariectomy is usually required for treatment of this condition [103]. Although it is rare in the mare, salpingitis may result from ascending infection of *Chlamydia* spp. as *Chlamidiaabortus* and *Chlamidia psittaci* after partum [74]. Salpingitis has been described in mares with CEM. Bilateral salpingitis in mares results in sterility [103].

http://dx.doi.org/10.5772/63741

5. Postpartum metritis

Postpartum uterine infections are of particular importance because of their severity and effect on the general health of the mare. The incidence of postpartum metritis—i.e., infection of the uterus within 7–10 days postpartum, sometimes involving the endometrium, myometrium, and perimetrium—in foaling mares is low but increases when birthing trauma and/or retained placenta occurs [2, 3]. Septic postpartum metritis is often a result of nonhygienic manipulation during foaling, obstetric manipulations, and retained placenta. Mares with postpartum may present severe systemic complications as endotoxemia and laminitis. The etiology of septic/toxic metritis is associated with uterine atony or inertia. Trauma to the uterus, autolysis of placental remnants, and excessive lochia accumulation likely contribute to rapid growth of gram negative as *E. coli* and *K. pneumoniae* bacteria and production of toxins, which may be absorbed into the bloodstream, particularly when expulsion of contents is delayed or when the normally intact uterine mucosal barrier is damaged. Disruption of the endometrial mucosal barrier occurs during dystocia or gradually progresses after retention of fetal membranes leading to bacterial overgrowth and absorption of produced toxins. This process normally develops septic/toxic metritis and/or laminitis. Treatment consists of daily uterine flushers, systemic antimicrobial therapy, and therapy for endotoxemia. Laminitis and dehydration should be immediately initiated in affected mares [3, 104].

Author details

K. Satué[1*] and J.C. Gardon[2]

*Address all correspondence to: ksatue@uchceu.es

1 Department of Animal Medicine and Surgery, Faculty of Veterinary, CEU-Cardenal Herrera University, Alfara del Patriarca, Valencia, Spain

2 Department of Animal Medicine and Surgery, Faculty of Veterinary and Experimental Sciences, Catholic University of Valencia "San Vicente Mártir", Valencia, Spain

References

[1] Samper JC, Tibary A. Disease transmission in horses. Theriogenology 2006;66:551–559.

[2] Tibary A, Pearson LK, Fite CL. Reproductive tract infections. In: Sellon DC, Long MT, editors. Equine infectious diseases, 2nd ed. St. Louis, Missouri: Saunders Elsevier; 2014; p. 84–105.

[3] Blanchard, TL. Postpartum metritis. In: McKinnon AO, Squires EL, Vaala WE, editors. Equine reproduction. Chichester, UK: Wiley-Blackwell; 2011; p. 2530–2536.

[4] Leblanc MM, McKinnon AO. Breeding the problem mare. In: McKinnon AO, Squires EL, Vaala WE, editors. Equine reproduction. Chichester, UK: Wiley-Blackwell; 2011; p. 2620–2642.

[5] Newcombe JR. Why are mares with pneumovagina susceptible to bacterial endometritis? A personal opinion. J Equine Vet Sci 2011;31(4):174–179.

[6] Bradecamp EA. Pneumovagina. In: McKinnon AO, Squires EL, Vaala WE, editors. Equine reproduction. Chichester, UK: Wiley-Blackwell; 2011; p. 2537–2544.

[7] Parrilla-Hernandez S, Ponthier J, Franck TY, Serteyn DD, Deleuze SC. High concentrations of myeloperoxidase in the equine uterus as an indicator of endometritis. Theriogenology 2014;81(7):936–940.

[8] McKinnon AO, Jalim SL. Surgery of the caudal reproductive tract. In: McKinnon AO, Squires EL, Vaala WE, editors. Equine reproduction. Chichester, UK: Wiley-Blackwell; 2011; p. 2545–2558.

[9] Sertichm PL. Cervix adhesions. In: McKinnon AO, Squires EL, Vaala WE, editors. Equine reproduction. Chichester, UK: Wiley-Blackwell; 2011; p. 2721–2723.

[10] Pollock PJ, Russell TM. Cervical surgery. In: McKinnon AO, Squires EL, Vaala WE, editors. Equine reproduction. Chichester, UK: Wiley-Blackwell; 2011; p. 2559–2563.

[11] Barrandeguy M, Thiry E. Equine coital exanthema and its potential economic implications for the equine industry. Vet J 2012;191(1):35–40.

[12] Arighi M. Developmental abnormalities of the male reproductive tract. In: McKinnon AO, Squires EL, Vaala WE, editors. Equine reproduction. Chichester, UK: Wiley-Blackwell; 2011; p. 1109–1112.

[13] Sijmons S, Vissani A, Tordoya MS, Muylkens B, Thiry E, Maes P, Matthijnssens J, Barrandeguy M, Van Ranst M. Complete genome sequence of equidherpesvirus 3. Genome Announc 2014;2(5):e00797-14.

[14] Barrandeguy M, Vissani A, Lezica FP, Salamone J, Heguy A, Becerra L, Olguin Perglione C, Thiry E. Subclinical infection and periodic shedding of equid herpesvirus 3. Theriogenology 2010;74(4):576–580.

[15] Lu K, Morresey PR. Infectious diseases in breeding stallion. Clin Tech Equine Pract 2007;6:285–290.

[16] Scacchia M, Cammà C, Di Francesco G, Di Provvido A, Giunta R, Luciani M, Marino AM, Pascucci I, Caporale V. A clinical case of dourine in an outbreak in Italy. Vet Ital 2011;47(4): 473–475.

[17] Robinson EM. Dourine infection in young equines. Onderstepoort J Vet Sci Anim Ind 1984;23:39–40.

[18] Timoney PJ. Contagious equine metritis. In: McKinnon AO, Squires EL, Vaala WE, editors. Equine reproduction. Chichester, UK: Wiley-Blackwell; 2011; p. 2399–2409.

[19] Pascucci I, Prowido A, Camma C, Di Francesco G, Calistri P, Tittarelli M, Ferri N, Scacchia M, Caporale V. Diagnosis of dourine outbreaks in Italy. Vet Parasitol 2013;193:30–38.

[20] Claes F, Agbo EC, Radwanska M, Tepas MF, Baltz T, De Waal DT, Goddeeris BM, Claassen E, Buscher P. How does *T. equiperdum* fit into the Trypanozoongenus?. A cluster analysis and multiplex genotyping approach. Parasitology 2003;126:425–431.

[21] Timoney PJ, Powell DG. Isolation of the contagious equine metritis organism from colts and fillies in the United Kingdom and Ireland. Vet Rec 1982;111(21):478–482.

[22] Breuil MF, Duquesne F, Leperchois E, Laugier C, Ferry B, Collin G, Petry S. Contagious equine metritis cases reported in France since 2006. Vet Rec 2015;177(13):340.

[23] Ricketts SW, Young A, Medici EB. Uterine and clitorial cultures. In: McKinnon AO, Voss JL, editors. Equine reproduction. Philadelphia, USA: Lea and Febinger; 1993; p. 234–245.

[24] Troedsson MHT. Endometritis. In: McKinnon AO, Squires EL, Vaala WE, editors. Equine reproduction. Chichester, UK: Wiley-Blackwell; 2011; p. 2608–2619.

[25] Aitken GJ. Subclinical fungal endometritis in an 8-year-old Hanoverian mare. Can Vet J 2012;53(2):196–198.

[26] Buczkowska J, Kozdrowski R, Nowak M, Raś A, Staroniewicz Z, Siemieniuch MJ. Comparison of the biopsy and cytobrush techniques for diagnosis of subclinical endometritis in mares. Reprod Biol Endocrinol 2014;4:12–27.

[27] Overbeck W, Witte TS, Heuwieser W. Comparison of three diagnostic methods to identify subclinical endometritis in mares. Theriogenology 2011;75(7):1311–1318.

[28] Christoffersen M, Söderlind M, Rudefalk SR, Pedersen HG, Allen J, Krekeler N. Risk factors associated with uterine fluid after breeding caused by *Streptococcus zooepidemicus*. Theriogenology 2015;84(8):1283–1290.

[29] Rohrbach BW, Sheerin PC, Cantrell CK, Matthews PM, Steiner JV, Dodds LE. Effect of adjunctive treatment with intravenously administered *Propioni bacterium acnes* on reproductive performance in mares with persistent endometritis. J Am Vet Med Assoc 2007;231:107–113.

[30] Cocchia N, Paciello O, Auletta L, Uccello V, Silvestro L, Mallardo K, Paraggio G, Pasolini MP. Comparison of the cytobrush, cottonswab, and low-volume uterine flush techniques to evaluate endometrial cytology for diagnosing endometritis in chronically infertile mares. Theriogenology 2012;77(1):89–98.

[31] Walter J, Neuberg KP, Failing K, Wehrend A. Cytological diagnosis of endometritis in the mare: Investigations of sampling techniques and relation to bacteriological results. Anim Reprod Sci 2012;132(3–4):178–186.

[32] Davies Morel MC, Lawlor ND. Equine endometrial cytology and bacteriology: Effectiveness for predicting live foaling rates. Vet J 2013;198(1):206–211.

[33] LeBlanc MM, Causey RC. Clinical and subclinical endometritis in the mare: Both threats to fertility. Reprod Domest Anim 2009;44(3):10–22.

[34] Woodward EM, Troedsson MH. Inflammatory mechanisms of endometritis. Equine Vet J 2015;47(4):384–389.

[35] Liu IK, Troedsson MH. The diagnosis and treatment of endometritis in the mare: Yesterday and today. Theriogenology 2008;70(3):415–420.

[36] Christoffersen M, Woodward EM, Bojesen AM, Petersen MR, Squires EL, Lehn-Jensen H, Troedsson MH. Effect of immunomodulatory therapy on the endometrial inflammatory response to induced infectious endometritis in susceptible mares. Theriogenology 2012;78(5):991–1004.

[37] Petersen MR, Skive B, Christoffersen M, Lu K, Nielsen JM, Troedsson MH, Bojesen AM. Activation of persistent *Streptococcus equi* subspecies *zooepidemicus* in mares with subclinical endometritis. Vet Microbiol 2015;179(1–2):119–125.

[38] Woodward EM, Christoffersen M, Horohov D, Squires EL, Troedsson MH. The effect of treatment with immune modulators on endometrial cytokine expression in mares susceptible to persistent breeding-induced endometritis. Equine Vet J 2015;47(2):235–239.

[39] Szóstek AZ, Lukasik K, Galvão AM, Ferreira-Dias GM, Skarzynski DJ. Impairment of the interleukin system in equine endometrium during the course of endometriosis. Biol Reprod 2013;89(4):79.

[40] Christoffersen M, Baagoe CD, Jacobsen S, Bojesen AM, Petersen MR, Lehn-Jensen H. Evaluation of the systemic acute phase response and endometrial gene expression of serum amyloid A and pro- and anti-inflammatory cytokines in mares with experimentally induced endometritis. Vet Immunol Immunopathol 2010;138(1–2):95–105.

[41] Gajos K, Kozdrowski R, Nowak M, Siemieniuch MJ. Altered secretion of selected arachidonic acid metabolites during subclinical endometritis relative to estrous cycle stage and grade of fibrosis in mares. Theriogenology 2015;84(3):457–466.

[42] Nash DM, Sheldon IM, Herath S, Lane EA. Markers of the uterine innate immune response of the mare. Anim Reprod Sci 2010;119(1–2):31–39.

[43] Rebordão MR, Galvão A, Szóstek A, Amaral A, Mateus L, Skarzynski DJ, Ferreira-Dias G. Physiopathologic mechanisms involved in mare endometriosis. J Reprod Immunol 2014;106:41–49.

[44] Troedsson MH, Liu IK, Thurmond M. Immunoglobulin (IgG and IgA) and complement (C3) concentrations in uterine secretion following an intrauterine challenge of *Streptococcus zooepidemicus* in mares susceptible to versus resistant to chronic uterine infection. Biol Reprod 1993;49(3):502–506.

[45] Troedsson MHT, Liu IKM, Thurmon M. Function of uterine and blood-derived polymorphonuclear neutrophils in mares susceptible and resistant to chronic uterine infection: Phagocytosis and chemotaxis. Biol Reprod 1993;49:507–514.

[46] Rebordão MR, Carneiro C, Alexandre-Pires G, Brito P, Pereira C, Nunes T, Galvão A, Leitão A, Vilela C, Ferreira-Dias G. Neutrophil extracellular traps formation by bacteria causing endometritis in the mare. Reprod Domest Anim 2014;49(4):82–87.

[47] Alghamdi AS, Foster DN, Carlson CS, Troedsson MH. Nitric oxide levels and nitric oxide synthase expression in uterine samples from mares susceptible and resistant to persistent breeding-induced endometritis. Am J Reprod Immunol 2005;53(5):230–237.

[48] Krumrych W, Danek J. Chemiluminescence of peripheral blood neutrophils in mares with endometritis. Bull Vet Inst Pulawy 2012;56:51–56.

[49] Brown AE, Hansen PJ, Asbury AC. Opsonization of bacteria by uterine secretions of cyclic mares. Am J Reprod Immunol Microbiol 1985;9(4):119–123.

[50] Causey RC. Making sense of equine uterine infections: The many faces of physiological clearance. Vet J 2006;172:405–421.

[51] Brinsko SP, Varner DD, Blanchard TL. The effect of uterine lavage performed four hours post-insemination on pregnancy rate in mares. Theriogenology 1991;35:1111–1119.

[52] Hurtgen JP. Pathogenesis and treatment of endometritis in the mare: A review. Theriogenology 2006;66(3):560–566.

[53] Da Costa R, Ferreira-Dias G, Mateus L, Korzekwa A, Andronowska A, Platek R, Skarzynski DJ. Endometrial nitric oxide production and nitric oxide synthases in the equine endometrium: Relationship with microvascular density during the estrous cycle. Domest Anim Endocrinol 2007;32(4):287–302.

[54] Strzemienski PJ, Do D, Kenney RM. Antibacterial activity of mare uterine fluid. Biol Reprod 1984;31:303–311.

[55] Johnson JU, Oxender WD, Berkhoff HA. Influence of estrogen on antibacterial and immunoglobulin secretory activities of uterine fluids from ovariectomized mares. Am J Vet Res 1994;55(5):643–649.

[56] Kolm G, Klein D, Knapp E, Watanabe K, Walter I. Lactoferrin expression in the horse endometrium: Relevance in persisting mating-induced endometritis. Vet Immunol Immunopathol 2006;114(1–2):159–167.

[57] Causey RC. Mucus and the mare: How little we know. Theriogenology 2007;68(3):386–394.

[58] Albihn A, Baverud V, Magnusson U. Uterine microbiology and antimicrobial susceptibility in isolated bacteria from mares with fertility problems. Acta Vet Scand 2003;44(3):121–129.

[59] Maeda Y, Ohtsuka H, Tomioka M, Tanabe T, Nambo Y, Uematsu H, Oikawa MA. Effect of progesterone on the in vitro response of peripheral blood mononuclear cells stimulated by *Escherichia coli* in mares. J Vet Med Sci 2012;74(5):629–632.

[60] Smit LI. Relationships between uterine microbiology, cytology and pregnancy rates in thoroughbred mares 2006–2013 [thesis]. Theses Master thesis. Faculty of Veterinary Medicine. Utrech University; 2015.

[61] Hamouda MA, Al-Hizab FA, Ghoneim IM, Al-Dughaym AM, Al-Hashim HJ. Assessment of endometritis in Arabian mare. J Anim Prod 2012;14(2):99–103.

[62] Rasmussen CD, Haugaard MM, Petersen MR, Nielsen JM, Pedersen HG, Bojesen AM. *Streptococcus equi* subsp. *zooepidemicus* isolates from equine infectious endometritis belong to a distinct genetic group. Vet Res 2013;44:26.

[63] Ricketts SW, Mackintosh ME. Role of anaerobic bacteria in equine endometritis. J Reprod Fertil Suppl 1987;35:343–351.

[64] Timoney JF, Artiushin CS, Boschwitz JS. Comparison of the sequences and functions of Streptococcus equi M-like proteins SeM and SzPSe. Infect Immun 1997;65(9):3600–3605.

[65] Nicholson ML, Ferdinand LR, Sampson JS, Benin A, Balter S, Pinto SW, Richard SF, Facklam R, Carlone GM, Beall B. Analysis of Immunoreactivity to a *Streptococcus equi* subsp. *zooepidemicus* M-like protein to confirm an outbreak of poststreptococcal glomerulonephritis, and sequences of M-Like proteins from isolates obtained from different host species. J Clin Microbiol 2000;38(11):4126–4130.

[66] Wittenbrink MM. Bacterial infections of the equine genital tract. Pferdeheilkunde 2012;28(1):30–32.

[67] Troedsson MH. Uterine clearance and resistance to persistent endometritis in the mare. Theriogenology 1999;52(3):461–471.

[68] LeBlanc MM. When to refer an infertile mare to a theriogenologist. Theriogenology 2008;70:421–429.

[69] Dascanio JJ, Schweizer C, Ley WB. Equine fungal endometritis. Equine Vet Educ 2001;13:324–329.

[70] Stefanetti V, Marenzoni ML, Lepri E, Coletti M, Proietti PC, Agnetti F, Crotti S, Pitzurra L, Del Sero A, Passamonti F. A case of *Candida guilliermondii* abortion in an Arab mare. Med Mycol Case Rep 2014;4:19–22.

[71] Beltaire KA, Cheong SH, Coutinho da Silva MA. Retrospective study on equine uterine fungal isolates and antifungal susceptibility patterns (1999–2011). Equine Vet J 2012;44:84–87.

[72] Stout TAE. Fungal endometritis in the mare. Pferdeheilkunde 2008;24(1):83–87.

[73] Rantala M, Attia S, Koukila-Kähkölä P, de Hoog S, Anttila M, Katila T. Cladophialophorabantiana as an emerging pathogen in animals: Case report of equine endometritis and review of the literature. J Clin Microbiol 2015;53(9):3047–3053.

[74] Wittenbrink MM. Aetiological significance of chlamydial infections in equine reproductive disorders. Pferdeheilkunde 1999;15(6):538–541.

[75] Threlfall WR, Carleton CL. Treatment of uterine infections in the mare. In: Morrow DA, editor. Current therapy in theriogenology. Philadelphia: W.B. Saunders Co.; 1986; p. 730–737.

[76] Vandeplassche M, Spincemaille J, Bouters R. Advanced pyometra with intact endometrial cups in a mare. Equine Vet J 1979;11:112–113.

[77] Kennedy PC, Miller RB. The uterus. In: Jubb KVF, Kennedy PC, Palmer N, editors. Pathology of domestic animals, 4th ed., vol. 3. San Diego, CA: Academic Press; 1993; p. 372–387.

[78] Abou-Gabal M, Hogle RM, West JK. Pyometra in a mare caused by Candida rugosa. J Am Vet Med Assoc 1977;170:177–178.

[79] Hughes JP, Stabenfeldt GH, Kindahl H, Kennedy PC, Edqvist LE, Neely DP, Schalm OW. Pyometra in the mare. J Reprod Fertil Suppl 1979;27:321–329.

[80] Timoney PJ. Aspects of the occurrence, diagnosis and control of selected venereal diseases in the stallion. In: Proceeding of the Stallion Reproduction Symposium Society Theriogenol, Baltimore MD, 1998; p. 76–83.

[81] Klug E, Sieme H. Infectious agents in equine semen. Acta Vet Scand 1992;88:73–81.

[82] Clement F, Vidament M, Guerin B. Microbial contamination of stallion semen. In: Proceeding of International Symposium on Equine Reproduction, Brazil, 1994; p. 199–200.

[83] Timoney PJ, Ward J, Kelly PA. A contagious genital infection of mares. Vet Rec 1977;101:103.

[84] Nakashiro H, Naruse M, Sugimoto C, Isayama Y, Kuniyasu C. Isolation of *Haemophilus equigenitalis* from an aborted equine fetus. Natl Inst Anim Health Q (Tokyo) 1981;21(4):184–185.

[85] Platt H, Atherton JG, Simpson DJ. The experimental infection of ponies with contagious equine metritis. Equine Vet J 1978;10:153–159.

[86] Timoney PJ. Contagious equine metritis. Comp Immunol Microb 1996;19:199–204.

[87] Powell DG. Contagious equine metritis. Adv Vet Sci Comp Med 1981;25:161–184.

[88] Schluter H, Kuller HJ, Friedrich U, Selbitz HJ, Marwitz T, Beyer C, Ullrich E. Epizootiology and treatment of contagious equine metritis (CEM), with particular reference to the treatment of infected stallions. Prakt Tierarzt 1991;72:503–511.

[89] Duquesne F, Pronost S, Laugier C, Petry S. Identification of *Taylorella equigenitalis* responsible for contagious equine metritis in equine genital swabs by direct polymerase chain reaction. Res Vet Sci 2007;82:47–49.

[90] Timoney PJ, McCollum WH. Equine viral arteritis. Vet Clin North Am Equine Pract 1993;9:295–309.

[91] Holyoak GR, Balasuriya UB, Broaddus CC, Timoney PJ. Equine viral arteritis: Current status and prevention. Theriogenology 2008;70(3):403–414.

[92] Metcalf ES. The role of international transport of equine semen on disease transmission. Anim ReprodSci 2001;68(3–4):229–237.

[93] LeBlanc MM. Uterine cytology. In: McKinnon AO, Squires EL, Vaala WE, editors. Equine reproduction. Chichester, UK: Wiley-Blackwell; 2011; p. 1922–1928.

[94] Nielsen JM. Endometritis in the mare: A diagnostic study comparing cultures from swab and biopsy. Theriogenology 2005;64(3):510–518.

[95] LeBlanc MM, Magsig J, Stromberg AJ. Use of a low-volume uterine flush for diagnosing endometritis in chronically infertile mares. Theriogenology 2007;68:403–412.

[96] Troedsson MH, Loset K, Alghamdi AM, Dahms B, Crabo BG. Interaction between equine semen and the endometrium: The inflammatory response to semen. Anim Reprod Sci 2001;68:273–278.

[97] Katila T. Uterine defence mechanisms in the mare. Anim Reprod Sci 1996;42:197–204.

[98] Betteridge KJ, Eaglesome MD, Mitchell D, Flood PF, Beriault R. Development of horse embryos up to twenty two days after ovulation: Observations on fresh specimens. J Anatomy 1982;135:191–209.

[99] Rambags BPB. Early pregnancy loss in aged mares: Probable causes and cures. Pferdeheilkunde 2003;19:653–656.

[100] Gores-Lindholm AR, LeBlanc MM, Causey R, Hitchborn A, Fayrer-Hosken RA, Kruger M, Vandenplas ML, Flores P, Ahlschwede S. Relationships between intrauterine infusion of N-acetylcysteine, equine endometrial pathology, neutrophil function, post-breeding therapy, and reproductive performance. Theriogenology 2013;80(3): 218–227.

[101] Bogh IB, Brink P, Jensen HE, Lehn-Jensen H, Greve T. Ovarian function and morphology in the mare after multiple follicular punctures. Equine Vet J 2003;35(6):575–579.

[102] Schlafer DH. Non-neoplastic abnormalities. In: McKinnon AO, Squires EL, Vaala WE, editors. Equine reproduction. Chichester, UK: Wiley-Blackwell; 2011; p. 2697–2706.

[103] Hawkins KL. Bilateral salpingitis, hydrosalpinx and oophoritis in a mare. Cornell Vet 1986;76(1):38–48.

[104] Blanchard TL, Varner DD, Scrutchfield WL, Bretzlaff KN, Taylor TS, Martin MT, Elmore RG. Management of distocia in mares: Retained placenta, metritis, and laminitis. Comp Cont Educ Pract Vet 1990;12:563–571.

Chapter 15

Endometritis and Infertility in the Mare – The Challenge in Equine Breeding Industry–A Review

Maria Pia Pasolini, Chiara Del Prete, Silvia Fabbri and Luigi Auletta

Additional information is available at the end of the chapter

http://dx.doi.org/10. 5772/62461

Abstract

Most major infertility problems are complex and several factors can cause failure to produce offspring. In the last few years, much of the efforts of practitioners and researchers working in equine breeding industry have been directed to individuate the pathophysiological mechanisms underlying poor reproductive performances in mares. Endometritis is on the talk in much of the recent research as the most frequent cause of subfertility in mares that cycle normally but do not conceive and in mares that cycle normally and conceive but then suffer early embryonic death. Post-breeding persistent endometritis, bacterial and other infective endometritis and poor uterine clearance have all been discussed in an attempt to define risk factors and a diagnostic algorithm. The aim of this chapter is to perform a thorough review of recent literature about endometritis. The diagnostic algorithms are carefully examined, highlighting pros as well as pitfalls of each diagnostic aid. Suggested therapeutic protocols are examined in the effort to detect what is actually recommended and what would better benefit from further corroboration. The idea that a better etiopathogenetical understanding of the endometritis remains the key to access to a correct diagnostic protocol and to a successful therapeutic plan will inspire this chapter.

Keywords: Endometritis, Mare, Diagnosis, Ultrasound, Therapy

1. Introduction

Every year many mares fail to become pregnant. These failures represent a substantial economic and genetic loss to the horse industry. Most major infertility problems are complex and several factors, singly or in combination, can cause failure to produce offspring. In the last few years, much of the efforts of practitioners and researchers working in equine breeding industry have been directed to individuate the pathophysiological mechanisms underlying poor reproductive performances in mares. To clarify, infertility includes three "problems" mares' types: mares that fail to cycle, mares that cycle normally but do not conceive and mares that cycle normally and conceive but then suffer early embryonic death. Endometritis is on the talk in much of the recent research as the most frequent cause of the last two conditions.

Post-breeding persistent endometritis, bacterial and other infective endometritis and poor uterine clearance have all been discussed in an attempt to define risk factors and a diagnostic algorithm, essential to reach a definitive diagnosis and to apply the appropriate therapeutic protocol. Breeding-induced endometritis is a normal physiological reaction in the horse, as it is believed that an inflammatory response is necessary for the effective removal of contaminating bacteria and excess spermatozoa introduced into the uterus. In a healthy uterus, the inflammation subsides within 48 hours, but the susceptible mares are not capable of resolving the inflammation triggered by sperm and develop persistent mating-induced endometritis (PMIE). A very strong relationship establishes between PMIE and infectious endometritis and a complex of mare (such as age, perineal conformation, uterine clearance and cervical competence) and microbial (such as induction of inflammation, epithelial adherence, resistance to phagocytosis and viscosity of secretion) factors contribute to the pathogenesis of endometritis. Traditionally, the mares that are prone to endometritis are called susceptible, in contrast to the "resistant" ones, not prone to uterine infection.

The aim of this chapter is to perform a thorough review of recent literature about endometritis. The cascades of inflammatory signals being complex and intertwined, the etiopathogenetical, diagnostic and prognostic roles of the recently studied inflammatory markers are discussed. In addition, the most common bacterial and fungal pathogens involved are reviewed, together with the recent advances in diagnostic procedures. In fact, the diagnostic algorithms are carefully examined, highlighting pros as well as pitfalls of each diagnostic aid. Suggested therapeutic protocols are examined in the effort to detect what is actually recommended and what would better benefit from further corroboration, with special attention to the correct use of antimicrobials and antibiotics, their common way of administration and contraindications. Consideration will be given to therapy alternatives such as proper breeding management, use of uterine lavage, oxytocin/prostaglandin administration and treatment of the biofilm formation. The idea that a better etiopathogenetical understanding of the endometritis remains the key to access to a correct diagnostic protocol and to a successful therapeutic plan will inspire this chapter.

2. Pathophysiology of endometritis in the mare

Endometritis is a major cause of infertility in the mare. It is an acute or chronic inflammation of the endometrium that can be classified based on both its etiology and pathophysiology. Susceptibility to persistent bacterial endometritis was characterized as early as 1969 [1]. Since then, the physiopathological mechanisms involved in persistent endometritis and its correlation with bacterial endometritis and infertility in the mare have been discussed in several studies [2–18]. Endometrium responds to the introduction of air, urine, semen, bacteria, fungi or yeasts through an inflammatory reaction that ultimately hesitates in restoring an environment suitable to receive the conceptus, as it migrates from the oviduct few days after the insemination. To induce endometritis in experimental conditions, either spermatozoa or bacteria such as *Streptococcus zooepidemicus* or *Escherichia coli* are commonly infused into the uterus. A subpopulation of mares, designated as susceptible, fails to resolve the endometritis and develops a persistent inflammatory condition, which affects fertility. Furthermore, if the mare is unable to clear bacteria that may have entered the uterus during breeding, a bacterial infection can develop [19, 20].

In conclusion, any difficulty in the physical clearance of inflammatory debris from the uterus after mating or foaling triggers the endometritis. Although the mechanisms for uterine clearance for different antigens are closely related, pathophysiology, clinical signs and therapy partially differ. For these reasons, breeding-induced endometritis and bacterial endometritis will be described separately.

2. 1. Transient and persistent mating-induced endometritis

The transient breeding-induced endometritis is a physiological reaction in the immediate hours after breeding. It is a local inflammatory response necessary to remove excess spermatozoa and bacteria introduced into the uterus [8]. This response is limited to local inflammation, because any hematological alteration in inflammatory parameters has not yet been detected during breeding-induced endometritis [21]. Furthermore, in healthy mares, the endometritis resolves within 24–48 hours, leaving the uterus clean and free from inflammation.

2. 1. 1. Mechanical clearance and inflammatory response

Semen and its extender play an important role in the induction of defense mechanisms, depending on seminal components and sperms numbers, concentration, viability and site of semen deposition. In mares mated, or artificially inseminated with fresh or cooled semen, seminal plasma activates the complement system that evokes massive migration of the polymorphonuclear leucocytes (PMNs), cytokines and mononuclear cells invasion that prepares the endometrium to recipe the embryo [11, 22]. During the cryopreservation process, an important mechanism of modulation of the inflammatory response is lost due to the removal of seminal plasma, so that a severe inflammation follows the insemination with frozen/thawed semen [13]. Furthermore, seminal plasma contributes to the transport and survival of viable spermatozoa and the elimination of non-viable spermatozoa from the uterus, suppressing binding between neutrophils and viable spermatozoa [23].

The complement activation cascade led to the formation of leukotriene B4, prostaglandin (PG) E and PGF2α and other arachidonic acid metabolites, which act as chemo-attractants for PMNs in the uterus [2–5, 7]. The PMNs, on their part, drive the inflammatory response to cleaning the uterus: spermatozoa and bacteria destruction is performed by way of phagocytosis and release of neutrophil extracellular traps, composed of extensions of DNA and histones with antimicrobial action [15]. The intrauterine fluid is composed of neutrophils, inflammatory mediators and plasma proteins, including immunoglobulin and enzymes [3–4, 6–7]. The release of PGF2α stimulates myometrial contractions combined with ciliary propulsion of the mucus blanket, promoting the elimination of bacteria and dead inflammatory cells via the cervix or the lymphatics [9, 12].

In "resistant" mares, uterine fluid is eliminated and inflammation resolves within 5 days post-insemination and the fertilized oocyte descends in a uterus ready to implantation [24]. On the contrary, susceptible mares are unable to resolve the physiological breeding-induced inflammation and they surrender to persistent post-insemination endometritis. The accumulation of intrauterine fluid persists over five days post-ovulation in susceptible mares [17]. Therefore, the success of getting the mare pregnant is compromised by an unprepared endometrium and by the development of concomitant bacterial infections.

It is likely that at the origin of both breeding-induced and bacterial endometritis, there are common failures in the physical mechanisms of uterine clearance by uterine contractions. Indeed, mechanical clearance plays a key role in the uterine response to the contamination, and deficits in myometrial contractility could have a major responsibility in the pathogenesis of delayed uterine clearance. The increase in myoelectric activity, indicating an increase in uterine contractions, observed in healthy mares after the insemination, resulted delayed by 2 hours in susceptible mares. Additionally, susceptible mares showed a sharp decline in activity, dropping below baseline levels after 12 hours [10]. Furthermore, it was observed that more radiocolloid was retained in the uterus of susceptible mares 2 hours after infusion than in resistant mares [25]. Impaired myometrial function could be related to the increased intrauterine accumulation of nitric oxide (NO), produced in excess by inducible NO synthase (iNOS) during inflammation in susceptible mares, as confirmed by an increased endometrial expression of iNOS mRNA after insemination [26–28]. The NO is a smooth muscle relaxant and myometrial tissue was unable to respond to electrical stimulus in the presence of NO, during in vitro experiments [29].

Reaction to the insemination could involve humoral and cellular mechanism, with differences between resistant and susceptible mares. Several studies produced contradictory findings, but most authors agree that immunoglobulins are involved mainly in the endometrial response to bacteria than to semen. However, there are no data to demonstrate that susceptibility is a direct cause of altered immunoglobulins in the uterus [30–32]. Similarly, it was suggested that in resistant and susceptible mares, different inflammatory cells were involved and that susceptibility to persistent endometritis was primarily caused by a dysfunction in the adaptive immune response. Until now, there are no data to prove these hypotheses, and just a decreased opsonizing ability of the uterine secretions in sub-fertile mares compared with normal mares was demonstrated [9].

The inflammatory response in endometritis is a complex process involving multiple signaling pathways, initiated by the cytokines, produced by a variety of cell types, to allow the recognition of antigens and the recruitment of inflammatory cells [33]. Specifically, the inflammatory response is modulated by a delicate balance between the expressions of pro- and anti-inflammatory interleukin (IL). Another important pro-inflammatory cytokine involved with the inflammatory response is interferon-γ. It promotes the migration of inflammatory cells through vessel walls and leads to the activation of microbicidal functions, and to an upregulation of iNOS [34]. Few studies focused on these inflammatory pathways in the mare so far, and they gave contradictory results in relation to the experimental protocol and the timing of evaluation [33, 35–37]. Specifically, timing is very important in the experimental design, since the difference between resistant and susceptible mares consist mainly in the persistence of the breeding-induced inflammatory response. Thus, results of the studies were sensibly different, measuring the expression of several IL at 24 hours or at 6 hours after breeding. However, an increased mRNA expression of IL8 and lower expression of IL10 were observed in susceptible mares compared to resistant mares 24 hours after insemination [38]. On measuring cytokines expression in mares at several time points within the first 24 hours after breeding, susceptible mares had lower expression of the inflammatory modulating cytokines IL10, IL1-receptor antagonist and IL6 when compared with resistant mares 6 hours after insemination. After 3–6 hours from breeding, there were no differences between resistant and susceptible mares in the degree of uterine inflammation, fluid retention, endometrial cytology and ultrasound imaging. However, on the basis of the differences in mRNA expression of cytokines observed, it was stated that a critical time in the development of persistent breeding-induced endometritis occurs around 6 hours after breeding [33].

2. 1. 2. Predisposing factors to persistent breeding-induced endometritis

Persistent endometritis has multifactorial pathogenesis, and properties of the bacteria and mare's characteristics are key components in the development and resolution of the inflammation [39]. Several predisposing factors are associated with the individual mare [17–18]. Young and fertile resistant mares and older and subfertile susceptible mares have been examined to clarify the differences in the ability to resolve uterine inflammation. Indeed, the aging and parity have been associated with altered systemic immune response [30–31]. Older mares present several predisposing factors to develop persistent uterine infections after breeding. Aging and parity influx on the ability of clearing debris, since mares develop over time anatomical or degenerative defects that interfere with uterine drainage. Other risk factors associated with persistent infections include the conformation or the acquired alteration of the internal and external reproductive organs. For example, not only poor vulvar conformation, incompetent vagino-vestibular sphincter, vaginal stretching or an incompetent cervix but also genital pathology, such as pneumovagina or vagino/cervical injuries can facilitate the entrance of pathogens, which normally lives over body surface [40]. Mares with cervical fibrosis secondary to a traumatic birth, or with the elongated, narrow cervix typical in aged maiden mares, accumulate uterine fluid easily because of the compromised cervical drainage [17]. Free fluid accumulation is also facilitated by a pendulous uterus or impaired lymphatic drainage and atrophy of endometrial folds [41–44].

Degenerative changes, such as an abnormal myometrium, periglandular fibrosis, vascular degeneration, lymphangiectasia, scarring and atrophy of endometrial folds or damage to the reproductive apparatus may also explain delayed uterine clearance of bacteria, fluid and debris [17]. The altered mucociliary activity does not impede the bacterial adhesion on the endometrium and expulsion of the inflammatory cells. Vascular degenerations inhibit hormones delivery to endometrium and disturb uterine drainage, reducing venous return in capillary beds. Prolonged endometrial edema and consequent persistent inflammation characterize the uterus of susceptible mares [43].

2. 2. Bacterial endometritis

The sexually transmissible disease in horses are caused by primary pathogens *Taylorella equigenitalis,* certain unspecified serotypes of *Pseudomonas aeruginosa* and *Klebsiella pneumoniae* capsule types 1, 2 and 5 [45]. The true venereal disease is caused by *T. equigenitalis* and is known as contagious equine metritis resulting in cervicitis, vaginitis and endometritis. Asymptomatic infected carrier stallions transmit the pathogens to the mares, which will present copious muco-purulent vaginal discharge within a week after breeding. However, this pathology is endemic in Europe and a more insidious form with minimal clinical signs has been recognized [46–47]. *P. aeruginosa* and *K. pneumoniae* inhabit the external genital of the stallion and infections are transmitted by coitus, insemination with infected semen and genital manipulations [48–49].

Contamination of the uterus by fecal and genital opportunistic flora may provoke an infection during mating or genital tract manipulations. A wide variety of opportunistic aerobic and anaerobic bacteria, fungi and yeasts, either alone or in synergy, have been occasionally implicated as causes of endometritis. In a report, *Streptococcus equi* subsp. *zooepidemicus* was responsible for approximately 65% of the cases while *Escherichia coli, K. pneumoniae* and *P. aeruginosa* accounted for approximately 10% [47]. The alteration of uterine defense mechanisms is attributed to individual microbial factors such as induction of inflammation, epithelial adherence, resistance to phagocytosis and viscosity of secretions [50]. Bacterial products can modify any properties of mucus, rendering cilia unable to expel uterine exudates. Changes in production, viscosity or elasticity of mucus and cilia function determinate the adverse effects on uterine clearance and hence, these can interfere with antibiotic penetration, resulting in treatment failure or antibiotic resistance [17].

2. 3. Chronic endometritis

Chronic infection and mixed population of microorganism cause severe, progressive and irreversible fibrotic condition that affects mare endometrium [51–54]. Long-standing influx of lymphocytes and plasmacells into the endometrium contribute to chronic degenerative changes, such as periglandular, perivascular or diffuse stromal fibrosis. This condition impairs endometrial function and future pregnancies, causing infertility [52–53].

3. Diagnosis of endometritis

The diagnosis of endometritis in the mare represents one of the crucial challenges for the equine clinical practice [55]. Equine practitioners have recently understood that the major cause of the progression from an acute to a chronic condition is the failure to identify the causative agent, given that affected mares do not always show evident clinical signs [55]. Hence, it is critical to make a correct etiological diagnosis, and to characterize the degree and the type of inflammation, in order to establish an effective treatment. Furthermore, it is not uncommon that mares with a long history of normal fertility can acquire post-breeding endometritis. In such cases, the clinician has no opportunity for prophylactic intervention [56].

The diagnostic algorithm for the identification of the causative agent comprises a detailed reproductive history and a complete clinical evaluation, including the transrectal palpation of the reproductive tract and the use of ancillary diagnostic aids [17, 57–58]. Among the latters, specific instrumental investigations, such as transrectal ultrasonography, vaginal and cervical exams, with both manual and endoscopic evaluation, and laboratory tools, such as uterine culture, endometrial cytology and biopsy, represent useful tools for the diagnosis of endometritis [17, 58]. Recently, myeloperoxidase has been investigated as a uterine inflammatory biomarker, but the relationship between its concentration and pathologic uterine conditions needs further studies [59]. To increase the pregnancy rates in "problem" mares, the practitioner should dispose a quick and reliable diagnostic technique to start the best treatment as soon as possible in the breeding season [56].

3. 1. Experimental identification of susceptible mares

Mares with endometritis begin to show intrauterine fluid accumulation following breeding, after the first three to four successful pregnancies. Uterine degenerative changes appear and worsen with age, the reproductive tract may become more pendulous and uterotonic drugs are no longer effective [57]. Furthermore, some reproductively normal, nulliparous as well as pluriparous mares exhibit an excessive uterine inflammatory response after being bred with frozen semen. The exuberant reaction may be a consequence of a low volume of seminal plasma and the lack of its beneficial action in decreasing the migration of neutrophils into the uterine lumen [57].

The delay in uterine clearance has an important role in the pathogenesis of uterine inflammation, since it influences the retention of endometrial inflammatory factors, whether they are bacterial or sperm-induced [60]. In fact, it was shown that mares susceptible to chronic uterine infections failed to clear adequately ^{51}Cr-labeled microspheres when compared with mares with normal uteri [37, 60]. The uterus, studied with scintigraphy in mares with a delayed uterine clearance, showed to be oriented vertically, while in reproductively normal mares it was oriented horizontally. Hence the "baggy" uterus contributes to fluid accumulation and low clearance [37, 57]. However, although scintigraphy has been proven to be a useful method for studying post-breeding endometritis, it seems not to be a functional diagnostic tool in a clinical setting [61]. In addition to the uterine position, the myometrial function plays an important role in uterine clearance, as confirmed by electromyographic recordings [60]. Nevertheless, not all mares susceptible to endometritis exhibit a delayed uterine clearance if cervical dilatation is appropriate [25].

3. 2. Clinical identification of susceptible mares

3. 2. 1. History

Mares susceptible to developing a persistent post-breeding endometritis are more often pluriparous, barren, older than 12 years of age and with a poor perineal conformation [57, 62]. Nonetheless, some maiden mares, which show an insufficient degree of relaxation of their cervix during estrus, may also develop persistent mating-induced endometritis, regardless of age. In such mares, the problem may be resolved with the first foal delivery [57].

3. 2. 2. Clinical examination

The mares' reproductive tract examination should include a body condition scoring and the notation of previous or existing foot problems [57]. Any changes in perineal, vulvar or cervical conformation should be evaluated before breeding [56–57, 63]. The two vulvar labia may not create a proper seal due to persistent relaxation of the vulva, and the rectum may be displaced cranially, stretching the vulva dorsally to the ischiatic arch and causing repeated fecal contamination of vulva and vestibule [56]. This kind of conformation is linked to the loss of fat in the perineal area due to a high level of fitness, and muscular fatigue and estrus exacerbate the perineal relaxation, but it can also be a heritable trait [63–64]. It is very important to check that the cervix opens properly in estrus and closes in diestrus [56].

3. 3. Clinical signs

Clinical signs of endometritis may be hidden, but vaginal discharge, short inter-estrus intervals and/or a shortened luteal phase and reduced fertility can be detected [17, 37, 65]. In bacterial endometritis, they can vary widely according to the pathogen, with symptoms markedly different between Gram-positive and Gram-negative bacteria [17]. A vaginal discharge may be seen more often during estrus [57]. However, the presence of evident clinical signs 48 hours post-breeding is of concern, since a non-inflammatory uterine environment is important for embryonic survival [16].

3. 4. Imaging of the reproductive system: ultrasonography

Ultrasonography (US) has always been considered an accurate and essential step in the diagnostic workup of endometritis [56, 59, 66]. The monitoring function of US is as important as the diagnostic one, since mares with subclinical endometritis require careful daily checking post-breeding [17]. Since its inception, the use of US has strongly impacted on the ability to detect the presence and to quantify the volume of uterine fluid accumulation, which is considered the main sign of endometritis, especially when observed after breeding; but this "hallmark" sign is not always present [17, 60, 67]. Intrauterine fluid presence has also been shown to be strongly related with low pregnancy rates, especially in mares older than 16 years, and to the biopsy score, revealing its diagnostic value in identifying the uterine inflammation [62, 67–68]. It may be detected as soon as 6 to 36 hours after breeding, but it can be noted at the pregnancy examination 14 to 16 days after breeding [57, 67]. Nonetheless, the more significant time to detect the uterine fluid collection is mid-to-late diestrus because the cervix is closed, and in a healthy uterus, fluid should be little or absent [68]. Intrauterine fluid has been also correlated to specific endometrial bacteria and cytological findings, with mares positive to non-pathogenic bacteria showing intra-uterine fluid in <40% of the US examinations [66–67]. The relevance of the uterine fluid accumulation can be evaluated by examining the depth, the echo-texture and persistence of the fluid [16]. Two or more centimeters of intra-uterine fluid during estrus, or between 6 and 36 hours post-breeding, are significant indices of susceptibility to mating-induced endometritis [62, 67]. A high echogenicity in the uterine fluid is associated with the presence of neutrophils and debris, thus indicative of inflammatory components [16]. Short, thick and hyperechoic lines within the uterus may represent air or exudates [17]. In Figure 1, some characteristic appearances of the equine uterus are depicted.

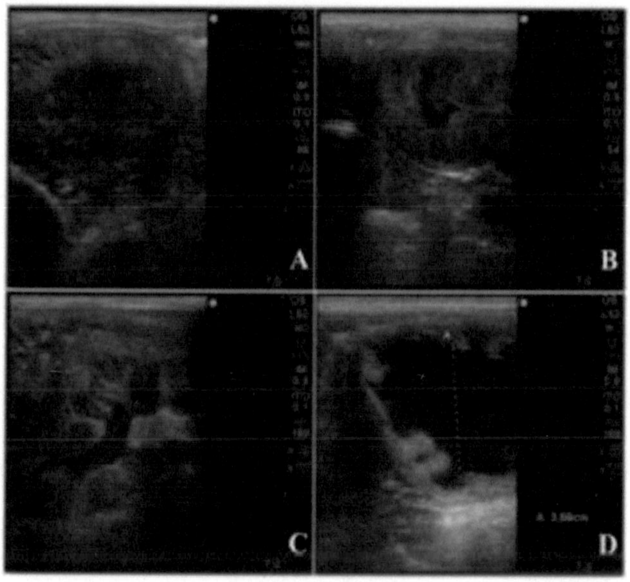

Figure 1. Trans-rectal ultrasonographic evaluation of the equine uterus with a linear transducer (bandwidth 5–10 MHz). In A: normal appearance of the uterus during early diestrus, 48 hours post-ovulation. In B: mild intrauterine fluid accumulation, with moderate edema of uterine folds during early estrus. In C: moderate intrauterine fluid accumulation, with severe edema of uterine folds during estrus. In D: severe (over 2 cm in depth) intrauterine fluid accumulation in diestrus, 13 days after ovulation, "hallmark" of equine endometritis.

Another important US sign of endometritis is abnormal edema [17]. Edema may occur physiologically due to lymphangiectasia and under influence of estrogen, i. e., during the early estrus. A modified version of the subjective system described by Samper has been developed to score uterine edema: grade 0 coincides with the absence of edema; grade I, in which it is difficult to identify uterine folds; grade II, characterized by some of the endometrial folds detectable and a cervix with a fish-bone aspect; grade III, with endometrial folds, easily identifiable and characterized by hyperechoic borders and hypoechoic centers (cartwheel); and grade IV for mares with "hyperedema", in which thickened and bulging endometrial folds are abnormally thick, with hyperechoic border and marked central hypoechogenicity, and the normal architecture of the cartwheel is lost [59]. Cervical incompetence, abnormal vascular reaction to estrogens, a lymphatic pathology or an altered myoelectric activity are all possible non-inflammatory causes of hyperedema [17, 59]. Thus, some edema patterns, such as excessive edema pre- or post-mating, or edema pattern that does not extend throughout the uterine wall, represent a pathological feature [17]. In particular, hyperedema has been considered the marker of uterine pathology when found during the estrus phase, independently from the positivity of a uterine cytology, but not during the early estrus [59]. Sometimes uterine fluid and edema are associated, probably due to the severity of drainage deficiency [59]. Furthermore, the appearance and dynamics of uterine cysts can be studied by US. Their effect on pregnancy rate seems to be a quantitative one, with only severely affected mares showing a reduction of fertility [68].

The use of more advanced US software, like Color-, Power-flow- and Pulse-Wave- Doppler applications, allows the evaluation of uterine vascularization. In humans, abnormal uterine blood flow and higher uterine artery impedance have been observed in women with recurrent pregnancy loss and different causes of infertility. Poor blood flow of the gravid uterus has been correlated with advanced age and diffuse endometrial degenerative changes during early pregnancy in mares. Furthermore, disturbed uterine blood flow has been recently associated to other uterine pathologies such as uterine cysts and endometrial elastosis in subfertile mares [69].

3. 5. Endoscopic evaluation of the reproductive system

After repeated mating in a season, mares may accumulate intrauterine fluid and display classic signs of inflammation on vaginoscopy. Endoscopic examination is the only way to establish the degree and the clinical significance of superficial intrauterine lesions and it is useful in several pathological conditions. It can be used in the mare suspected of having subclinical endometritis due to focal lesions, intra-uterine adhesions and endometrial cups retention. It has proven to be useful in mares with a history of silent heats, which may display endometrial scarring or loss of endometrial folds [17]. The best time to perform endoscopy is during diestrus or early estrus, since it is easier to perform than in other phases. Before the examination, the uterine lumen is dilated with air or saline, but the best visibility is obtained with air. It is important to remember to discard air out of the uterus after the procedure, with a catheter or a pump, because of possible irritation [17].

3. 6. Sampling techniques for bacteriological, cytological and histological evaluation: uterine swab, cytobrush, low volume flush and endometrial biopsy

The diagnostic methods used to characterize endometritis are the uterine swab, the cytobrush, low volume flush and the endometrial biopsy [37, 70]. As always, the clinician must interpret the data resulting from such techniques together with the clinical signs and bearing in mind how the results of each technique vary, depending on the pathogen [17, 58, 61, 65, 70–73]. All the procedures described thereafter assume that the mares are restrained in an examination stock, the tail is wrapped in an examination glove and suspended to the stock, and the whole perineal area is cleaned and disinfected to avoid contamination from the environment [16, 58, 71]. Each method has its pro and cons and many comparisons of the different techniques have been indeed performed [58, 65, 70–73]. Histologic evaluation of endometrial biopsies is the "gold standard", to which each technique has been compared to calculate the sensitivity and specificity [17, 65, 71]. Nevertheless, it should be remembered that all techniques can yield false-negative results if not conducted by expert clinician [37].

3. 6. 1. *Uterine swab*

The uterine swab collection methods for bacteriologic and cytological analysis are the mainstay for the diagnosis of acute endometritis in the mare [74]. Through this technique, bacteria as well as inflammatory cells can be collected and examined by culturing it, or smearing the swab for cytology [70, 74]. Uterine swabs are the most commonly used procedure because of low costs, ease of collection and safety of use; hence, routine pre-breeding uterine swabs should be always obtained from mares "at risk" [56, 65].

The double-guarded swab technique implicates the use of a double sheath, which allows minimizing vaginal contamination [16, 70–71]. The tip of the double-guarded swab is kept covered and free from lubricant as it is introduced into the reproductive tract. Then, it is advanced through the cervix into the uterus and the inner sheath is pushed through the outer sheath. The examiner starts moving the swab to sample the endometrial surface using a pushing and rolling motion for up to 1 min, redirecting the swab into different areas of the uterus. At the end of the sampling, the swab is pulled within the inner sheath, which is drawn back into the outer sheath, and the entire unit is then removed from the reproductive tract [16, 70–71].

Another kind of guarded uterine instrument is the Knudsen catheter that can be autoclaved and used repeatedly. It consists of a metal tube of 87 cm in length and an inner spiral metal rod, and it has a small hole at the tip, to allow advancing a cotton swab. The tube includes a thickened area, the olive, which marks the point of the catheter that should be placed at the outer cervical orifice [74].

For the classic uterine swab, cytological smears are prepared by gently rolling the side of the swab, and by pushing the end on a sterile slide. The swab is sent to laboratory for microbiological tests, including the tip in a transport container [16, 70–71]. On the other hand, the Knudsen catheter use provides the cotton swab for bacteriology, whereas the cytological sample is obtained by gently removing the material on the spiral rod [74]. Even if this technique, when properly adopted, is ideal for bacteriology, it leads to contrasting results for the cytological sampling. The use of this technique decreased strongly the number of mares improperly treated, but it may lead to cells deformation depending on the pressure applied during the smearing procedure [70, 74]. Nevertheless, too little pressure during the rolling procedure may lead to clumping of cells [74]. Moistening and gentle rolling have been proven to relief distortion and fragmentation of the collected cells [70]. Furthermore, this method can yield false negative results. In fact, about half of the cases of infectious endometritis resulted negative, since the microorganisms were located in the most pendulous part of uterus that is not easily reached. Conversely, false positive results can be associated with a contaminated sampling [55]. Furthermore, it collects a small superficial endometrial area, resulting in a small amount of total cells [70].

Otherwise, the degree of cellularity obtainable with the Knudsen catheter is influenced by the level of uterine secretion. Indeed, the contact of the smooth surface of the metallic spiral with a dry endometrial surface provides poor cellularity, whereas in case of abundant secretions, samples obtained show an excellent cellularity due to the larger surface area, without cells distortion and with infrequent red blood cells [74].

3. 6. 2. Cytobrush

Uterine brushes have been used for uterine cytology in humans, as well as in the equine species [60]. As described for the uterine swabs, a guarded technique is used, and the properly lubricated guarding tube is passed through the vagina to the base of a uterine horn or into the uterine body. Once in the area selected for the sampling, the outer tube is retracted far enough to expose the brush, and the cytobrush is rotated in a clockwise direction while in contact with the uterine wall [70]. The instrument is then retracted into the tube prior to removal from the uterus and then rolled on slides.

Cytobrush has been considered superior to the other methods for cytological sampling, since it is easier, more consistent and produces samples with higher cellularity than other techniques, but a gentle preparation of smear is mandatory to reduce the cells distortion [70, 74]. Cells fragmentation has been frequently observed in cytobrush smears probably due to the rigid fibers that damage the cells, as well as the common occurrence of red blood cells, which is an index of its invasiveness [70]. Proteinaceous material may contaminate the smears obtained with this technique, as well [70]. Nonetheless, it allows collecting cells both from the surface and from the depth of endometrium, up to glandular cells [70]. Such technique could preferentially be used to detect subclinical endometritis in field practice, for its inexpensiveness and safeness, particularly in comparison to endometrial biopsy [58, 65].

3. 6. 3. Low volume flush

The low volume flush is a method for uterine fluid collection [55]. It is almost as efficient as endometrial biopsy for microorganisms' isolation and can be performed during estrus or diestrus [55]. The procedure involves the use of a low volume (60 to 150 ml) of phosphate-buffered saline (PBS) or lactated Ringer's solution or physiological saline injected into the uterus. The practitioner, properly gloved, advances a sterile insemination pipette, or a Bivona catheter, *per vaginam* into the uterus, through which the solution is injected. Thus, the uterus is transrectally massaged to distribute the fluid evenly throughout the uterine lumen. Meanwhile, the pipette is moved back and forth and suction is applied to trap cells in the pipette. Finally, the effluent fluid is recovered in a sterile container. If the mare is in estrus, intravenous administration of 10 IU of oxytocin is suggested, to facilitate the release of fluid trapped in the edematous endometrial folds [16, 55, 70, 72].

The fluid is first evaluated macroscopically, holding the sample up to the light, for cloudiness and amount of mucus. The efflux is graded as clear, cloudy or clear with mucus strains. Both mucus and cloudiness are strongly correlated to the presence of *Streptococcus β haemolyticus* and *E. coli* [55, 72]. The recovered fluid is then centrifuged at 400 rpm for 10 min, the supernatant is discarded and the pellet is aliquoted in two parts, one for microbiological culture and the other one is resuspended in 1 ml of PBS and drops of the suspension are spilled onto slides for cytological evaluation [16, 55, 70, 72].

The low volume flush is a suitable method to collect cells over a larger surface area and provide more information about cells, mucus and/or exudates than other techniques [70]. It has been showed to be twice as sensitive as swab culture [71–72]. Indeed, it allows quick identification of Gram-negative bacteria, e. g. , *E. coli* [55, 72]. Even if low volume flush requires a larger equipment to be performed than other procedures, it is considered rapid and accurate, and it may prove to be valuable for subclinical endometritis in the chronically infected mare. Nevertheless, this method may cause irritation of the endometrial mucosa and it may be more likely source of contamination from vaginal flora [60, 72]. Such contamination may yield false positive culture results; hence, other indices of endometritis should be added to improve the diagnostic power, such as a rise in pH or presence of debris [70, 72]. Moreover, the samples may show a high number of blood red cells, probably due to the transrectal manipulation of uterus and the scraping effect of the tip of the catheter [70].

Recently, a double-guarded low volume flush technique has been developed, with improved sensibility and specificity in identifying endometritis in the mare [18]. Overall, this new method represents a valid alternative to the classic low volume flush and seems to decrease the risk of contamination during sampling procedure. Furthermore, the availability of a disposable lavage tube and of a closed fluid-tubing system is favorable to be used on field and allows the execution by only one person [18]. On the other hand, the technique showed a poorer ability to find PMNs compared to biopsy [18].

3. 6. 4. *Endometrial biopsy*

The endometrial biopsy is a very helpful tool for diagnosing the cause of subclinical endometritis, always relating the microscopic lesions to mares' age and reproductive history [17]. Its results about the changes within the endometrium are considered the most reliable. Indeed, it is used to look for degenerative and inflammatory changes, which are classified using both the histologic grading system proposed by Kenney & Doig and modified by Schoon and coll. and the classification of Ricketts [17, 65]. Endometrial biopsies are collected using a sterilized dedicated biopsy instrument, which is passed through the cervix within the uterine lumen. One arm is then inserted into the rectum to guide the biopsy forceps to the desired location, usually at the base of one uterine horn [58, 71]. Once the forceps is closed, it is withdrawn and the sample is macroscopically evaluated for consistency and size, and immediately put in the selected media, depending on its further use.

Bacteriological culture and cytology from endometrial biopsy were demonstrated to be superior to culture swabs, both for sensitivity and for positive predictive value [71]. Endometrial biopsy is safe, but it is not particularly practical [58]. A practical disadvantage is the time between sampling and histologic results, while bacteriological and cytological results are achievable in a short time [58]. Moreover, it is objectively more invasive than other techniques and needs specific equipment, requires further processing, such as shipping to skilled laboratories, time for examination and transmission of results. Hence, it takes longer to have final diagnosis [65, 71].

3. 7. Endometrial cytology

Endometrial cytology is an inestimable tool in assessing the endometrial inflammation, mainly through the detection of PMNs. Unfortunately, an agreement on the classification and interpretation of cytological results has not yet been reached and different interpretative cut-offs were proposed [16, 70, 74–75]. Indeed, some authors record the number of PMNs as a percentage of all cells seen on a slide and the cut-off value for positive to endometritis ranges from 0. 5 to 5%, according to the guidelines of Brook [16, 71]. The latter classification system categorizes cytological samples as: non-inflammatory (PMNs < 5%), mild inflammation (PMNs 5–15%), moderate inflammation (PMNs 15–30%) and severe inflammation (PMNs > 30%)[16, 70, 75]. Other authors record the amount of PMNs seen per microscopic high power field (HPF) examined. In details, cytological smears are graded as not inflammatory (0–2 neutrophils/field), moderate inflammation (2–5 neutrophils/field), severe inflammation (>5 neutrophils/field) or hypocellular (scant epithelial cells and no neutrophils) [70, 75]. The presence of uterine fluid during estrus has been found to be associated with an increased number of PMNs, and mares with intrauterine fluid on the second–third day of estrus were 1. 4 times more likely to have more than 5 PMNs per HPF than those with no or mild inflammation [66–67]. Recently, it has been suggested to evaluate endometrial cytology using the percentage of PMNs in relation to epithelial cells, rather than counting the number of PMNs per HPF, when using the cytobrush for sampling [73]. Nonetheless, the number of PMNs per HPF was found to be inversely proportional to the pregnancy rate, i. e., mares without inflammation had pregnancy rates 1. 3 and 3 times higher than those of mares exhibiting moderate or severe inflammation, respectively [75].

The amount of PMNs detectable is affected by various factors. Samples obtained in early estrus may not contain inflammatory cells, since PMNs' migration into the uterine lumen during the period of waning progesterone dominance is lower than during maximal estrogen dominance [70, 75]. Nonetheless, the time post-ovulation does not seem to display any effect on endometrial cytological parameters in non-bred mares. Moreover, a small resident amount of PMNs in the endometrium has been demonstrated from 24 to 96 hours after ovulation as well as during pro-estrus, in healthy mares [16, 65, 70–71]. The PMNs number increases in the uterine stratum compactum, but not in low volume flushes, after infusion of semen extenders, saline or seminal plasma, which are known to have an inflammatory effect [65].

Other important parameters useful to interpret the cytological sample are: the background content of the slides, i. e., if it is proteinaceous, contaminated with red blood cells, or clear; the quality of the cells harvested, i. e. , if they are intact, distorted, or fragmented; the total cellularity, that is the number of cells per HPF; the ratio between PMNs and uterine epithelial cells; the presence of other inflammatory cells, e. g. , eosinophils and monocytes, and their number per HPF; the presence and the number per HPF of vaginal epithelial cells; and the eventual presence of bacteria [55, 70].

Cytology is at the top among the diagnostic techniques, since it is a relatively inexpensive method to obtain results in a short time [73]. However, this method has a relatively high rate of false negative results and it does not provide information about the cause of the inflammation [58, 70]. That is why it should always be conducted together with bacteriology, as the detection of PMNs together with potential pathogens is a stronger indicator of endometritis, and the number of mares identified as positive to endometritis is significantly higher than with either technique alone [58, 65, 70–71]. Furthermore, cytological samples supported by positive cultures show on average twice neutrophils than those associated with negative cultures,

http://dx.doi.org/10. 5772/62461

regardless of the virulence of the bacteria individuated [74]. Nonetheless, mares may have positive cytology with negative culture, and *vice versa* [55, 65]. Various interpretations have been made to explain the absence of a correlation between the two techniques, in particular to justify negative cultures, such as that uterine swabs may miss focal infections, the presence of antimicrobial preparations in the uterus, deep-seated infection or non-infectious irritation [65].

3. 8. Endometrial microbiology

A positive uterine culture before breeding is among the causes of infertility linked to endometritis [17, 75]. If a mare does not spontaneously eliminate an infection in 2 to 4 days, she is considered either persistently infected or on her way of becoming persistently infected, as supported by the study on uterine clearance of bacteria in healthy mares [60]. Mares are classified as resistant when able to clear intrauterine fluid, inflammatory cells, and bacteria within 48 hours from breeding, otherwise they are considered susceptible [61]. In addition, the mares may change their susceptibility over subsequent breeding seasons, in a gradual manner. Some of them exhibit a decreased endometrial quality, while others show a floating resistance [61]. Most susceptible mares exhibit minimal signs of inflammation prior to the first breeding of the year, likely because of prolonged sexual rest [57]. Although uterine culture may yield false positive or false negative results, aerobic endometrial culture is still the most common method for diagnosing infectious endometritis [65, 71]. Indeed, although bacteria may be recovered indicating an infectious endometritis, the underlying problem may be a persistent post-breeding endometritis, either not managed or treated suitably [57]. Bacteria and other microorganisms (yeast or fungi) may be found on cytological smears, free or phagocytized within neutrophils or macrophages, and should be scored based on their number per HPF [16]. Cultures may be positive for one or more bacterial species, but mixed cultures of more than three pathogens are usually considered as the result of contamination [58, 65, 71].

Various correlations have been demonstrated between endometrial bacteria and different US and endometrial cytological findings. Mares with intrauterine fluid were 1. 4 times more likely to have 5 PMNs per HPF on cytological specimens than those with no or mild fluid [66]. Intrauterine fluid was more commonly detected when *hemolytic Streptococcus, Klebsiella* species, *Enterobacter cloacae* or yeast were isolated, compared with *E. coli, Staphylococcus aureus* and *Pseudomonas* species [66, 72]. Also intrauterine fluid and a cytology containing 2 PMNs per HPF were more commonly associated to *hemolytic Streptococcus* than *E. coli* [66]. Nevertheless, less than 40% of mares from which were isolated *E. coli, S. aureus, Pseudomonas* spp. , or non-pathogen bacteria, such as *Micrococcus* spp. , *Alpha Streptococcus* or *Bacillus* spp. , had intrauterine fluid at US, immediately before the uterine culture was done [66]. Intrauterine fluid was seen more frequently, in 45–55% of the US examinations, when *β-hemolytic Streptococcus, K. pneumoniae, E. cloacae* or yeast were isolated [66]. However, intrauterine fluid, especially during estrus, was not always associated with bacterial endometritis [66]. Furthermore, pathogens associated with uterine fluid were more likely to coincide to neutrophils findings on cytology and vice versa [67]. Hence, the uterine fluid indicates an acute inflammation, but not necessarily a bacterial infection. This is confirmed by the presence of other causes of acute and neutrophilic intrauterine collection, such as pneumovagina, irritating effect of semen, urine reflux into the uterus and excessive production of endometrial mucus [67]. Moreover, not all microbes cause a neutrophilic response and the amount of cytological specimens graded as positive for inflammation varied among the microbial findings [75]. Indeed, *β-hemolytic Streptococcus* or *Klebsiella* yield more often positive uterine cytology, whereas *E. coli, S. aureus* and *Pseudomonas* spp. had fewer positive cytological results [66, 75]. Presence of PMNs was strongly associated with *S. equi* subsp. *zooepidemicus*, rather than *E. coli*[71, 74–75]. Among the main pathogens, *β-hemolytic Streptococcus*, in particular *S. equi* subsp. *zooepidemicus*, a Gram-positive bacteria, is more likely to cause an endometrial inflammatory response and it was more often associated with positive cytology, differently from other pathogens [74].

Various bacterial species have proven to be pathogenic in the mares' uterine environment, and each species have been isolated in different percentage. Most frequently isolated bacteria, the relative percentage, the sampling techniques adopted and the geographical area in which the study was conducted are summarized in Table 1. In general, *β-hemolytic Streptococcus* is strongly related to a rise in pH in the low volume flush efflux, probably due to super antigens, released by the bacteria itself, which beckon pro-inflammatory mediators into the uterine lumen [72]. They were reported as the most common microorganisms isolated from mares' uterus [71–72, 75]. The double-guarded low volume flush allowed to isolate more *β-hemolytic Streptococcus*, even if uterine lavage seems to be not proper to detect it, probably due to its deep localization in the endometrium [18]. Furthermore, in some *S. equi* subsp. *zooepidemicus* strains, a clear ability to form persistent cells, highly tolerant to penicillin, has been demonstrated. The prevalence of subclinical *S. zooepidemicus* endometritis in the mare is still to be determined, and in subfertile mares the prevalence has been determined to be as high as 64%. The activation of dormant bacteria, using bacterial growth mediums like *bActivate*, may improve significantly the sensitivity of traditional diagnostics [76].

On the other hand, *E. coli*, a Gram-negative bacteria, was associated neither with cytological evidence of inflammation nor with increased pH [65, 71–72, 74–75]. The absence of correlation between *E. coli* and positive cytology may be due to its inability to attract PMNs into the uterine lumen [18]. In fact, the pathogen–host relationship, and consequently the uterine inflammatory response, of *E. coli* appears to be different from that of *β-hemolytic Streptococcus* [72]. On the other hand, it appears to associate with moderate to heavy debris on cytological smears. The interpretation of cultures positive for *E. coli* is difficult, since only pure cultures and large numbers of colonies are considered significant, and an increased sensitivity seems obtainable by culturing low volume flush [71–72, 74]. *E. coli*is sometimes considered a contaminant, but it is believed to cause subfertility in the mare [65], and it has been associated with focal infections, in the form of granulomatous plaques identified with endoscopic evaluation in two mares [72]. Another pathogen is *P. aeruginosa*, a Gram-negative bacteria, which produces a biofilm, i. e. , an adhesive matrix that harbors bacterial microcolonies and resists as well to antibiotics as to the immune system [67]. *P. aeruginosa* is believed to be cause of chronic and persistent infections [67].

The role of non-pathogenic bacteria isolated from the mares' uterus is still unknown, but they may be the cause of decreased pregnancy rates [75]. Mares with bacteriological positivity but no cytological evidence of PMNs may be affected by contaminants [58, 72, 75]. However, their pregnancy rate resulted lower than those of the mares without any positivity to the tests. For example, *Bacillus* and *Micrococcus* are skin commensals that are not usually the cause of lowered pregnancy rates, but in barren and older mares with weakened physical barriers they may play a role in decreased fertility [75]. Even if *S. zooepidemicus* is a commensal and common bacterium of the caudal reproductive tract, the cervix has been considered an efficient barrier maintaining a sterile uterine environment. Trans-cervical medical procedures, particularly when involving instillation of substances that may possibly favor bacterial growth, represent a risk of iatrogenic contamination of the uterus with bacteria from the micro-flora of the caudal reproductive tract [76].

Bacterial Species	Prevalence (%)	SamplingMethod	Area	Reference
S. equi subsp. *zooepidemicus*	28.3	Cotton Swab /	Kentucky	[66]
E. coli	20.5	Low Volume Flush		
S. equi subsp. *zooepidemicus*	34	Cotton Swab	Kentucky	[75]
E. coli	17			
Pseudomonas spp.	11.7			
Non-pathogens (Micrococcus, α-Streptococcus, Bacillus)	11.3			
E. coli	27.6	Low Volume	Kentucky	[72]
Mixed	14.6	Flush		
S. equi subsp. *zooepidemicus*	20.9			
Mixed	16.7			
S. equi subsp. *zooepidemicus* + *E. coli*	7.8			
S. equi subsp. *zooepidemicus*	39	Cotton Swab		
E. coli	16			
S. equi subsp. *zooepidemicus*	19	Endometrial	Denmark	[71]
S. aureus	1	Biopsy		
E. coli	1	Cotton Swab		
S. equi subsp. *zooepidemicus*	31.7	Cotton Swab	Italy	[103]
E. coli	19.6			
Non-hemolytic	18.4			
Hemolytic	1.2			
E. coli		Cotton Swab	Sweden	[101]
Hemolytic	3			
Non-hemolytic	64			
S. equi subsp. *zooepidemicus*	20			
Gramnegative *Coccus*	8			
E. coli	30	Low Volume	Denmark/	[18]
S. equi subsp. *zooepidemicus*	11	Flush	Kentucky	
E. coli + *β-Streptococcus*	20			
E. coli	21	Swab		

Bacterial Species	Prevalence (%)	SamplingMethod	Area	Reference
S. equi subsp. *zooepidemicus*	8			
E. coli + *β-Streptococcus*	4			
E. coli	12	Endometrial		
S. equi subsp. *zooepidemicus*	7	Biopsy		
E. coli + *β-Streptococcus*	3			
S. equi subsp. zooepidemicus	Not Specified	Cotton Swab / Low Volume Flush	Canada	[16]
Bacillus spp.	10	Cytobrush	Poland	[58]
S. equi subsp. *zooepidemicus*	6			
E. coli	5			
Bacillus spp.	11	Endometrial		
S. equi subsp. *zooepidemicus*	8	Biopsy		
E. coli	5			
E. coli	10.9	Cotton Swab /	Germany	[65]
S. equi subsp. *zooepidemicus*	9.1	Cytobrush /Endometrial Biopsy		
E. coli	Not	Knudsen	Germany	[74]
Non hemolytic	Specified	Catheter		
S. equi subsp. *zooepidemicus*				
Klebsiella spp.	Not			
Pseudomonas spp.	Specified			
S. equi subsp. zooepidemicus	Not	Cytobrush		
E. coli	Specified			
Non-hemolytic				
Klebsiella spp.	Not			
Pseudomonas spp.	Specified			
E. coli	Not	Cotton Swab		
Non-hemolytic	Specified			
S. equi subsp. *zooepidemicus*				
Klebsiella spp.	Not			
Pseudomonas spp.	Specified			

Table 1. Prevalence of the most common bacterial species isolated from mares' uterus in various geographical areas

3. 9. Endometrial histology

In brief, the histological grading system for the endometrium ranges from I to III. Grade I is an essentially normal endometrium with minimal alterations. Grade II is a wide category, often divided into subcategories, IIA and IIB, from mild to moderate pathologic conditions. Grade

III includes severe and widespread inflammatory and/or degenerative changes of the endometrium [77]. This technique is considered the "gold standard" to diagnose endometritis, in particular the detection of PMNs infiltrating the luminal epithelium and the stratum compactum [71]. Grade IIB and III mares have also shown an increased incidence of intrauterine fluid retention, compared to grade I and IIA mares [61].

The endometrial lesions are further classified as inflammatory, i. e., acute, sub-acute or chronic, and non-inflammatory lesions, e. g. , hypoplasia, hyperplasia or chronic degenerative conditions. The acute inflammatory lesions are characterized by at least one PMN per 5 HPF, whereas the chronic ones by lymphocytes are often accompanied by eosinophils [58, 71]. Anyway, the number of PMNs is affected by the phase of the estrus cycle, with more neutrophils especially during estrus, regardless the cause of endometritis, breeding as well as bacterial-induced. Degenerative processes are the sclerosis of uterine vessels, i. e. , "angiosis" also known as "pregnancy sclerosis" in humans, which increase with parity, the lymphangiectasia, secondary to vascular degeneration or persistent inflammation, the loss of epithelium and the epithelial hyperplasia, which are highly influenced by ageing, hormones and parity [57, 61, 70]. Even if the age combined with parity has been related with endometrial degeneration, and that increased parity is clearly positively correlated with increased age, old maiden mares may display much more marked changes than expected for their age [17, 61]. Sports mares differ in regard to their endometrial pathology from equine populations of nearly exclusively non-sports mares, i. e., sports mares have a much higher prevalence of endometrial periglandular fibrosis [78]. An irregular glandular differentiation may occur physiologically during the transitional cycles, but when these findings are seen during the breeding season, they represent a pathological alteration correlated with a permanent or temporary reduced fertility [78].

In mares susceptible to post-breeding endometritis, findings may differ depending on when the examination is performed [57]. Prior to the first breeding of the year, endometrial biopsy score may be a category IIA, with pathological findings of mild, focal, subacute inflammation with or without lymphangiectasia [57]. Bacteria and PMNs are usually absent. After repeated mating in a season, these mares accumulate intrauterine fluid and may have interstitial edema within the uterine wall after ovulation. At this time, the endometrial biopsy score may worsen to a category IIB, with the primary lesions of diffuse, moderate, subacute inflammation, lymphangiectasia, and moderate to severe edema [57]. Then, positive uterine culture and neutrophilic uterine cytology can be observed [17].

3. 10. Novel and old biomarkers for endometritis: myeloperoxidase and nitric oxide

Myeloperoxidase is a pro-oxidant enzyme stored in and released by neutrophils during degranulation or after lysis [59]. In horses, myeloperoxidase has been demonstrated in different biological samples, such as plasma and broncho-alveolar lavage fluid, reaching variable concentrations. Its presence has been recently confirmed in the uterine lumen, both in physiological conditions, like during estrus, and it seems to be related to uterine inflammation [59]. Samples were collected by low volume flush and stored in tubes with EDTA, since it prevents coagulation and consequently degranulation of neutrophils, thus stabilizing myeloperoxidase concentration. It has been noted that its concentration is high in mares affected by endometritis, showing a positive correlation both with positive cytological results and with the presence of intrauterine fluid [59]. Further studies to establish the threshold between normal and pathologic uterine concentrations of myeloperoxidase are needed.

Another intriguing biomarker is NO, a smooth muscle relaxant able to compromise the uterine contractility and, consequently, its clearance [60]. A higher amount of NO and a higher NOS expression in uterine biopsies were found in susceptible mares 13 hours after insemination, compared with resistant ones [26]. Although it is not clear whether the higher NO concentration in susceptible mares is the cause or the result of a delayed uterine clearance, the difference between the susceptible and the resistant mares suggests a possible role for it either directly or through a NO-associated pathway [26].

4. Treatment of endometritis

The purpose of the treatment protocol is always to prepare the endometrium for embryo descent, which happens about 6 days after-mating, but the choice of the exact management depends on the specific etiological diagnosis [56]. The main objective is to resolve endometrial inflammation by restricting the bacterial contamination and by improving uterine physical clearance. This goal is reached through the control of post-mating inflammation length and degree, and/or through the identification and the elimination of the microorganism involved in the uterine infection [67]. Resolution of underlying problems is necessary to succeed in endometritis treatment.

Any anatomical defects, which may contribute to development of infections and impairs the post-insemination fluid drainage, should be corrected with surgery, e. g. , Caslick's vulvoplasty or urethral extension [79]. Traditional therapy to improve physical clearance of uterine fluid is uterine irrigation, associated to the administration of ecbolic, either oxytocin (10–25 UI i. v. or i. m.) or cloprostenol (250 μg i. m.), 4 to 8 hours after breeding [44, 80–86]. In case of infectious endometritis, the key to resolve the pathology is the antimicrobial therapy, either with systemic or intrauterine administration. Mucolytic irrigations have been recommended before the antimicrobial infusion, in order to eliminate bacterial biofilm and to improve drugs absorption by the uterine mucosa [17].

New treatment strategies are being developed, thanks to the growth of knowledge about persistent uterine infection pathophysiology. For example, immunomodulatory therapy has been proven effective in modulating the impaired uterine inflammatory response in susceptible mares. Different biological products such asheterologous or autologous plasma, platelet-rich plasma infusions, autologous conditioned serum and mesenchymal stem cells have been tested [87–92]. Corticoids and *Mycobacterium* cell wall extract or *Propionibacterium acnes* have been confirmed to be useful to treat endometritis [93]. At the end of the treatment, its efficacy should be controlled. A clinic examination should always be performed and culture swab and/or a biopsy sample should be collected at 3–4 weeks from the beginning of the treatment.

4. 1. Uterine flushing

The uterine lavage is helpful to remove debris, microbes, neutrophils and other substances that interfere with the mucosal absorption of antimicrobial and with neutrophils action. This also improves the clearance by stimulating uterine contractility. The lavage contrasts infectious agents by mechanical irritation of endometrium, which helps recruitment of neutrophils and opsonins [17].

The choice to treat or not a mare with uterine lavage relies on the presence of post-mating intrauterine fluid and on the degree of edema. An US examination is performed 4 to 8 hours post-mating: when no or little edema or slight accumulation of fluid is detected, the lavage is not performed. Otherwise, when the intrauterine fluid is more than 2 cm in depth, the mare is treated with immediate uterine irrigation [17]. To avoid the interference with conception, the best timing for uterine flushing is 4 hours post-breeding [94]. Thus, a further US examination is advisable 24 hours post-breeding to evaluate if additional uterine irrigations are needed. Whenever US results are impracticable, a preventive uterine lavage between 4 and 12 hours after breeding should be performed [47].

The procedure for a therapeutic uterine lavage is identical to that described for the low volume uterine flush, except for that a large-bore (e. g., 8 mm inner diameter × 11 mm outside diameter) Bivona catheter with a balloon cuff is used, and that a volume of 1 to 2 liters of warm solution is typically infused and then removed by gravity [95]. The warm uterine flushing should be combined with uterine massage per rectum to uniformly diffuse the fluid and to stimulate the myometrium contraction. Lavage is generally repeated until the effluent results are clear or not too turbid.

Uterine infusions are performed with isotonic saline solution or other balanced electrolytes solutions, such as lactated Ringer's solution. A low volume, 5–10 ml, of povidone-iodine solution can be added to 1 L of saline as preventive antimicrobial and antifungal treatment. This management is cost-effective and easy to be prepared, stored and delivered. However, it has been reported that intrauterine administration of1% povidone-iodine solution during days 0 and 2 post-ovulation in healthy mares did not induce the histological changes of endometritis, but altered progesterone concentrations and reduced the expression of endometrial progesterone receptors, without affecting estrogen receptors. It was suggested that these changes could reduce embryo survival [96]. Ecbolics are administered as described to eliminate completely the infused fluids [17].

4. 2. Antibiotic treatment

Identifying and destroying bacterial infections might be the key to resolve some chronic reproductive problems. On the other hand, the decision to use antibiotics should rely on clear diagnostic evidences, which is not always the case. Hence, the key factor in treating endometritis with antibiotics is to confirm the presence of a true bacterial infection [97]. In endometritis, the infection is frequently limited to the endometrium and intrauterine infusion of antimicrobials is the most common approach treatment. However, the analysis of uterine biopsies showed that *Streptococcus zooepidemicus* was present deep within the endometrial tissue in infertile mares [98]. In these cases, treatments limited to intra-uterine infusions may be unsuccessful, especially if the antibiotic did not achieve deep-tissue concentrations, adequate to kill the microorganism [97]. Infectious endometritis must be treated by intrauterine infusion, during estrus, with the appropriate antimicrobial administered daily for 3 to 7 days and after uterine irrigations, which eliminate organic material that may interfere with the antibiotic function. Intrauterine infusion volumes of antibiotics from 30 to 200 ml have been suggested to achieve distribution throughout the uterine lumen [99]. The infusion of small volumes is advisable, since larger volume infusions result in reflux through the cervix and inadequate distribution over the endometrium. Anyhow, the solution should be water-soluble and non-irritant.

Due to the increased spread of antimicrobial resistance, the choice of the antibiotic should be made considering the susceptibility pattern obtained from uterine culture [67]. Sometimes it is not possible to obtain a culture, either because the owners refuse the procedure or because there is no time to wait for results. In these cases, broad-spectrum antibiotics are the first choice to treat endometritis. Criteria for the choice are based on the consideration of the most common bacteria isolated from mares' reproductive tract: *S. equi* subsp. *zooepidemicus* (Gram positive), *E. coli* (Gram negative), *K. pneumoniae* (Gram negative), *P. aeruginosa* (Gram negative), *S. aureus* (Gram positive), and *Bacteroides* spp. (Gram negative, anaerobe) [19, 71, 100–103].

The effect of various antibiotics has been evaluated with controversial results. Gentamicin (1-2 g) or Amikacin (1-2 g) Gram-negative coveragehave both been demonstrated to significantly reduce the activity of neutrophils [17]. On the basis of the results of an online survey of veterinarians concerning antibiotic use in equine reproduction, the most common antimicrobials used for intrauterine infusions in the mare before receiving culture/ antibiotic sensitivity results were ceftiofur (21%), followed by gentamicin (19%), ticarcillin with clavulanic acid (13%), ampicillin (12%), other (12%), procaine penicillin (5%), amikacin (5%), potassium penicillin (3%) and ticarcillin (3%). The category "other" included combination of penicillin and gentamicin (2%), penicillin and neomycin (2%), ampicillin and gentamicin (1%), oxytetracycline, framomycin, framycetin, cefquinome, cefazolin or chloramphenicol [97]. Dosages for antibiotics and antimicotics commonly administered either systemically or through intrauterine irrigation to treat endometritis are summarizedin Table 2.

Antibiotic intrauterine infusion in the estrus cycle may be realized either before or after breeding, preferably after ovulation is confirmed. The use of antimicrobial that may potentially have spermicidal properties onthe day of insemination/mating generates controversial opinions. The uterine lavage or infusion is executed at least 4 hours after the insemination, so that the oviduct colonization with the sperm is not compromised. Then, 2 days after ovulation the progesterone levels increase, and the uterine defense mechanisms efficiency consequently decrease. For this reason, performing the infusion between 4 hours after insemination and 2 days after ovulation is considered to be harmless for the conception [104]. On the other hand, the antimicrobial uterine infusion in progesterone phase has been associated with increased incidence of resistant bacterial and fungal infection [105–106].

During acute endometritis, the time length of the antimicrobial treatment should depend on the degree of endometritis, according to endometrial biopsy. In slightly endometritis 3 days,

http://dx.doi.org/10. 5772/62461

in moderate one 5 days and in severe endometritis 7 days are necessary [99]. Concerns about inducing secondary fungal infections and/or antibiotic resistance are some of the reasons why the intrauterine antibiotic infusions have been reduced. Indeed, uterine lavages with saline associated to the use of ecbolics are now commonly accepted, and antibiotic therapies are more targeted at specific isolated organisms, in conjunction with methods to disrupt biofilms [97].

The combination of local and systemic antimicrobial treatment must be performed when clinical examination results in evident general illness, in case of infection or inflammation involving the deeper layers of the uterus, when repeated antimicrobial intrauterine infusions fail to cure, and when the recontamination is alarming. Systemic therapy during diestrus is preferable, since it is associated to lower fluctuation in antibiotic tissue levels and further contamination of the uterus should not happen. Trimethoprim-sulfa, ampicillin, penicillin and gentamicin are commonly used as systemic therapy. Oral administration of enrofloxacin at 5 mg/kg is recommended twice daily, to reach endometrial levels above the minimum inhibitory concentration of many endometritis-associatedbacteria. In adequate doses repetition or drug interaction may create resistant microorganism and superinfections, such as yeasts or fungal overgrowth, which makes it particularly difficult to treat.

Molecule	**Dosage (mg/kg)**	**Route**	**Intrauterine Dosage**	**Bacterial Susceptibility**	**Ref.**
Amikacin	10 q24h	IV/IM	1–2 g	Gram negative	[128]
Ampicillin	29 q12–24h	IV/IM	1–3 g	Gram positive & negative, *E.coli*	[128]
Carbenicillin			2–6 g	Gram negative	[97]
Ceftiofur	2—4 q12–24h	IV/IM	1 g	Gram positive, some Gram negative, *S. zooepidemicus*	[128]
Doxycyline	10 q12h	OS		Broad-spectrum	[97]
Enrofloxacin	5.5 q24h 7.5 q24h 4.0 q12h	IV slow OS OS		Gram negative, Resistant bacteria	[128]
Gentamicin	6.6 q24h	IV/IM	1–3 g	Gram negative	[128]
Kanamycin			1–3 g	*E. coli*	[97]
Metronidazole	15–25 q24h	OS		Anaerobic Gram negative	[97]
Neomycin			2–4 g	Gram negative, *E .coli*	[97]
Oxytetracycline	6.6 q12h	IV slow			[97]
K-penicillin	22,000 IU/kg q6h	IV	5×10^6 UI	Gram positive, *S. zooepidemicus*	[128]

Molecule	Dosage (mg/kg)	Route	Intrauterine Dosage	Bacterial Susceptibility	Ref.
Procaine penicillin	22,000 IU/kg q12h	IM	4.5–6 × 10^6 UI	Gram positive	[128]
Ticarcillin			3–6 g	Gram positive, *Pseudomonas*	[97]
Ticarcillin + clavulanic acid			3–6 g /200 mg	Broad spectrum [*Staphylococcus, Enterobacter, Bacillus*]	[97]
Trimethoprim sulfa	30 q12h		OS	*S. aureus, E. coli, Klebsiella* spp., *Proteus*, some *Nocardia* spp.	[128]
Amphotericin B	0.3–0.9 q24-48h	IV	100–200 mg q24h	Broad spectrum	[128]
Clotrimazole			400–700 mg q24h	Yeast	[128]
Fluconazole	14 loading then 5 q24h	IV/OS	100 mg q24h	Yeast	[128]
Itraconazole	5 q12–24h	IV/OS		Broad spectrum	[128]
Ketokonazole	20 q12h	Via Nasogastric intubation in 1–2 h		Broad spectrum	[128]
Miconazole			500–700 mg q24h	Broad spectrum	[128]
Nystatin			0.5–2.5 × 10^6 UI q24h	Yeast	[128]

Table 2. Most commonly used antibiotics and antimicotics to treat equine endometritis, dosages for either systemic or intrauterine use, and bacterial susceptibility

4. 3. Mucolytics and chelating agents

Persistent endometritis could be associated with hypersecretion of mucus by endometrial epithelium and the presence of exudate renders aminoglycosides chemically inert and generally interferes with antibiotic penetration. Some Gram-negative and positive bacteria or fungi produce biofilm that confers antibiotic resistance [107–108]. The pathogens confirmed to produce biofilm include *S. epidermis, E. coli, E. cloacae* and the most potent biofilm producer *P. aeruginosa.*

Administration of mucolytic drugs is used to eliminate excessive mucus and exudates for the negative effect of the latters both on intrauterine antibiotics and on sperm transport to the oviduct. Despite controversial viewpoints, intrauterine effects of mucolytic oral administration have not been confirmed. However, it was stated that oral N-acetylcysteine (NAC) treatment, even if it does not reduce the viscosity of uterine mucus, has an anti-inflammatory effect on the equine endometrium [109]. Different kinds of intrauterine mucolytics are used and include NAC, dimethyl sulfoxide (DMSO) and kerosene.

http://dx.doi.org/10. 5772/62461

The NAC is a mucolytic agent that disrupts disulfide bonds between mucin polymers, thereby reducing mucus viscosity, and in addition possesses antioxidant and possibly antimicrobial properties [110–112]. Furthermore, its properties help the sperm transport to the oviduct. Intrauterine post-breeding infusion of 3. 3% solution of NAC did not result to be harmful to mares' endometrium, and it decreased the extracellular mucus thickness and staining intensity in healthy mares, but not in mares with active bacterial endometritis. The same NAC protocol applied in mares repeatedly bred and with a history of mucus hypersecretion, combined with post-mating uterine lavage, oxytocin, and infusion of an antibiotic, was correlated to good pregnancy rates [113]. The safety of NAC on mucosal surfaces is clear, based on its use as a mucolytic for respiratory disease in humans and treatment for meconium impaction in foals [113]. Interestingly, some recent findings demonstrate that intrauterine application of NAC in healthy mares in estrus may reduce the endometrial response to irritants [114]. The intrauterine administration of 0. 6% NAC solution, prepared by adding30 ml of 20% NAC to 150 ml of sterile saline, performed 48 hours before breeding, improves the pregnancy rates [110]. The effect of post-breeding intrauterine infusion of 30% DMSO solution showed to be effective in improving the endometrial biopsy score, and it lead to higher pregnancy rates compared with mares infused with saline [115]. The improvement of the pregnancy rate, following the infusion of 50 ml of commercial kerosene, operates differently from the other mucolytics. The mechanisms hypothesized were that kerosene activates endometrial glands and reduces the mucus through the destruction of the uterine epithelium. A moderate to severe endometritis results from kerosene uterine administration, with severe edema and production of serum-like exudates. Half of the treated mares manifest necrosis of the endometrium [116].

Advanced strategies include uterine infusion of buffered chelating agents. Their mechanism of action is not completely clear, but they alter the integrity and permeability of the bacterial cell wall by chelation of the calcium and/or magnesium on the outer membrane. To explicate this action, the chelating agents have to be indirect contact with the bacterial cell wall [67]. Recommended treatment is the infusion of 200 to 500 ml of the first-generation *Tris-EDTA* (ethylenediaminetetraacetic acid 3. 5 M plus tromethamine 50 mM) or third-generation *Tricide* (8 mM disodium EDTA dehydrate plus 20 mM 2-amino-2-hydroxymethyl-1, 2-propanediol) [117–120]. After 12–24 hours, the uterus should be flushed to remove debris and accumulated dead cells. The efflux should be examined; and if it is cloudy or mucus is present, the chelating treatment should be repeated one more time [58].

4. 4. Ecbolics

Uterine irrigation should be associated with systemic administration of ecbolic drugs, which increase clearance of the fluid through cervix, stimulate myometrial contraction and impair lymphatic drainage from the uterus. Oxytocin is an equine uterine ecbolic commonly utilized in doses ranging from 10 to 25 IU i. v. or i. m. Higher doses should be avoided, since it may impair pregnancy rates [86]. The administration of oxytocin, in estrus and 48 hours post-breeding, induces high-amplitude uterine contractions lasting from 30 minutes to 1 hour. However, oxytocin half-life is very short and repeated administrations enhance treatment effectiveness [81, 121–122].

These drugs may be ineffective in aged maiden mares in which the cervix often fails to dilate. In such cases, oxytocin therapy should be associated with topical application to the cervical epithelium of misoprostol, a synthetic PGE1 analogue, before breeding, or substituted by cloprostenol administration to sustain low-amplitude uterine contraction for 2 to 4 hours. Intramuscular administration of cloprostenol or PGF2α at a dosage of 250μgis recommended, before the ovulation or within 12 hours. However, administration post-ovulation is not advisable, since it decreases serum progesterone concentration and consequently the pregnancy rates. The cloprostenol-induced contractions last longer; therefore, cloprostenol is more suitable for mares with lymphatic stasis. Side effects, such as sweating and abdominal cramping, are minimal, transient, inconstant and dose-dependent [123].

The best timing for ecbolic administration after uterine lavage associated to the antimicrobial infusion has not been established, yet. When treating anxious or excitable mares, sedatives with α2-adrenergic agonist action, such as xylazine or detomidine, should be used. These sedatives optimize oxytocin effect and increase the intrauterine pressure, where as acepromazine, aα1-adrenergic antagonist, can cause a reduction of uterine contractions after oxytocin treatment [47].

4. 5. Immunomodulators

Higher levels of anti-inflammatory cytokines were observed in resistant mares compared with susceptible ones. The rationale for using immunomodulators is to equilibrate the expression of pro- and anti-inflammatory cytokines in susceptible mares and to rehabilitate the homeostasis of the local inflammatory response.

Glucocorticoids have been demonstrated to suppress the immune response, decreasing gene expressions of the pro-inflammatory cytokines, IL-1α, IL-6, IL-8, while enhancing defense mechanisms and stimulating a higher anti-inflammatory response. Thus, short-term steroid therapy maybe beneficial for treating post-mating endometritis in the mare [124]. An increase of pregnancy rates after single injection of dexamethasone within 1 hour post-mating, approximately 0. 1 mg/kgi. v. , associated with routine therapy, has been demonstrated in mares with history of fluid accumulation after breeding. Oral administration of 9-alpha-prednisolone acetate at 0. 1 mg/kg twice daily for 4 days, beginning 48 hours before breeding, and the association of dexamethasone, administered within 1hour after mating, and prednisolone, administered once daily before and after mating, were confirmed to be efficacious only in susceptible mares, decreasing uterine edema, and reducing and clarifying intra-uterine fluid [125–126].

Other immunomodulatory treatments have been tested to elicit a general increase in immune system activity by means of non-specific cell-mediated response and modulating the release of cytokines [127]. *Mycobacterium phlei* wall extractand *Propionibacterium acnes* were reported to be efficient in uterine infectioncaused by *S. equi* and *S. zooepidemicus* and in chronic endometritis, respectively [17, 93]. In 2014, mesenchymal stem cells and autologous conditioned serum were used to modulate successfully the uterine inflammatory response to spermatozoa in healthy mares [90]. However, the former seems to be more reliable than the latter, and additional studies are ongoing to determinate the effects of mesenchymal stem cells on "problem" mares. Preliminary data on small volume intrauterine infusion of platelet-rich plasma, either before or after insemination, suggest an improvement in conception rate, probably due to a more appropriate uterine environment for embryo survival. Both the efficacy and the exact mechanisms of action of these treatments need further elucidation, but they seem to be triggered through activating platelets, cytokines and growth factors, and they seem to regulate cell migration, attachment, proliferation and differentiation, and to promote extracellular matrix accumulation [89, 91–92, 128].

5. Fungal endometritis

Whereas a rich literature describes the etiopathogenesis of equine microbial endometritis, few papers are dedicated to the role of fungi as responsible for uterine inflammation in the mare. The incidence of fungal infection in mares affected by endometritis is probably significantly lower than the incidence of bacterial infection, but fungal endometritis is more challenging to treat and is associated to a guarded-to-poor prognosis for future fertility [129]. Fungal growth was demonstrated in different rates, ranging from 1 to 7%, considering either the total number of reproductive cultures submitted to laboratories or the percent of cultures positive for fungal compared to the total number of mares affected by endometritis [130–134]. The term "fungi" is referred to heterotrophic, aerobic or facultative anaerobic, non-motile organisms widely distributed in the environment [132]. They could have characteristics of both yeasts, round to oblong single-cell organisms, and molds, that are long, branched, filamentous structures [135]. The filamentous cells are also named hyphae and are often organized in small masses, called mycelia, sometimes isolated in fluid from uterine lavage. Cytological and histological specimens may demonstrate both yeasts, most adapted to grow in liquids, and hyphae, better suited to penetrate deeper inside the endometrial tissue [136].

5. 1. Aetiology

The most common organisms isolated during equine fungal endometritis are *Candida* spp. , *Aspergillus* spp. and *Mucor* spp. [137]. However, many other organisms have been reported (Table 3). Recently, *Cladophialophora bantiana* has been isolated in a 15-year-old Standard bred mare that displayed infertility and uterine fluid accumulation with numerous black, hairy granules. *C. bantiana* is an emerging pathogen, causing cerebral phaeohyphomycosis in humans, while animal cases are rare [138]. The inflammatory mechanisms associated with these types of endometritis have not been clarified until now, and probably endometritis involving fungus or yeast will be feared as long as the inflammatory mechanisms associated will not be studied [134].

The most common source of fungi causing reproductive disease in the mare is probably from skin or fecal origin and the primary reservoir for infectious agents is the caudal reproductive tract, vagina and external genitalia [132]. Fungal elements that cause reproductive disease are generally opportunistic and their growth is considered to be secondary to underlying factors impairing the local humoral and, particularly, cell-mediated immunity. Mares with uterine fungal infections may have predisposing conditions such as: anatomical defects, i. e. , an incompetent vulvar seal from multiple Caslick's procedure or trauma, or a tilted vulvar conformation; cervical trauma and inadequate closure of the cervix due to dystocia or fetotomy; immunosuppression; malnutrition; endocrine diseases; a history of antibiotic treatment; veterinary manipulations due to frequent artificial inseminations and intrauterine treatments [132, 137–139]. Even if fungal endometritis has been reported also in mares without the history of previous uterine therapies, this pathology has been more often documented in older multiparous mares, treated for bacterial endometritis in the past [136].

One of the most discussed predisposing factors is the prolonged use of antibiotics, which is believed to modify the normal flora of the caudal reproductive tract, disrupting the biological barriers and allowing yeast overgrowth. Alteration of the vaginal flora may also destroy organisms producing anti-fungal substances and/or competing for available nutrients, interfere with the local microbial synthesis of vitamins or change vaginal pH [132]. Intrauterine antibiotics reach the vagina when cleared by the increased myometrial tone or through passive leakage, affecting the vaginal flora and the fungal colonization. Repeated reproductive manipulations, such as mating, or inseminations, or infusions and irrigations during the estrus may transfer microorganism from the caudal reproductive tract into the uterus. In mares in which deficit of uterine clearance mechanisms exist, opportunistic fungi find an endometrial environment favorable to their proliferation [132]. Administration of progesterone may be another predisposing factor due to reduction of neutrophilic phagocytic ability, decreased myometrial activity and increased cervical tone. Furthermore, a moist environment, the exposure to large numbers of fungi and the presence of necrotic, ischemic or infected foci may contribute to the fungal infection [132]. Fungal endometritis due to *Cladophialophora bantiana* was diagnosed in an infertile mare with a history of dystocia, fetotomy and cervical laceration [138]. Nevertheless, subclinical fungal endometritis was also demonstrated in an 8-year-old Hanoverian mare at her first breeding, with no further reproductive available history [140].

Fungi have been isolated from urethral cultures (*Mucor* spp.), fresh semen (*Absidia* spp.) and extended semen (*Candida* spp.) from stallions [141]. The transmission of fungal infection through the natural coitus or artificial insemination has not been demonstrated until now, in the horse. However, in humans, there is some evidence that the male may harbor fungi as asymptomatic carriers. This can cause the re-infection of the sexual partner. Thus, when multiple mares are diagnosed with fungal endometritis, cultures of the stallion's penis, prepuce and semen should be performed [136].

5. 2. Diagnosis of fungal endometritis

History of mares affected may reveal the presence of predisposing factors to fungal infections. Frequently, mares are presented with a history of infertility and of repeated use of intrauterine diagnostic and therapeutic procedures [132]. Clinical signs range from subclinical infection to profuse vaginal discharge [138]. Sometimes, at the physical examination, a gray vulvar discharge is evident [132]. The presence of mycelia, as granules, in the fluid from uterine lavage is strongly indicative. The diagnosis of fungal endometritis relies on endometrial cytology, uterine culture or uterine biopsy [136]. Microscopic examination of uterine fluid or uterine

http://dx.doi.org/10. 5772/62461

Fungi	Reference
Actinomyces spp.	[132]
Aspergillus fumigatus	
*Aspergillus*spp.	
Aureobasidium pullulans	
Candida albicans	
Candida spp.	
Rhodotorula spp.	
Coccidiodes immitis	
Trichosporon beigelii	
Fusarium spp.	
Hansenula spp.	
Monosporium spp.	
Mucor spp.	
Nocardia spp.	
Paecilomyces spp.	
Penicillium spp.	
Rhodotorula spp.	
Scedosporium apiospermum	
Saccharomyces cerevisiae	
Torulopis candida	
Cryptococcus neoformans	
Trichisporon spp.	
Cladophialophora bantiana	[138]

Table 3. Most common fungi isolated from the mares' uterus

swab cytology is an important diagnostic tool for fungal endometritis [138]. Cytological smears may show yeast or hyphae. Yeasts appear as 3 to 5 μm round-to oval single-cell organism and often have a capsule surrounding them that exclude dyes. This capsule is visible by altering the focal point when viewing the microscope slide and is considered a protective barrier against phagocytosis. Hyphae are less common and appear as subtle filamentous multicellular organisms [132, 136]. Yeasts are usually associated to superficial infections; on the contrary, hyphae are generally associated to deeper-seated fungal infections, requiring a longer treatment. Fungi should be always isolated and identified by cultures, to allow for antifungal drug sensitivities to be performed. They may be cultured initially on blood agar, and then passed on Sabaroud's agar [132]. Time for their growth is sensibly higher than bacteria and the laboratory should be aware that a search for fungal organism is requested. Otherwise, after the routine time of observation for microbial growth, the culture could be deemed negative, because of the early reporting of the results [142]. A microculture system, Dermatobac®, originally developed for the isolation of fungi in human medicine, was recently tested to evaluate its sensitivity in the diagnosis of equine fungal endometritis. Dermatobac® proved to be efficient, showing conclusive information after only 24 hours of culture [139]. A rapid, sensitive and repeatable quantitative polymerase chain reaction assay (qPCR) was also developed for the detection of fungal DNA from equine endometrial samples. The qPCR assay identified fungal DNA in samples from 12 of 17 mares suspected of having fungal endometritis and proved to be potentially useful as an adjunct to microbial culture and cytological examination in clinical situations to provide identification of fungal organisms in a timely manner [143]. The clitoral fossa and vaginal mucosa should be cultured in addition to the uterine lumen because they could be the reservoir for fungal organism, allowing recontamination after successful uterine treatments [132].

Equine fungal endometritis is usually accompanied by bacteria, among which *β-hemolytic Streptococci* group C and *E. coli* are the most common species. The underlying factors impairing the local immunity, which promote the fungal growth, may favor the microbial growth as well [138]. Especially if bacteria are in low number, they can be missed at the culture, confounding the diagnosis. In these cases, after the treatment with antifungal drugs, in the absence of other concurrent microorganisms, a bacterial endometritis develops, and infertility persists. It is also possible that the microbial infection has its origin in the alteration of the vaginal microflora due to the antifungal treatments. For these reasons, it is important for early identification of mixed fungal and bacterial infection at either the cultural or the cytological examinations [136]. Endometrial biopsy may also be used in the diagnosis of fungal endometritis, when cytology is inconclusive or to confirm the successful treatment of uterine infection. Fungal elements may be observed either adherent to the luminal surface, within endometrial gland lumens or within the endometrium [132].

5. 3. Therapy of fungal endometritis

Many difficulties can prevent a successful treatment of mares affected by fungal endometritis, due to invasive forms that are not exposed to intrauterine therapies, poor uterine clearance mechanism, inadequate immune response or to recontamination from posterior reproductive tract sources, mixed or chronic infections. Therapy for fungal endometritis is made of a combination of predisposing factors correction, uterine lavage and intrauterine infusion of antifungal agents [137]. Any defect in the physical barriers to uterine infection, at the level of perineum, vulva, vulvo-vaginal folds and cervix, must be surgically corrected whenever possible [136]. All the tissue of the reproductive tract that may harbor the fungal elements should be treated. These include the clitoris, clitoral fossa, vagina, cervix and uterus.

Large volume uterine lavage may be used with the aim to decrease the overall fungal number, increase the infiltration of inflammatory cells and the myometrial tone and expose organism to antifungal solutions. Some substances and drugs are usually added to saline, which may interfere with the fungal growth by means of different mechanisms. The use of DMSO is

http://dx.doi.org/10. 5772/62461

reported at concentrations of 10–20%, because of its in vitro activity against the growth of *Candida albicans* [132]. A potential antifungal effect has been attributed to diluted iodine (0. 05–1%) and to acetic acid (vinegar, 2% – 20 ml of white vinegar in 1 L of 0. 9% saline) [136]. Intrauterine iodine should be used with caution, because of the danger of tissue damage and adhesions in particularly sensitive mare, even if it was demonstrated that a 1% povidone-iodine infusion during days 0 and 2 post ovulation in healthy mares did not induce histological changes compatible with endometritis [96]. Ecbolic drugs, such as oxytocin (10-20 IU intramuscularly or intravenously) or prostaglandins may be administered after the lavage to facilitate the expulsion of residual uterine fluid [136]. After the uterine lavage, the treatment should be completed with the intrauterine and/or systemic administration of an antifungal drug, ideally chosen on the basis of the results of cultural examination and susceptibility [136].

The two main categories of antifungal agents are the polyene and the imidazole drugs, which interfere with the formation of fungal ergosterol, resulting in an increased permeability of the cell wall and eventual cell death. The polyene antibiotics include amphotericin B, nystatin and natamycin, whereas clotrimazole, econazole, ketoconazole, fluconazole and itraconazole are the most used azole derivatives [132]. Clotrimazole, miconazole and ketoconazole have two nitrogen molecules; fluconazole and itraconazole are called triazoles because of the presence of three nitrogen atoms in an azole ring [137]. Common antifungal agents used in the treatment of fungal endometritis are reported in Table 2. Amphotericin B (100–200 mg), clotrimazole (300–600 mg) and miconazole (500–700 mg) are active against *Candida* spp. , *Aspergillus* spp. and other dimorphic fungi, and are the antifungal drugs generally in use by intrauterine infusion. Nystatin (0. 5–2. 5 million UI) and fluconazole (100 mg) are active only against *Candida* spp. [97]. Although many antifungal agents are available for intrauterine therapy, few data are available about the disposition of antifungal drugs in endometrial tissue after oral administration. A recent study showed that the oral administration of fluconazole (14 mg/kg once, followed by 5 mg/kg every 24 hours) resulted in mean plasma and endometrial tissue levels above the minimal inhibiting concentration for *Candida Albicans* for the entire treatment period, without potential sequel. Thus, oral fluconazole can be considered in a multimodal and multidrug treatment protocol to treat fungal endometritis in the mare [137]. Knowledge of commonly encountered fungi infecting the mare's reproductive tract and their respective drug susceptibilities should improve treatment efficacy in mares with fungal endometritis, when culture results are not available or incomplete. A study reports that the spectrum of fungal isolates from uterine samples from mares with reproductive problems includes 99 to 100% of organisms susceptible to the polyenes, while response to the azoles varied from 47 to 81%. Yeast isolates were 100% susceptible to the polyenes and least susceptible to miconazole (48%) while isolates of mold with septated hyphae were most susceptible to natamycin (100%) and least susceptible to fluconazole (0%). Results from this study suggest that polyenes are effective against uterine fungal isolates in vitro and may be the empiric treatment of choice for fungal endometritis, when cultural and susceptibilities examination are lacking. Furthermore, resistance to specific azoles was also observed increasing over time [129].

The study about the potential use of chitin inhibitors for the treatment of fungal infections in the horse gave contradictory results. These substances have insecticidal properties due to their ability to inhibit chitin synthesis, polymerization and deposition. It was supposed that they might interfere with the formation of new chitin in the cell wall, but have no effect on the fungal cell walls that have already formed. Thus, their potential effect may consist in the prevention of a new fungal growth and, thus, reinfection. Lufenuron is an insecticide chitin inhibitor that was evaluated as a treatment for endometrial fungal infections. Preliminary results were promising, and intrauterine lavages, performed with lufenuron suspended in sterile saline solution, were effective in eliminating fungal endometritis in four mares [144]. However, further studies did not confirm the efficacy against *Aspergillus* spp. or *Fusarium* spp. in vitro and indicated that very low concentrations in whole blood of horses were achieved after oral administration [145]. Further investigations about the efficacy of chitin inhibitors are necessary before they can be indicated for the treatment of fungal endometritis in the horse [136].

Another suggested protocol consists in morning lavage with 2% acetic acid solution followed by intrauterine irrigation with the specific antifungal antibiotic in the afternoon. The length of this therapy should be of 7–10 days. If uterine culture and cytology obtained in the first day of the next estrus are negative, the mare is bred with the minimum number of insemination and using sterile techniques and double-guarded pipette, to prevent accidental seeding with organisms from reservoir sources [136].

The prognosis for future fertility of mares affected by fungal endometritis is guarded to poor. The success of the therapy relies on the timely identification and treatment of delayed uterine clearance, poor perineal conformation, or fungal colonization of the more distal reproductive tract, the correct length of the treatment period, the appropriate choice and dosage of the antifungal [132]. The uterine biopsy for many of these mares indicates significant fibrosis, probably due to fungal infection, as well as to a previous bacterial infection and age-related changes. Once the fungal infection is resolved, a uterine biopsy may be advised to quantify the resulting uterine damage [136].

6. Conclusions

Endometritis is the butler of the equine reproduction, and it is the main suspect in all cases of impaired fertility of the mare. Every year the literature is enriched by new interesting reports about this subject, which throw even more light on the knowledge of its pathogenesis. The events occurring during the uterine inflammatory response are complex and intertwined. A thorough understanding of the physiological response to uterine contamination, which is necessarily correlated with the act of the insemination, may allow timely identification of susceptible mares, in which these mechanisms get jammed within the first hours after breeding. Type and dose of treatments, as well as timing of administration, should be correctly targeted towards susceptible and/or affected mares to optimize the results and reduce the cost and the resources used. Continued research is welcome in this area of equine medicine, so that treatment strategies can be further improved.

Author details

Maria Pia Pasolini[1], Chiara Del Prete[1], Silvia Fabbri[1] and Luigi Auletta[2*]

*Address all correspondence to: lauletta@sdn-napoli. it

1 Department of Veterinary Medicine and Animal Productions, University of Napoli Federico II, Napoli, Italy

2 IRCCS SDN, Napoli, Italy

References

[1] Hughes J, Loy R. Investigations on the effect of intrauterine inoculations of Streptococcus zooepidemicus in the mare. In: Proceedings of the AAEP American Association of Equine Practitioners; 1–3 December 1969; Houston, Texas. pp. 289-292

[2] Lees P, Dawson J, Sedgwick AD. Eicosanoid and equine leukocyte locomotion in vitro. Equine Veterinary Journal. 1986;18:493-497

[3] Watson ED, Stokes CR, Bourne FJ. Cellular and humoral defence mechanisms in mares susceptible and resistant to persistent endometritis. Veterinary Immunology and Immunopathology. 1987;16:107-121

[4] Watson ED, Stokes CR, Bourne FJ. Influence of arachidonic acid metabolites in vitro and in uterine washings on migration of equine neutrophils under agarose. Research in Veterinary Science. 1987;43:203-207

[5] Pycock JF, Allen WE. Pre-chemotactic and chemotactic properties of uterine fluid from mares with experimentally induced endometritis. Veterinary Record. 1988;123:193-195

[6] Katila T, Lock TF, Hoffmann WE, Smith AR. Lysozime alkaline phosphatase and neutrophils uterine secretions of mares with differing resistance to endometritis. Theriogenology. 1990;33:723-732

[7] Pycock JF, Allen WE. Inflammatory components in uterine fluid from mares with experimentally induced bacterial endometritis. Equine Veterinary Journal. 1990;22:422-425.

[8] Troedsson MH, Liu I. Uterine clearance of non-antigenicmarkers (51Cr) in response to a bacterial challenge in mares potentially susceptible and resistant to chronic uterine infections. Journal of Reproduction and Fertility, Supplement. 1991;44:283-288

[9] Troedsson MH, Liu IK, Thurmond M. Function of uterine and blood-derived polymorphonuclear neutrophils in mares susceptible and resistant to chronic uterine infection: phagocytosis and chemotaxis. Biology of Reproduction. 1993;49:507-514

[10] Troedsson MHT, Liu IK, Ing M, Pascoe J, Thurmond M. Multiple site electromyography recordings of uterine activity following an intrauterine bacterial challenge in mares susceptible and resistant to chronic uterine infection. Journal of Reproduction and Fertility. 1993;99:307-313

[11] Troedsson MHT, Ibrahim NM, King VL, Foster DN, Crabo BG. Post-breeding endometritis: the role of seminal components. Pferdeheilkunde. 1997;13:542

[12] Troedsson MHT. Uterine clearance and resistance to persistent endometritis in the mare. Theriogenology. 1999;52:461-471

[13] Burns T, Pierson RA, Card CE. Subjective and quantitative assessments of endometrial changes in mares inseminated with cryopreserved semen. Proceedings of the Society for Theriogenology. 2000. p. 47

[14] Troedsson MHT, Loset K, Alghamdi AM, Dahms B, Crabo BG. Interaction between equine semen and the endometrium: the inflammatory response to semen. Animal Reproduction Science. 2001;68(3):273-278

[15] Brinkmann V, Reichard U, Goosmann C, Fauler B, Uhlemann Y, Weiss DS. Neutrophil extracellular traps kill bacteria. Science. 2004;303:1532-1535

[16] Card C. Post-breeding inflammation and endometrial cytology in mares. Theriogenology. 2005;64(3):580-588

[17] LeBlanc MM, Causey RC. Clinical and subclinical endometritis in the mare: both threats to fertility. Reproduction in Domestic Animals. 2009;44(3):10-22

[18] Christoffersen M, Söderlind M, Rudefalk SR, Pedersen HG, Allen J, Krekeler N. Risk factors associated with uterine fluid after breeding caused by Streptococcus zooepidemicus. Theriogenology. 2015;84(8):1283-1290

[19] Ricketts SW, Mackintosh ME. Role of anaerobic bacteria in equine endometritis. Journal of Reproduction and Fertility, Supplement. 1987;35:343-351

[20] Madsen M, Christensen P. Bacterial flora of semen collected from Danish warmblood stallions by artificial vagina. ActaVeterinariaScandinavica. 1995;36:1-7

[21] Tuppits U, Orro T, Einarsson S, Kask K, Kavak A. Influence of the uterine inflammatory response after insemination with frozen-thawed semen on serum concentrations of acute phase proteins in mares. Animal Reproduction Science. 2014;146:182-186

[22] Amulic B, Hayes G. Neutrophil extracellular traps. Current Biology. 2011;21(9):R297-298. DOI: 10. 1016/j. cub. 2011. 03. 021

[23] Troedsson MH, Desvousges A, Alghamdi AS, Dahms B, Dow CA, Hayna J, Valesco R, Collahan PT, Macpherson ML, Pozor M, Buhi WC. Components in seminal plasma regulating sperm transport and elimination. Animal Reproduction Science. 2005;89:171-186

[24] Katila T. Onset and duration of uterine inflammatory response of mares after insemination with fresh semen (monograph). Biology of Reproduction. 1995;1:515-517

[25] LeBlanc MM, Neuwirth L, Asbury AC, Tran T, Mauragis D, Klapstein E. Scintigraphic measurement of uterine clearance in normal mares and mares with recurrent endometritis. Equine Veterinary Journal. 1994;26:109-113

[26] Alghamdi AS, Foster DN, Carlson CS, Troedsson. MHT. Nitric oxide levels and nitric oxide synthase expression in uterine samples from mares susceptible and resistant to persistent breeding-induced endometritis. American Journal of Reproductive Immunology. 2005;53:230-237

[27] Woodward E, Christoffersen M, Campos J, Horohov D, Scoggin K, Squires E, Troedsson MHT. An investigation of uterine nitric oxide production in mares susceptible and resistant to persistent breeding-induced endometritis and the effects of immunomodulation. Reproduction in Domestic Animals. 2013a;48:554-561

[28] Khan FA, Scholtz EL, Chenier TS. The Nitric Oxide System in Equine Reproduction: Current Status and Future Directions. Journal of Equine Veterinary Science. 2015;35:481-487

[29] Liu I, Rakestraw PA, Coit C, Harmon F, Snyder J. An in vitro investigation of the mechanism of neuromuscular regulation in myometrial contractility. Pferdeheilkunde. 1997;13:557

[30] Asbury AC, Halliwell RE, Foster GW, Longino SJ. Immunoglobulins in uterine secretions of mares with differing resistance to endometritis. Theriogenology. 1980;14:299-308

[31] Mitchell G, Liu IK, Perryman LE, Stabenfeldt GH, Hughes JP. Preferential production and secretion of immunoglobulins by the equine endometrium–a mucosal immune system. Journal of Reproduction and Fertility. 1982;32:161-168

[32] Williamson P, Dunning A, O'Connor J, Penhale WJ. Immunoglobulin levels, protein concentrations and alkaline phosphatase activity in uterine flushings from mares with endometritis. Theriogenology. 1982;19:441-448

[33] Woodward EM, Christoffersen M. , Campos J, Betancourt A, Horohov D, Scoggin KE, Squires EL, Troedsson MHT. Endometrial inflammatory markers of the early immune response in mares susceptible or resistant to persistent breeding induced endometritis (PBIE). Reproduction. 2013;145(3):289-296

[34] Schroder K, Hertzog PJ, Ravasi T, Hume DA. Interferon-gamma: an overview of signals, mechanisms, and functions. Journal of Leukocyte Biology. 2004;75:163-189

[35] Tilg H, Trehu E, Atkins MB, Dinarello CA, Mier JW. Interleukin-6 (IL-6) as an anti-inflammatory cytokine: induction of circulating IL-1 receptor antagonist and soluble tumor necrosis factor receptor p55. Blood. 1994;83:113-118

[36] Fumuso E, Giguere S, Wade J, Rogan D, Videla-Dorna I, Bowden RA. Endometrial IL-1beta, IL-6 and TNF-alpha, mRNA expression in mares resistant or susceptible to post-breeding endometritis. Effects of estrous cycle, artificial insemination and immunomodulation. Veterinary Immunology and Immunopathology. 2003;96:31-41

[37] Woodward EM, Troedsson MH. Equine Breeding-induced Endometritis: a Review. Journal of Equine Veterinary Science. 2013;33:673-682

[38] Fumuso E, Aguilar G, Giguere S, David O, Wade J, Rogan D. Interleukin-8 (IL-8) and 10 (IL-10) mRNA transcriptions in the endometrium of normal mares and mares susceptible to persistent post-breeding endometritis. Animal Reproduction Science. 2006;94:282-285

[39] LeBlanc MM. When to refer an infertile mare to a theriogenologist. Theriogenology. 2008;70:421-429

[40] Ricketts SW. The treatment of equine endometritis in studfarm practice Pferdeheilkunde. 1999;6:588-593

[41] Bracher V, Allen WR. Videoendoscopic evaluation of the mare's uterus: I. Findings in normal fertile mares. Equine Veterinary Journal. 1992;24:274-278

[42] LeBlanc MM, Johnson RD, Calderwood-Mays MB, Valderrama C. Lymphatic clearance of India ink in reproductively normal mares and mares susceptible to endometritis (monograph). Biology of Reproduction. 1995;1:501-506

[43] LeBlanc MM, Neuwirth L, Jones L, Cage C, Mauragis D. Differences in uterine position of reproductively normal mares and those with delayed uterine clearance detected by scintigraphy. Theriogenology. 1998;50:49-54

[44] Pycock JF. Breeding management of the problem mare. In: Samper JC, editor. Equine Breeding Management and Artificial Insemination. St Louis: Saunders Elsevier; 2009. pp. 139-164

[45] Platt H, Atherston JG, Orskov I. Klebsiella and enterobacter organisms isolated from horses. Journal of Hygiene (Cambridge). 1977;77:401-408

[46] Watson ED. Post-breeding endometritis in the mare. Animal Reproduction Science. 2000;60-61:221-232

[47] Brito LFC, Barth AD. Endometritis in mares. Large Animal Veterinary Rounds. 2003;3(9). https://www. researchgate. net/publication/213858523_Endometritis_in_mares

[48] Merkt H, Klug E, Gunzel AR. Control of equine venereal diseases, Klebsiella and Pseudomonas. In: Proceedings of the International Symposium on Equine Venereal Diseases; 1980; Newmarket, UK. pp. 50-53

[49] Ozgur N, Bagcigil A, Ikiz S, Kilicarslan M, Carioglu B. Isolation of Klebsiella pneumoniae from mares with metritis and stallions, detection of biotypes and capsule types. Turkish Journal of Veterinary and Animal Science. 2003;27:241-247

[50] Causey RC. Making sense of equine uterine infections: the many faces of physical clearance. Veterinary Journal. 2006;172:405-421

[51] Kenney RM. The aetiology, diagnosis, and classification of chronic degenerative endometritis. In: Proceedings of the John P. Hughes International Workshop on Equine Endometritis; August 1992; Davis. Equine Veterinary Journal. 1993;25:184-193

[52] Hoffmann C, Bazer FW, Klug J, Aupperle H, Ellenberger C, Schoon HA. Immunohistochemical and histochemical identification of proteins and carbohydrates in the equine endometrium. Expression patterns for mares suffering from endometrosis. Theriogenology. 2009a;71:264-274

[53] Hoffmann C, Ellenberger C, Mattos RC, Aupperle H, Dhein S, Stief B, Schoon HA. The equine endometrosis: new insights into the pathogenesis. Animal Reproduction Science. 2009b;111:261-278

[54] Aresu L, Benali S, Giannuzzi D, Mantovani R, Castagnaro M, Falomo ME. The role of inflammation and matrix metalloproteinases in equine endometriosis. Journal of Veterinary Science. 2012;13:171-177

[55] Cadario ME. Revisiting the diagnosis and the treatment options for an old problem: Chronic and post-breeding endometritis in the mare. The Practitioner. 2014;1:21-25

[56] Maischberger E, Irwin JA, Carrington SD, Duggan VE. Equine post-breeding endometritis: A review. Irish Veterinary Journal. 2008;61(3):163-168

[57] LeBlanc MM. Persistent Mating Induced Endometritis in the Mare: Pathogenesis, Diagnosis and Treatment. In: Ball BA, editor. Recent Advances in Equine Reproduction. Ithaca: International Veterinary Information Service; 2003.

[58] Buczkowska J, Kozdrowski R, Nowak M, Raś A, Staroniewicz Z and Siemieniuch M. Comparison of the biopsy and cytobrush techniques for diagnosis of subclinical endometritis in mares. Reproductive Biology and Endocrinology. 2014;12:27. DOI: 10. 1186/1477-7827-12-27

[59] Parrilla-Hernandez S, Ponthier J, Franck TY, Serteyn DD, Deleuze SC. High concentrations of myeloperoxidase in the equine uterus as an indicator of endometritis. Theriogenology. 2014;81:936-940

[60] Liu IKM. The diagnosis, causes and treatment of persistent endometritis in the mare. RevistaBrasileira de Reproducao Animal. 2011;35(2):256-261

[61] Woodward EM, Christoffersen M, Campos J, Squires EL, Troedsson MH. Susceptibility to persistent breeding-induced endometritis in the mare: relationship to endome-

trial biopsy score and age, and variations between seasons. Theriogenology. 2012;78(3):495-501. DOI: 10. 1016/j. theriogenology. 2012. 02. 028

[62] Barbacini S, Necchi D, Zavaglia G, Squires EL. Retrospective study on the incidence of postinsemination uterine fluid in mares inseminated with frozen/thawed semen. Journal of Equine Veterinary Science. 2003;23:493-496

[63] Hemberg E, Lundeheim N, Einarsson S. Retrospective study on vulvar conformation in relation to endometrial cytology and fertility in thoroughbred mares. Journal of Veterinary Medicine A. 2005;52:474-477

[64] Hurtgen JP. Pathogenesis and treatment of endometritis in the mare: a review. Theriogenology. 2006;66:560-566

[65] Overbeck W, Witte TS, Heuwieser W. Comparison of three diagnostic methods to identify subclinical endometritis in mares. Theriogenology. 2011;75:1311-1318

[66] Burleson MD, LeBlanc MM, Riddle WT, Hendricks KEM. Endometrial microbial isolates are associated with different ultrasonographic and endometrial cytology findings in thoroughbred mares. Animal Reproduction Science. 2010;121:103

[67] LeBlanc MM. Advances in the diagnosis and treatment of chronic infectious and post-mating-induced endometritis in the mare. Reproduction in Domestic Animals. 2010;45(s2):21-27

[68] Adams GP, Kastelic JP, Bergfelt DR, Ginther OJ. Effect of uterine inflammation and ultrasonically - detected uterine pathology on fertility in the mare. Journal of Reproduction and Fertility, Supplement. 1987;35:445-454

[69] Ferreira JC, Canesin HS, Ignácio FS, Rocha NS, Pinto CR, Meira C. Effect of age and endometrial degenerative changes on uterine blood flow during early gestation in mares. Theriogenology. 2015;84:1123-1130

[70] Cocchia N, Paciello O, Auletta L, Uccello V, Silvestro L, Mallardo K, Paraggio G, Pasolini MP. Comparison of the cytobrush, cottonswab, and low-volume uterine flush techniques to evaluate endometrial cytology for diagnosing endometritis in chronically infertile mares. Theriogenology. 2012;7:89-98

[71] Nielsen JM. Endometritis in the mare: a diagnostic study comparing cultures from swab and biopsy. Theriogenology. 2005;64:510-518

[72] LeBlanc MM, Magsig J, Stromberg AJ. Use of a low-volume uterine flush for diagnosing endometritis in chronically infertile mares. Theriogenology. 2007;68:403-412

[73] Kozdrowski R, Sikora M, Buczkowska J, Nowak M, Ras A, Dzieciol M. Effects of cycle stage and sampling procedure on interpretation of endometrial cytology in mares. Animal Reproduction Science. 2015;154:56-62

[74] Walter J, Neuberg KP, Failing K, Wehrend A. Cytological diagnosis of endometritis in the mare: Investigations of sampling techniques and relation to bacteriological results. Animal Reproduction Science. 2012;132:178-186

[75] Riddle WT, LeBlanc MM, Stromberg AJ. Relationships between uterine culture, cytology and pregnancy rates in a Thoroughbred practice. Theriogenology. 2007;68(3): 395-402

[76] Petersen MR, Skive B, Christoffersen M, Lud K, Nielsen JM, Troedsson MHT, Bojesen AM. Activation of persistent Streptococcus equi subspecies zooepidemicus in mares with subclinical endometritis. Veterinary Microbiology. 2015;179:119-125

[77] Perkin NR, Chopin JB. Mare breeding soundness examination. In: Reed SM, Bayly WM, Sellon DC, editors. Equine Internal Medicine. 3rd ed. St. Louis: Saunders Elsevier; 2010. p. 1008-1016

[78] Kilgenstein HJ, Schöniger S, Schoon D, Schoon H-A. Microscopic examination of endometrial biopsies of retired sports mares: An explanation for the clinically observed subfertility? Research in Veterinary Science. 2015;99:171-179

[79] Rambags BPB, Colenbrander B, Stout TAE. Early pregnancy loss in aged mares: probable causes and possible cures. Pferdeheilkunde. 2003;19:653-656

[80] Brinsko SP, Varner DD, Blanchard TL. The effect of uterine lavage performed four hours post insemination on pregnancy rate in mares. Theriogenology. 1991;35(6): 1111-1119

[81] LeBlanc M, Neuwirth L, Mauragis D, Klapstein E, Tran T. Oxytocin enhances clearance of radiocolloid from the uterine lumen of reproductively normal mares and mares susceptible to endometritis. Equine Veterinary Journal. 1994;26:279-282

[82] Troedsson MH, Scott MA, Liu IK. Comparative treatment of mares susceptible to chronic uterine infection. American Journal of Veterinary Research. 1995;56:468-472

[83] Combs GB, LeBlanc MM, Neuwirth L, Tran TQ. Effects of prostaglandin F2a, cloprostenol and fenprostalene on uterine clearance of radiocolloid in the mare. Theriogenology. 1996;45:1449-1455

[84] Pycock JF, Newcombe JR. Assessment of the effect of three treatments to remove intrauterine fluid on pregnancy rate in the mare. Veterinary Record. 1996;138:320-323

[85] Rasch K, Schoon HA, Sieme H, Klug E. Histomorphological endometrial status and influence of oxytocin on the uterine drainage and pregnancy rate in mares. Equine Veterinary Journal. 1996;28:455-460

[86] Knutti B, Pycock JF, van der Weijden GC, Kupper U. The influence of early postbreeding uterine lavage on pregnancy rate in mares with intrauterine fluid accumulations after breeding. Equine Veterinary Education. 2000;5:346-349

[87] Asbury AC. Uterine defense mechanisms in the mare: the use of intrauterine plasma in the management of endometritis. Theriogenology. 1984;21:387-393

[88] Liu IKM, Troedsson M. The diagnosis and treatment of endometritis in the mare: yesterday and today. Theriogenology. 2008;70:415-420

[89] Metcalf ES, Scoggin K, Troedsson MH. The effect of platelet-rich plasma on endometrial pro-inflammatory cytokines in susceptible mares following semen deposition. Journal of Equine Veterinary Science. 2012;32:498. DOI: http://dx. doi. org/10. 1016/j. jevs. 2012. 06. 065

[90] Ferris RA, Frisbie DD, McCue PM. Use of mesenchymal stem cells or autologous conditioned serum to modulate the inflammatory response to spermatozoa in mares. Theriogenology. 2014;82:36-42

[91] Metcalf ES. The effect of platelet-rich plasma (PRP) on intraluminal fluid and pregnancy rates in mares susceptible to persistent mating-induced endometritis (PMIE). Journal of Equine Veterinary Science. 2014;34:128

[92] Reghini MFS, Bussiere MCC, Neto CR, Castro-Chaves MMB, Resende HL, Fioratti E, Farras MC, Alvarenga MA. Effect of use of platelet rich plasma on post-breeding uterine inflammatory response of mares. Journal of Equine Veterinary Science. 2014;34:127

[93] Christoffersen M. , Woodward EM. , Bojesen AM, Petersen MR, Squires EL, Lehn-Jensen H, Troedsson MH. Effect of immunomodulatory therapy on the endometrial inflammatory response to induced infectious endometritis in susceptible mares. Theriogenology. 2012;78:991-1004

[94] Brinsko SP, Varner DD, Blanchard TL, Meyers SA. The effect of post-breeding uterine lavage on pregnancy rate in mares. Theriogenology. 1990;33:465-475

[95] Pycock JF. How to maximize the chances of breeding successfully from the older maiden mare. In: Proceedings of the AAEP American Association of Equine Practitioners; 2–6 December 2006; San Antonio. pp. 245-249

[96] Kalpokas I, Perdigón F, Rivero R, Talmon M, Sartore I, Viñoles C. Effect of a povidone-iodine intrauterine infusion on progesterone levels and endometrial steroid receptor expression in mares. ActaVeterinariaScandinavica. 2010;52(1):66. DOI: 10. 1186/1751-0147-52-66

[97] Dascanio JJ. How and when to treat endometritis with systemic or local antibiotics. In: Proceedings of the AAEP 57th Annual Convention of the American Association of Equine Practitioners; 18–22 November 2011; San Antonio. pp. 24-31

[98] Petersen MR, Nielsen JM, Lehn-Jensen H, Bojesen AM. Streptococcus equi subspecies zooepidemicus resides deep in the chronically infected endometrium of mares. Clinical Theriogenology. 2009;1:393-409

[99] Perkins NR. Equine reproductive pharmacology. Veterinary Clinics of North America Equine Practice. 1999;15:687-704

[100] Brook D. Uterine culture in mares. Modern Veterinary Practice. 1984;65:A3-A8

[101] Albihn A, Baverud V, Magnusson U. Uterine microbiology and antimicrobial susceptibility in isolated bacteria from mares with fertility problems. ActaVeterinariaScandinavica. 2003;44:121-129

[102] Riddle WT, LeBlanc MM, Pierce SW, Stromberg AJ. Relationships between pregnancy rates, uterine cytology, and culture results in a Thoroughbred practice in central Kentucky. In: Proceedings of the AAEP 51st Annual Convention of the American Association of Equine Practitioners; 3–7 December 2005; Washington. pp. 51-54

[103] Frontoso R, De Carlo E, Pasolini MP, van der Meulen K, Pagnini U, Iovane G, De Martino L. Retrospective study of bacterial isolates and their antimicrobial susceptibilities in equine uteri during fertility problems. Research in Veterinary Science. 2008;84:1-6. DOI: 10. 1016/j. rvsc. 2007. 02. 008.

[104] Pycock JF. Management of the problem breeding mare. In: Proceedings of the Annual Conference of the Society of Theriogenology; 1999; Nashville. pp. 79-89

[105] Hinrichs K, Spensley M, McDonough P. Evaluation of progesterone treatment to create a model for equine endometritis. Equine Veterinary Journal. 1992;24:457-461

[106] McDonnell AM, Watson ED. The effect of transcervicaluterine manipulations on establishment of uterine infectionin mares under the influence of progesterone. Theriogenology. 1992;38:945-950

[107] Causey RC, Ginn P, Katz B, Hall B, Anderson KJ, LeBlanc MM. Mucus production by endometrium of reproductively healthy mares and mares with delayed uterine clearance. Journal of Reproduction and Fertility. 2000;56:333-339

[108] Lambert PA. Mechanisms of antibiotic resistance in Pseudomonas aeruginosa. Journal of the Royal Society of Medicine. 2002;95(s41):22-26

[109] Witte TS, Melkus E, Walter I, Senge B, Schwab S, Aurich C, Heuwieser W. Effects of oral treatment with N-acetylcysteine on the viscosity of intrauterine mucus and endometrial function in estrous mares. Theriogenology. 2012;78(6):1199-1208

[110] Zuin R, Palamidese A, Negrin R, Catozzo L, Scarda A, Balbinot M. High-dose N-acetylcysteine in patients with exacerbations of chronic obstructive pulmonary disease. Clinical Drug Investigation. 2005;25:401-408

[111] Estany S, Palacio JR, Barnadas R, Sabes M, Iborra A, Martinez P. Antioxidant activity of N-acetylcysteine, flavonoids and alpha-tocopherol on endometrial cells in culture. Journal of Reproductive Immunology. 2007;75:1-10

[112] Duru M, Nacar A, Yonden Z, Kuvandik G, Helvaci MR, Koc A, Akaydin Y, Oksuz H, Sogut S. Protective effects of N-acetylcysteine on cyclosporine-A-induced nephrotoxicity. Renal Failure. 2008;30:453-459

[113] Gores-Lindholm AR, LeBlanc MM, Causey R, Hitchborn A, Fayrer-Hosken RA, Kruger M, Vandenplas ML, Flores P, Ahlschwede S. Relationships between intrauterine infusion of N-acetylcysteine, equine endometrial pathology, neutrophil function, post-breeding therapy, and reproductive performance Theriogenology2013;80:218-227

[114] Melkus E, Witte TS, Walter I, Heuwieser W, Aurich C. Investigations on the endometrial response to intrauterine administration of N-acetylcysteine in oestrus mares. ReprodDomestAnim 2013;48(4):591-597.

[115] Ley WB, Bowen JM, Sponenberg DP, Lessard PN. Dimethyl sulfoxide intrauterine therapy in the mare: effects upon endometrial histological features and biopsy classification. Theriogenology. 1989;32:263-276

[116] Bracher V, Neuschaefer A, Allen WR. The effect of intra-uterine infusion of kerosene on the endometrium of mares. Journal of Reproduction and Fertility. 1991;44:706-707

[117] Wooley RE, Blue JL. In-vitro effect of edta-tris-lysozyme solutions on selected pathogenic bacteria. Journal of Medical Microbiology. 1975;8:189-194

[118] Wooley RE, Jones MS. Action of EDTA-Tris and antimicrobial agent combinations on selected pathogenic bacteria. Veterinary Microbiology. 1983;8;271-280

[119] Ashworth CD, Nelson DR. Antimicrobial potentiation of irrigation solutions containing tris-(hydroxymethyl)-aminomethane-EDTA. Journal of the American Medical Association. 1990;197:1513-1514

[120] Farca AM, Nebbia P, Re G. Potentiation of the in vitro activity of some antimicrobial agents against selected gramnegative bacteria by EDTA-tromethamine. Veterinary Research Communications. 1993;17:77-84

[121] Paccamonti DL, Pycock JF, Taverne MA, Bevers M, Van Der Weijden GC, Gutjahr S, Schams D, Blouin D. PGFM response to exogenous oxytocin and determination of the half-life of oxytocin in nonpregnant mares. Equine Veterinary Journal. 1999;31:285-288

[122] Gutjahr S, Paccamonti DL, Pycock JF, Taverne MA, Dieleman SJ, van der Weijden GC. Effect of dose and day of treatment on uterine response to oxytocin in mares. Theriogenology. 2000;54:447-456

[123] Blanchard TL, Varner DD, Love CC, Brinsko SP, Rigby SL, Schumacher J, editors. Manual of Equine Reproduction. 2nd ed. St Louis: Mosby; 2003. 272 p.

[124] Wolf CA, Maslchitzky E, Gregory RM, Jobim MI, Mattos RC. Effect of corticotherapy on proteomics of endometrial fluid from mares susceptible to persistent post breeding endometritis. Theriogenology. 2012;77:1351-1359

[125] Bucca S, Carli A, Buckley T, Dolci G, Fogarty U. The use of dexamethasone administered to mares at breeding time in the modulation of persistent mating induced endometritis. Theriogenology. 2008;70:1093-1100.

[126] Papa FO, Dell'aqua JA Jr, Alvarenga MA, Melo CM, Soares Zahn F, Lopes MD. Use of corticosteroid therapy onthe modulation of uterine inflammatory response in mares after artificial insemination with frozen semen. Pferdeheilkunde. 2008;24:79-82

[127] Cox WI. Examining the immunologic and hematopoietic properties of an immunostimulant. Veterinary Medicine, Small Animal Clinician. 1988;6:424-428

[128] LeBlanc MM, McKinnon. Breeding the Problem Mare. In: McKinnon AO, Squires EL, Vaala WE, Varner DD, editors. Equine Reproduction. 2nd ed. Philadelphia:John Wiley&Sons; 2011. pp. 2620-2642

[129] BeltaireKA, CheongSH, Coutinhoda Silva MA. Retrospective study on equine uterine fungal isolates and antifungal susceptibility patterns (1999–2011). Equine Veterinary Journal. 2012;44(s43):84–87

[130] Elvinger F, Roberts AW. Equine Genital Tract Isolates. Georgia Veterinary Diagnostic Laboratories Newsletter. 1995. pp. 3

[131] Elvinger F, Roberts AW. Equine Genital Tract Specimens. Georgia Veterinary Diagnostic Laboratories Newsletter. 1996. pp. 5

[132] Dascanio JJ, Schweizer C, Ley WB. Equine fungal endometritis. Equine VeterinaryEducation. 2001, 13(6):324-329

[133] Albihn A, Baverud V, Magnusson U. Uterine microbiology and antimicrobial susceptibility in isolated bacteria from mares with fertility problems. Acta VeterinariaScandinavica. 2003, 44:121-129

[134] Coutinho da Silva MA, Alvarenga MA. Fungal endometritis. In:McKinnon AO, Squires EL, Vaala WE, Varner DD editors. Equine Reproduction. 2nd ed. Philadelphia:John Wiley&Sons; 2011. pp. 2643-2651

[135] Tortora GJ, Funke BR, Case CL. Fungi, algae, protozoa, and multi-cellular parasites. In:Tortora GJ, Funke BR, Case CL, editors. Microbiology, An Introduction. Menlo Park:Addison Wesley Longman, Inc; 1998. pp. 320-358

[136] Dascanio JJ. Treatment of Fungal Endometritis. In: Samper JC, PycockJ, McKinnon AO, editors. Current therapy in Equine Reproduction. St Louis: Saunders Elsevier; 2007. pp. 116-120

[137] Scofield DB, Wittenburg LA, Ferris RA, Gustafson DL, McCue PM. Equine endometrial tissue concentration of fluconazole following oral administration. Journal of Equine Veterinary Science. 2013, 33:44-50

[138] RantalaM, AttiaS, Koukila-KähköläP, de HoogS, AnttilaM, KatilaT. Cladophialophorabantiana as an emerging pathogen in animals: casereport of equine endometritis and review of the literature. Journal of Clinical Microbiology. 2015, 53(9): 3047-3053. DOI: 10. 1128/JCM. 00728-15

[139] de Oliveira Tongu EA, Taborda CP, Vieira Marques SA, Gomes GM, de Macedo-Gomes LP, da CunhaPeixoto Jr. K, CrespilhoAM. Sensibility of microcultivation assay Dermatobac® for fungal endometritis diagnosis in mares. Ciência Animal Brasileira. 2015, 16(4):598-607

[140] Aitken GJ. Subclinical fungal endometritis in an 8-year-old Hanoverian mare. Canadian Veterinary Journal. 2012;53:196-198

[141] Malmgren L, Olsson Engvall E, Engvall A, Albihn A. Aerobic bacterial flora of semen and stallion reproductive tract and its relation to fertility under field conditions. ActaVeterinariaScandinavica. 1998;39:173-182

[142] Freeman KP, Roszel JF, Slusher SH, Payne M. Mycotic infections of the equine uterus. Equine Practice. 1986;8:34-42

[143] Ferris RA, Dern K, Veir JK, Hawley JR, Lappin MR, McCue PM. Development of a broad-range quantitative polymerase chain reaction assay to detect and identify fungal DNA in equine endometrial samples. American Journal of Veterinary Research. 2013;74(1):161-165

[144] Hess MB, Parker NA, Purswell BJ, Dascanio JD. Use of lufenuron as a treatment for fungal endometritis in four mares. Journal of the AmericanVeterinay Medical Association. 2002;221(2):266-267

[145] Scotty NC, Evans TJ, Giuliano E, Johnson PJ, Rottinghaus GE, Fothergill AW, Cutler TJ. In vitro efficacy of lufenuron against filamentous fungi and blood concentrations after PO administration in horses. Journal of Veterinary Internal Medicine. 2005;19:878-882

Chapter 16

Pregnancy Loss in Mares

K. Satué and J.C. Gardon

Additional information is available at the end of the chapter

http://dx.doi.org/10.5772/63742

Abstract

The reasons concerning losses during the first months of pregnancy has special importance in equine reproduction. Most of these losses occur early in pregnancy and around 15-20% of mares that conceive will lose the embryo before day 50. Early pregnancy loss is generally characterized by the sudden disappearance of the embryonic vesicle and is due to different reasons. Several etiologies factors involving both the mother and the embryo as, inflammatory and non-inflammatory endometrial disease, progesterone insufficiency, maternal age, lactation, site of intrauterine fixation of the embryonic vesicle, stress, plane of nutrition, season or climate, chromosome abnormalities or oocyte quality are some of the factor listed. Abortion occurs from the first month of pregnancy to full term and may be have an infectious or not origin. Causes of abortion include viral or bacterial infections, ingestion of mycotoxins, stress, gene mutations, Mare Reproductive Loss Syndrome, lack of sufficient nutrients and umbilical cord abnormalities. Some mares will show signs of impending abortion but other mares will abort without warning. Premature labor, discomfort, unusual activity or having a vulvar discharge of the mare require immediate attention. Pregnancy failure in mares represents a serious economic damages, expectations, and potential genetic improvement. Therefore is absolutely important that all losses are assessed for giving an appropriate treatment, and for preventing current and future losses.

Keywords: equine, mare, pregnancy, fetal loss, abortion

1. Introduction

1.1. Pregnancy loss in mares

In equine normal pregnancy, parameters include a gestation length of 330–340 days, an umbilical cord with a length of 36–84 cm and a placental weight (thoroughbred) of 5.7 ± 0.08 kg, or 11% of the foal's body weight. The fail of fertilized eggs to result in a live foal about 11 months later is one of the more frustrating aspects of horse breeding [1, 2].

In mares, abortion is defined as the failure of the fetus before it reaches the 300-day gestation period. A dead foal, either during or at the end of the pregnancy, may result from a diversity of reasons. Infectious agents, such as bacteria, viruses or fungi, or other "causes", can attack the fetus or fetus membranes, causing fetal death and expulsion. These "causes" are attributable to the mare, fetus, or external factors, including twinning, hormonal deficiencies, congenital anomalies, ergot alkaloid toxicity, or ingestion of tent caterpillar setae [3, 4].

Most of the losses occur in the first 35 days of pregnancy and the embryo is resorbed, after which the mare may come back into heat at a longer interval after the last estrus. In fact, around 20% of mares that conceive will lose the embryo before day 50. Older mares and mares with uterine inflammation have an increased risk of early embryonic loss. Stress and other diseases also may increase the rate of early embryonic loss. If the embryonic loss is detected, the mare can be served again later in the breeding season [5, 6].

If the abortion cause is bacterial, fungal, viral, hormonal, stress-induced, or the result of twinning, will appear to be spontaneous with symptoms of the contributing cause, which sometimes, do not have time to develop fully. Therefore, premature labor, discomfort, unusual activity, bagging up or having a vulvar discharge of the mare require immediate attention, and actions should be taken to safeguard the health of the mare and, if possible, the foal [7].

1.2. Early embryonic loss

In the mare, early pregnancy failure corresponds to the time of transition from the embryo stage to the fetal stage of conceptus development [6]. Early pregnancy loss is generally characterized by the sudden disappearance of the embryonic vesicle between ultrasound examinations. However, signs of impending embryonic loss can be detectable with transrectal ultrasonography. Usually, there are different signs which include the following: irregular shape of an embryonic vesicle, prolonged mobility of a vesicle beyond day 16, excessive endometrial edema, an undersized vesicle, loss of embryonic heartbeat, detachment of a vesicle with fluid loss, increased echogenicity of fluid within the conceptus, or abnormal development of the embryonic membranes [5].

Ultrasonography provided an early diagnosis of pregnancy (day 12th–14th postovulation) and important information about the development of embryo and embryonic death. Thus, under field conditions, this method allows direct assessment of the conceptus viability during approximately three-quarters of the interval when early embryonic loss occurs. The incidence of embryonic loss is generally in the range of 5–15%; however, foaling rates decline with maternal age after 14–16 years[8]. Thus, in mares over 18 years of age, the highest embryonic loss rates (20–30%) can be detected[9].

During the first stages of embryo development (fertilization to day 10th), several studies estimate that the embryonic loss rate were 9% for young mares compared to 60–70% for aged mares[10–12]. Thus, blastocysts recovered from the uterus of aged mares have more morphological defects, and fewer of them survive after embryo transfer to healthy recipient mares [13, 14].

The interval between day 2 and 4 might represent a critical period in pregnancy failure in aged mares. This finding indicates that pregnancy rates at day 2 were similar in young and aged mares; by 4 days after fertilization, there was a significant reduction in pregnancy rates in aged mares [10]. The equine embryo resides in the oviduct for 6 days and reaches morula or early blastocyst stage of development before entering the uterus. Therefore, there are a number of important events that occur during oviductal transit that could affect embryonic survival. During this time, early blastomeres cleavage progresses to further differentiation resulting in compaction, blastulation, and initial formation of the inner cell mass and trophoblast. Likewise, the embryonic genome is activated, and the transition from maternal to embryonic control of development has been proposed as a critical juncture in embryonic development [15]. Differences in proteins synthesized and secreted in vitro by explanted oviductal tissue have been reported and demonstrated that both qualitative and quantitative differences in the patterns of proteins from oviductal epithelium were detected between young and aged mares [16].

Several etiology factors have been described as responsible for early embryonic loss in mares. Vanderwall[9] discussed several etiology factors involving both the mother and the embryo. Thus, inflammatory and non-inflammatory endometrial disease, progesterone insufficiency, maternal age, lactation, site of intrauterine fixation of the embryonic vesicle, stress, plane of nutrition, season or climate, chromosome abnormalities, and oocyte quality are some of the factor listed.

Related to oocyte quality, mare age-related decline in oocyte quality is a major factor in the reduced fertility. In an in vitro studies [15], oocytes from aged mares reached metaphase II at a much lower rate than did oocytes from younger mares, with more oocytes from older mares arresting at metaphase I. This suggests that meiotic division of oocytes from older mares is more likely to be abnormal. In a report of Carnevale and Ginther[17], using gamete intrafallopian transfer studies, oocytes were collected from both young and aged mares and transferred into the uterine tube of young recipient mares. The results of this experiment inform that oocytes from aged mares resulted in significantly fewer pregnancies than those from young mares after transfer to the uterine tube of a young recipient mare. Mitochondria from in vitro matured oocytes from aged mares also demonstrated more ultrastructural abnormalities, suggesting that it may be an important underlying factor associated with reduced oocyte quality[18].

Prolongation of the follicular phase in aged mares is associated with an elevation of both Follicle Stimulating Hormone (FSH) and Luteinizing Hormone (LH), and this prolonged follicular development is related with an increased incidence of abnormal oocytes[19]. Different reports show that in mares, aging of the oocyte subsequent to ovulation results in a decline in pregnancy rates, a delayed embryonic development, and possibly an increased rate of subsequent embryonic loss [20, 21].

Endocrine factors, such as progesterone, have also been cited as a potential factor contributing to reduced fertility or early embryonic loss in mares[16, 22, 23, 24]. Progesterone is the hormone whose function is to prepare the uterus for the reception and development of the fertilized egg. In most animals, this hormone is produced primarily by the corpus luteum of pregnancy. The corpus luteum is constituted of specialized cells (small and large cells) that produce progesterone. In the horse, in case of pregnancy, the corpus luteum produces enough progesterone to maintain the gestation for only 40–50 days. Around this time, the "endometrial cups" develop in the uterus. These structures produce and secrete equine chorionic gonadotropin (eCG), a hormone that stimulates the production of additional progesterone by the ovary. These "extra" progesterone is required to maintain pregnancy into the fourth or fifth month of gestation[25]. Until day 40 of the embryonic period, progesterone is produced solely by the primary corpus luteum that is formed at the time of the initial ovulation. Minimal accepted concentrations of serum progesterone vary according to the laboratory or study reported; however, values between 2.0 and 4.0 ng/mL are typically used as the minimal serum progesterone concentration during early gestation [22, 26].

Maternal recognition of pregnancy involves an interaction between the conceptus and the uterine environment, which lead early conceptus development and implantation. Also is used to refer to the physiological process by which the lifespan of the corpus luteum is prolonged. During the estrus cycle, an increase in the secretion of prostaglandin can be observed 14 days after ovulation, which promotes lysis of the corpus luteum[27]. According to this, the pregnancy recognition signal has to be present on or before day 14 of pregnancy. In this regard, a study conducted with conceptuses collected 14 days after ovulation were placed in dialysis bags permeable for substances of different molecular weights and co-incubated with endometrial explants. These results indicate that prostaglandin inhibitory factor is a low molecular mass (3-10 kDa) proteinase K-resistant substance that may be adsorbed by dextran-coated charcoal [28].

Lysis of the corpus luteum associated with failure of maternal recognition of pregnancy can lead to early embryonic death[29, 30]. Failure of the embryo to block luteolysis has been identified in mares with embryonic loss prior to day 20 and was characterized by the presence of embryonic vesicles that were too small for days of age and by failure of fixation. In these mares, serum progesterone concentrations were lower at days 12, 15, and 18[31].

1.3. Abortions

Causes of abortion in mares include viral diseases, ingestion of poisonous plants, mycotoxins, bacterial infections, stress of either the mare or the fetus, gene mutations, mare reproductive loss syndrome (MRLS), and lack of sufficient nutrients to support the fetus, especially in the case of twins [32, 33].

Umbilical cord abnormalities also cause abortion. Those abnormal conditions of the cord, which can produce potentially lethal problems in the fetus, are usually associated with excessive length and include strangulation of the amniotic portion of the cord around parts of the fetus and excessive torsion of the amniotic part of the cord with urachal and vascular obstruction [34].

1.3.1. Infectious causes of abortion

Over the past 6 years, infectious abortions have accounted for approximately one-third of all abortions diagnosed. Equine herpesvirus (EHV-1) is the major infectious agent, accounting for 18% of all abortion diagnoses [35].

1.3.1.1. Viral abortion

Equine herpesviruses

Five, equid herpesviruses (EHV) have been identified and are known to infect the horse. Of these, equid herpesviruses 1 and 4 are the most important for horse industries worldwide based on their veterinary medical and economic consequence. Equid herpesvirus 1 (EHV-1) or abortion virus is most often related with abortions, whereas equid herpesvirus 4 (EHV-4) or rhinopneumonitis virus is associated with respiratory disease in colts. Beyond, both virus subtypes have the potential to cause respiratory disease and abortion [36].

Equid herpesvirus 3 is the cause of equine coital exanthema. This is contagious venereally transmissible disease affecting the external genitalia of the stallion and the mare, but there is no evidence implicating the virus in infertility or abortion in the mare [37, 38]. Equid herpesviruses 2 and 5 are gammaherpesviruses that have been associated with different clinical manifestations in the horse, such as upper and lower respiratory disease [39], keratoconjunctivitis[40], chronic follicular pharyngitis, and poor performance [41].

Equid herpesviruses 1 and 4 were originally considered subtypes of one virus EHV-1[42]. For both viruses, the natural host species is the horse and in this situation both are genetically stable[43]. However, EHV-1 can infect cattle, cervids, camelids, and laboratory mice [44, 45]. Likewise Equid herpesvirus 1 is considered as the principal cause of contagious abortion in mares in many countries [43]. Another clinical outcome of EHV-1 infection is a neurological syndrome, specifically a myeloencephalopathy[46] and also has been linked to a fatal non-neurological syndrome characterized by a multisystemic vasculitis, severe pulmonary edema, and a mild enterotyphocolitis[47].

Transmission of EHV-1 and EHV-4 takes place primarily by the respiratory route. This is consequence of direct or indirect contact with nasal or conjunctival secretions of infected animals, aborted fetuses, placental membranes, and fluids. Transplacental transmission may occur in the case of EHV-1 and not often for EHV-4. In the case that these type of transmission occurs, usually result in abortions in the last trimester of pregnancy [48].

Most abortions due to this virus occur between 8 and 11 months of gestation, although they may occur as early as 5 months. Once the virus reaches the pregnant uterus, it infects endothelial cells of the uterine vascular layer causing endometrial vasculitis. This causes the damage of the endometrium and the chorioallantoic membrane. At the same time, this leads to thrombosis of the affected vessels of the placenta[3, 49, 50].

The severity and the extent of thrombosis determine whether the abortion occurs or not. In those areas where thrombotic lesions are focal and not widespread, the virus is transmitted to the fetus by infected fetal leukocytes, causing widespread in many tissues necrotic lesions. At the same time, a local edema develops in the maternal-fetal interface, resulting in premature separation of the chorioallantoic membrane from the endometrium. The final result is abortion with the fetus and placenta positive for the virus. However, in cases of extensive thrombotic lesions, placental ischemia occurs rapidly with premature separation of the placenta and abortion. In such circumstances, the virus has not had enough time to invade the fetus and therefore the placenta, but not the fetus is positive for the virus[51].

Infected mares during early pregnancy, no induction of abortion before the fifth month of pregnancy is attributed to the fact that endometrial vascular changes and expression of viral antigen on endothelial cells, are significantly lower than those observed in mares infected later in pregnancy [52]. Mares exposed very late in pregnancy to EHV-1, may not abort, however, will give birth to a congenitally infected live foal. In some cases, the foal will be born alive at term and will die shortly after birth due to infection by the virus. The abortion rate may approach 100% in a herd of susceptible mares [36].

Abortion due to EHV-1 or EHV-4 has no adverse effect on the subsequent fertility of the mare. Viruses cannot be detected in the mare's uterus beyond 48 hours after abortion of an infected fetus. Mares rarely abort from virus in successive years but may abort later in their reproductive life if reinfected during pregnancy [53, 54].

The family of herpesviruses has the ability to persist in the body of its host in a latent state as a carrier no apparent after primary infection. In a time that can vary from months or years after primary infection, latent herpesvirus can manifest itself again with renewed replication and with the possibility of starting new outbreaks of the disease in their host, as well as stable mates susceptible. Consequently, it is the existence of these latently infected carrier horses, from which the virus is reactivated by stress-induced circumstances and provides the means to infect other individuals, which starts a new occurrence of this disease[36].

Equine arteritis virus

Equine viral arteritis (EVA) is an infectious disease of equids that is caused by equine arteritis virus (EAV). EVA occurs throughout much of the world, although the prevalence varies greatly between countries and among horses of different breeds [55]. EAV is the prototype virus in the family Arteriviridae, a grouping that also includes porcine reproductive and respiratory syndrome virus, simian hemorrhagic fever virus, and lactate dehydrogenase-elevating virus of mice [56, 57].

EAV was first isolated in 1953 from the lung of an aborted fetus after an extensive outbreak of respiratory disease and abortion on Standardbred mares. EVA was distinguished from equine influenza and equine herpesviruses type 1 and type 4 [58, 59]. EVA was identified as an etiologically distinct disease after isolation of the EAV and description of characteristic vascular lesions [60].

The majority of EAV infections are subclinical, but occasional are characterized by any combination of influenza-like illness in adult horses, abortion in pregnant mares, and interstitial pneumonia in young foals [35, 61]. Abortion after infection of pregnant mares EAV is the result of a lethal fetal infection. This is actually that leads to expulsion of the fetus, rather than myometritis or damage to the placenta that affects the synthesis of progesterone. Aborted fetus tissues contain high titers of virus than mares which aborted, indicating that substantial virus replication occurs in the fetus. Is thought to the stress that results from fetal infection is responsible for activating the hypothalamus-pituitary axis fetal, which induces abortion [62].

In pregnant mares, EAV-infected abortions are not preceded by premonitory signs and can occur late in the acute phase or early in the convalescent phase infection. In the past after natural or experimental infection, abortions have been documented at 3 months to over 10 months of gestation [55, 59, 63, 64]. Abortion rates in outbreaks of EVA have varied from less than 10% to more than 60%. While the abortive potential of different strains of EAV has not been adequately compared, it appears that abortigenic strains differ in their potential as well as their virulence characteristics [55].

During acute infection, stallions may undergo a period of temporary infertility associated with decreased libido. Ejaculates may have decreased sperm motility, concentration, and percentage of morphologically normal cells. These changes can persist for 6–7 weeks after infection and considered to be the result of increased testicular temperature instead of any pathological effect induced by the virus. Semen quality is apparently normal in persistently infected stallions, despite active shedding of virus into the semen [55, 65].

Transmission of EAV between horses occurs through either respiratory or venereal routes[55, 66]. EAV can also be transmitted by aerosol from urine and other body secretions of acutely infected horses, infected respiratory tract secretions, aborted fetuses, and their membranes [67]. Another important route of natural transmission of the virus is in the semen of stallions that are either acutely or chronically infected. Persistently infected carrier stallions are the essential reservoir responsible for perpetuation and maintenance of EAV in equine populations [66, 68].

Mares that become infected following natural or artificial insemination with semen collected from shedding stallions can readily transmit the virus by the respiratory route to susceptible partners in close proximity [69]. Also it has been demonstrated that under experimental conditions, EAV can be transmitted to a recipient mares through embryo transfer from a donor mare inseminated with EAV infective semen[70]. In mares infected with EAV in late gestation, congenital infection of foals after transplacental transmission frequently develops a rapidly progressive, fulminating interstitial pneumonia, and fibronecrotic enteritis [71, 72].

EAV appears to be restricted to the reproductive tract during persistent infection of carrier stallions [55, 73]. Virus in semen is associated with the sperm-rich fraction and not with the pre-ejaculatory fluid, and the titers of virus in sequential ejaculates vary little from the same stallion. The mechanism of persistence of EAV in the male reproductive tract is not clear. However, persistence of EAV in stallions is testosterone-dependent.

It has been shown that carrier stallions are clearly responsible for the generation of genetic heterogeneity in field strains of EAV. Some reports indicate that sequence analyses of the variable gene of strains of EAV present in the semen of carrier stallions showed that the EAV acts as a population of genetically related viral variants during persistent infection. This involves both genetic and phenotypic divergence virus[66, 74].

1.3.1.2. Bacterial abortions

Several species of bacteria have been implicated as causative agents of abortion and infertility in mares. The most common causative agent of bacterial abortion in mares, belongs to the group of streptococci. However, we have identified other groups of bacteria from aborted fetuses, which include *Leptospira, Nocardia, Klebsiella,* and Staphylococcal species. Bacteria can be introduced at breeding, ascend through the cervix. Cervical incompetence and/or pneumovagina can predispose the mare to an ascending bacterial infection and abortion. The bacterial infection may extent to the fetus itself and infect and damage a range of organs. Abortion occurs following fetal death either from septicemia or by progressive placentitis and subsequent placental insufficiency [75, 76].

As a consequence to bacterial abortion, retention of the placenta is often common as well as the infection of the uterus (endometritis and/or metritis). Before a successful breeding, treatment of the mare is often required. A good practice is to swab mares before breeding to determine whether dangerous bacteria are present in the uterus. The veterinarian can advise on the need to lavage the mare's uterus with or without an antibiotic [7].

Streptococcal infections

The streptococci are Gram-positive, catalase-negative, facultative anaerobic, coccoid, or ovoid bacteria. The numerous species of streptococci may be as α-hemolytic, β-hemolytic, and nonhemolytic species. From all of them, *Streptococcus equi* subsp. *zooepidemicus, S. equi* subsp. *equi,* and *S. dysgalactiae* subsp. *equisimilis* assume greater importance in equine medicine[77].

Streptococcus equi subsp. *equi* is the agent responsible for strangles, which is a highly contagious infection of the upper respiratory tract and associated lymph nodes [78]. This streptococci enter through the mouth or nose and attach to cells in the crypt of the tonsil and adjacent superficial lymphoid nodules. Nasal shedding usually begins after a latent period of 4–14 days and ceases between 3 and 6 weeks after the acute phase [79, 80]. Horses in the nearest postconvalescent phase are resistant to experimental challenge even with numbers of *S. equi* exceeding those required to produce the original infection[78]. Thus, almost 75% of horses develop a solid immunity to strangles following recovery from the disease [81].

Streptococcus equi subsp. *zooepidemicus* shares very high DNA homology (>98%) with its clonal derivative *S. equi* but differs in their biology and pathogenicity. Normally is a mucosal commensal that opportunistically produces disease in situations of virus infection, heat stress, or tissue injury. *S. zooepidemicus* is the most frequently isolated pathogen from the uterus of the mare[82]. The clitoral fossa, clitoral sinuses, and the vagina have been suggested as possible bacterial reservoirs [82, 83]. *S. zooepidemicus* is able to reach the uterus and pass the vulva, the vestibulovaginal sphincter, and the cervix. Poor anatomical conformation of the internal and external reproductive organs may impair these barriers and allow bacteria to ascend into the uterus. Consequently, endometritis is caused by an ascending infection in a random manner primarily governed by the uterine defense mechanisms of the mare [3, 84, 85]. Uterine infection has been described to depend on factors related to the uterine defense mechanisms as well as mare with advanced age, repeated history of unsuccessful foaling results also called "high-risk mares"[84, 86]. Virulence factors, such as fibronectin-binding proteins [87], hyaluronic capsule [88], M-like proteins [89], and Fc receptors, have also been identified [90].

A recent study of Rasmussen et al. [91] indicates that *S. zooepidemicus*-associated endometritis in mares belongs to a genetically distinct subpopulation. These findings add a new perspective to the pathogenesis of equine infectious endometritis. In this regard, it could not be caused by rather probable pathogenic strains of more specialized endometrium random contamination

S. zooepidemicus in the reproductive tract but flow. This indicates that not only the efficiency of uterine defense mechanisms to determine if *S. zooepidemicus* establish an infection, but rather to the interaction between strain of *S. zooepidemicus* and uterine defense mechanisms involved. Contamination of the uterus also takes place during live mounting, artificial insemination, or iatrogenically[86].

The normal habitat of *Streptococcus dysgalactia* subsp. *equisimilis* appears to be the skin and mucosal surfaces. Therefore, it was considered to be an infrequent bacterium isolated from horses and has been reported in horses from aborted placenta [75]. However, in a retrospective study Erol et al. (2012), repot that *Streptococcus equisimilis* was recovered, fetal tissues, umbilical cord and genital tracts of both foals and adult horses. These data comprise 74.8% of total sites isolated for *S. equisimilis*. This records strongly suggests that S. *equisimilis* is mostly a reproductive system agent. Also the results show that both *S. equisimilis* and *S. zooepidemicus* have an ability to invade sterile organs such as brain, kidney, and joints suggesting they have similar pathogenesis and tissue tropism.

Placentitis

Placentitis in mares is a potential threat because of the involvement of fetal and neonatal viability. This disease is normally caused by bacteria rising through the vagina. The most common pathogens implicated in equine placentitis are *Streptococcus equi* subspecies *zooepidemicus, Escherichia coli, Klebsiella pneumonia,* and *Pseudomonas aeruginosa*[93]. *S. zooepidemicus* and *E. coli* are able to cause acute placentitis with bacteremia during early and midgestation in foals[34, 94].

Usually bacterial infection initiates disease; however, a work from an experimental model of placentitis in pony mares showed that premature delivery may happen secondary to inflammation of the chorion instead of as a consequence of fetal infection. It was suggested that these inflammatory processes result in PGE2 and PGF2α, production and stimulation of uterus contractility, resulting in premature delivery [95].

In some cases of placentitis (chronic cases), foals will suffer a faster fetal maturation. As a consequence, these foals will be delivered prematurely, but will be mature enough to survive. It has been demonstrated that, in humans, the indirect stimulation of the fetal HHG axis by proinflammatory cytokines is responsible for advanced fetal maturation [96]. If this assumption is true for equine fetuses, then the possibility of delaying preterm delivery sufficiently to allow fetal maturation can improve survival rates colt. To achieve this goal, it is necessary to diagnose and treat disease. Transrectal ultrasonographic examination of reproductive tract has become a routine diagnostic tool for placentitis. This method allows direct examination of the cervical region and also allows for evaluation of fetal activity, fetal fluid character, and subjective amniotic evaluation. In the normal pregnant mare, the area visualized in the region of the cervical is the combined uterine and placental unit.

Renaudin et al. [97, 98] developed the technique for evaluation of the combined thickness of the uterus and placenta (CTUP) and established normal values in light-horse mares throughout gestation. Thus, for 271–300, 301–330, and >330 days of gestation, normal concentrations for CUTP were <8, <10, and <12 mm, respectively. However, during placental infection or inflammation, CTUP measures have increased, or membranes are separated from the endometrium. Additionally, purulent material may accumulate in pouches between the chorioallantois and the endometrium. Thickening of the amnion is also indicative of inflammation. Throughout the gestation, the allantoic fluid is hypoechoic, whereas amniotic fluid is slightly more echodense. Normal, fetal activity can shake cellular material and change the characteristics of the fluid. Fluids that persistently increased echodensity have increased cellularity due to infection or inflammation. For that reason, successive ultrasound examinations are essential to determine whether fluid character changes are pathologic or not [99].

Placental membrane integrity and thickness and fetal fluid are evaluated using transabdominal ultrasonography. Since the chorioallantois is intimately associated with the endometrium, it cannot be easily identified as a separate structure from the transabdominal procedure. Mares with normal pregnancies should have a minimum CTUP of 7.1±1.6 mm and a maximal CTUP of 11.5±2.4 mm[100]. Evaluation of the caudal allantochorion is inaccurate using the transabdominal approach. However, transabdominal assessment of fetal membranes is useful for recognizing placental abnormalities in mares with placentitis. Thus, mares infected with bacteria will often exhibit placental separation and purulent debris at the base of the gravid horn [101].

Ultrasound techniques, combined with endocrinological assays, provide additional tools for early diagnosing and progression of placentitis in mares. Pregnant mares with signs of placentitis should be treated with systemic broad spectrum antibiotics and anti-inflammatories. Different researchers [99, 102] informed that the administration of penicillin (22,000 IU/kg, q 6 hours), gentamicin (6.6 mg/kg, q 24 hours), and trimethoprim sulfamethoxazole (30 mg/kg, BID) resulted in inhibitory concentrations (MIC) of these drugs in allantoic fluid and placental tissue of pregnant pony mares. Similarly, another observation suggests that long-term therapy with a combination altrenogest (0.088 mg/kg), flunixin meglumine (1.1 mg/kg BID), and pentoxifylline (8.4 mg/kg BID) and antibiotics have a positive influence on pregnancy outcome with delivery of healthy foals [103].

Most placental lesions are observed by transrectal ultrasonography as over 90% of cases are caused by ascending infections. In cases of Nocardioform placentitis, changes in the placental unit may be seen transrectally or transabdominally by ultrasound, especially in the cervical region. The CTUP should be measured in the ventral portion of the uterus, just cranial to the cervix. The CTUP increases from a mean of 4.0 mm between 4 and 8 months of gestation to 1.0–1.2 cm at term [104]. A CTUP greater than 1.2 cm at 9 months of gestation or a CTUP greater than 1.5 cm at 11 months should be associated with placentitis[105, 106]. Usually, the fetal membranes may separate from the uterus and pus may be visualized swirling between the membranes and uterus [107]. In case that mares show premature udder development without a vaginal discharge should be evaluated by transabdominal ultrasonography for twins and Nocardioform placentitis. Uterine infections caused by Nocardioform bacteria, an organism that resides in the soil, frequently result in abortion or premature delivery [108].

Mares with placental pathology may have increased plasma concentrations of progestagens as a result of stress to the fetal placental unit. Fetal–placental progesterone is rapidly metabolized to 5α-pregnanes. Unfortunately, 5α-pregnanes are not readily assayed in a commercial setting, so diagnosis of placental disease using 5α-pregnane concentrations is not possible.

This progestins cross-react with the progesterone antibody used in commercial radioimmunoassay and enzyme-linked immunosorbent assays and can be measured in the maternal circulation in late gestation [109, 110]. Also, subnormal plasma relaxin concentrations were detected in mares with abnormal pregnancies [111]. Mares with clinical signs of placentitis and mares exhibiting signs of fescue toxicosis had suppressed plasma relaxin concentrations. Furthermore, sensitivity assays can be improved when combined with evidence of placental thickening as detected using transrectal ultrasonography [112].

Unfortunately, many mares do not exhibit classical signs of infection, premature udder development, and a vaginal discharge, so infections are commonly missed. Mares having vaginal discharge with or without udder development should be examined ultrasonographically[108]. A weak foal resulting for a premature delivery is devastating to horse owners. Most of these foals, if they live, never have productive performance, even if they receive the best neonatal care. The most important cause of premature delivery is placentitis due to it accounts for nearly a third of late-term abortions and fetal mortality during the first day after foal[113]. Placentitis affects approximately 3–7% of pregnant mares, the value of the foals, both economically and emotionally, makes this an important disease to study [108].

Mares most commonly afflicted are pluriparous. Many have anatomical defects of the caudal reproductive tract, such as pneumovagina, vestibule-vaginal reflux or cervical fibrosis, tears, or adhesions. Some, but not all mares, exhibit a vaginal discharge and develop an udder premature in response to placentitis. Management of mares at risk of abortion owing to placentitis is directed at prolonging pregnancy because chronic placentitis has been associated with accelerated fetal maturation. A foal may be born significantly premature and survive with limited neonatal care, if premature birth can be delayed for a few weeks after placentitis develops [107, 114].

Treatment protocols designed for prolonging gestation and for producing viable foals are currently being studied in experimental models [114, 115]. Induction of parturition prematurely with the expectation of delivering a mature foal is not an option because fetal maturation only occurs in the last 5 days of gestation and gestation length varies widely from 320 to 365 days. Removing the fetus from its dam's uterus before its final maturation will result in a premature foal that usually will not survive even with the best of neonatal care. So inducing precocious maturation of the fetus with corticosteroids has been considered a risk and not reliable in mares. Although data are limited, large doses (100 mg q 24 hours for 3 days) are necessary, and laminitis can be an important sequel [116].

Leptospira infections

Leptospirosis is a bacterial disease of worldwide distribution caused by spirochetes of the genus *Leptospira*. The first report of naturally occurring leptospirosis in horses was done in Russia by Lubashenko and Novikova in 1947. *Leptospira* infection in horses is manifested as either abortion or recurrent uveitis although sporadic cases of renal and hepatic disease have also been reported [117, 118].

Leptospires are motile bacteria called spirochetes. The order Spirochaetales includes two families of spiral bacteria, *Spirochaetaceae* and *Leptospiraceae*, which share unique morphologic and functional features. The genus *Leptospira* includes a large number of both pathogenic and nonpathogenic bacteria. Morphologically, all the leptospires are flexible, tightly coiled, unicellular bacteria and can be are grouped into serogroups, serovars as well as genotypes based on DNA homology. The serovars *pomona, grippotyphosa, hardjo, bratislava, canicola,* and *icterohaemmorhagiae* are the ones we are most interested in. Leptospires are very common in domestic and wild animals and can also infect humans. Leptospirosis is maintained in nature by subclinically infected maintenance hosts, also known as reservoir hosts or definitive hosts, such as deer, raccoons, or rodents [119, 120]. Leptospires can invade the mucous membranes and/or damaged skin and migrate to various body organs of an incidental host[121].

Leptospirosis has been confirmed as a significant cause of abortion, stillbirth, and perinatal death in horses in locations worldwide [36, 122]. For most serovars of *Leptospira*, horses are incidental hosts. Although there are evidence suggesting that as in other farm animals (cattle and pigs), horses may be a maintenance host for *L. interrogans* serovar Bratislava [123].

Multiple serovars of *Leptospira* have been associated with abortion, with serovar Pomona type kennewicki being among the most common[124, 125]. In this regard, some reports indicate that the genotype kennewicki of the pomona serogroup was responsible for 86% of the abortions. However, the genotype grippotyphosa was responsible for only the 8% of abortion in mares [126]. The authors indicated that mammal of the raccoon family (Procyonidae) is the maintenance host for grippotyphosa, whereas the maintenance host for kennewicki has not been determined. Also mixed infections with multiple serovars have been reported[127].

Most leptospiral abortions occur between 6 and 9 months of gestation. The affected placenta is thick, edematous, hemorrhagic and could be covered with a brown mucoid material on the chorionic surface. However, occasionally, the affected placenta lacks detectable gross lesions. In some cases, a green discoloration or cystic adenomatous hyperplasia of the allantois is observed, and it has also been described funisitis or inflammation of the umbilical cord [119, 128]. Several serovars of *Leptospira* have been isolated from aborted equine fetuses. The fetus may present with mild to moderate icterus and liver enlargement. Fetal histopathologic lesions may include various degrees of nephritis and hepatitis[119, 129].

Clinical presentation of bacterial abortion is preceded by vaginal discharge and premature lactation. Mares with these symptoms should be considered high risk and should be required for detailed fetoplacental evaluations. The appearance of the placenta following a bacterial abortion can vary from minimal alterations in acute cases to a thickened, edematous placenta, either generally or in localized areas. The chorionic surface is often brown and covered in exudate [130].

1.4. Noninfectious abortion

1.4.1. Abortion due to twinning

In horse breeding, twins are not good news and are well known that the birth of healthy twin foals is unusual. The origin of equine twins is almost exclusively dizygotic originated from two separate fertilized oocytes with two different spermatozoa. A strong association between twinning rate and breed, age, reproductive status, season, use of drugs to control ovulation

http://dx.doi.org/10.5772/63742

has been reported. Twinning also appears to have a high degree of repeatability and heritability [131].

Compared with other breeds, more twins are diagnosed per cycle in Thoroughbreds mares [132]. Twinning rate is also more common in older mares than younger mares[133]. Similarly, fewer multiple ovulations are expected on the first postpartum estrus compared to other cycles [6]. As well as multiple pregnancies are more commonly detected when ovulation induction was used [134].

It is generally accepted that the inability of a mare to successfully carry twin foals to term is due to placental insufficiency. In twin pregnancies usually, one fetus develops more rapidly, progressively assuming the major portion of the maternal blood supply and causing the other fetus to die from lack of blood. In other words, insufficient fetal membranes are produced to accommodate and provide nutrition to two developing fetus. Therefore, the death of one fetus usually results in the abortion of both. Abortion due to twinning is most common between the 5th and 9th months [135].

Most twin pregnancies terminate in early fetal resorption or loss, late-term abortions, or the birth of small growth retarded foals. The mare is very efficient at reducing twins to a single pregnancy. In some cases, one twin dies and becomes mummified, allowing the other twin to continue to develop and be maintained to term. In case of resorption, the reduction is reached by a competitive absorption of nutrients that is related to size and position of the early pregnancy and later to orientation of the embryo proper within the developing conceptus[6]. However, the resolution of twins by the application of any nonintervention program depends on the age at identification, the orientation of the vesicles, and any disparity in size[136].

With the common use of ultrasound in equine practice, twin pregnancies are now commonly detected early and dealt with. Mares with a history of producing twins should have an ultrasound pregnancy test preferably between 14 and 16 days after the last service, and then one embryo can be destroyed so that the other can continue to develop normally. The mare is very efficient at reducing twins to a single pregnancy. Due to this, sometimes one twin will fail to develop and be resorbed without any veterinary intervention[6].

Mares aborting twins in late gestation frequently have foaling difficulties, damage their reproductive tracts, and are difficult to rebreed. Few twins can carry to term and survive. Complications that can arise with late-term abortion of twins or delivery of twins at term include dystocia, retained placenta, delayed uterine involution and metritis, and death of one or both twins [137]. If foals born alive, they are frequently small, demonstrate the effects of intrauterine growth retardation, and have a poor survival rate, with many needing expensive sophisticated critical care[93].

1.4.2. *Umbilical cord torsion*

Primary umbilical torsion is the most commonly diagnosed condition of the noninfectious causes of abortion [35]. Torsion, or strangulation of the umbilical cord, is said to be the cause of fetal deaths and abortions in the later stages of pregnancy. Excessive twisting or wrapping of cord around the limb of the fetus cause vascular obstruction in the umbilical cord resulting in the death of the fetus. Equine fetuses are extraordinarily active and their movements can result in 360° twisting of the amniotic and/or the allantoic parts of the cord[138]. Umbilical torsion was observed in 19% of 515 cases submitted to the Animal Health Laboratory over six breeding seasons[35]. Statistical reviews from Ricketts et al.[139] showed that umbilical cord torsions resulting in vascular compromise and fetal death involved the 35.7% of abortion and neonatal deaths and 46.2% of pre-term abortions, respectively.

In equine fetuses, sudden vascular compression/cord torsions tended to occur before signs of urachal dilatation (urinary retention) developed at twist sites (5.5–7.5 months). Where urachal dilatations had developed the pregnancies tended to continue up to 6–10 months [34, 35]. Fetuses dying in utero due to vascular obstruction in the umbilical cord are not usually aborted immediately, so the tissues display variable degrees of autolysis when aborted. Cord lesions include local intimal or medial vascular wall tears and associated intramural and stromal hemorrhages, local edema even sufficient to cause 'stretch tears' at the amniotic surface, and small aneurysmal dilatations[34].

1.4.3. Fungal abortions

Fungal abortions are caused by fungi that produce mycotoxins in the class of chemicals called "ergot" or "ergopeptine alkaloids".

1.4.3.1. Ergot alkaloid toxicity in the late gestation

Different mycotoxins called ergot or ergopeptine alkaloids are produced for number of fungi, both saprophytic and endophytic. Among the different animal species, sensitive to ergopeptine alkaloids is dissimilar. While mares are sensitive to at levels as low as 50–100 ppb, cattle do not show visible signs until 1000–2000 ppb. These alkaloids have toxic effects on the reproductive tract and mammary gland of the mare, and also they have been associated with depression of serum prolactin (PR) and progestagens (P4), prolonged gestation, thickened edematous placenta, and agalactia. The ergopeptine interfere with the normal rise of P4 and PR in the last 40 days of gestation. The normal P4 levels increase from 300 days to birth (4.8 ± 1.5 to 22.7 ± 2.7 ng/mL). Foals born without the normal increases in progestagens suffer hypoadrenocortical function with the consequence of being born smaller, weak, or stillborn[140].

1.4.3.2. Fescue toxicosis

Fescue toxicosis in horses is caused by an endophytic fungus infection of tall fescue grasses (*Festuca arundinacea*). Fescue toxicity is the form of ergot alkaloid toxicity by the endophytic fungus *Neotyphodium coenophialum* (formerly called Acremonium coenophialum). It lives inside the plant, between the cells, and produces ergot alkaloids, resulting in the disease condition called fescue toxicity [141].

Ergotism is the clinical syndrome of ergot poisoning caused by *Claviceps purpurea* fungus. It is a saprophytic fungus that infects cereals, using the plant's nutrients. *Claviceps purpurea* can live on a variety of hays and pasture grasses, including bluegrass, barley, and cereal rye [141]. It

http://dx.doi.org/10.5772/63742

has been demonstrated that three classes of alkaloids, including the ergovaline, lolines, and peramine, are produced by the fungus and play a potential role in affecting animal performance [142].

Signs commonly associated with mares consuming infected fescue are prolonged gestation, agalactia, increased foal and mare mortality, dystocia, tough and thickened placentas, weak and dysmature foals, reduced serum progesterone and prolactin, and increased serum estradiol-17β. These chemicals cause dystocia in mares and deaths of foals. An early study by Garrett et al. [143] shows the relative incidence of 38% prolonged gestation, 18% abortion, and 9% thickened placentas in mares with fescue toxicosis.

In cattle and horses, toxins have vasoconstrictive effects on the vascular system. The ergopeptine alkaloids are agonists of the dopamine D2 receptors. Thus, under the reproductive point of view, the consequence of dopamine is the inhibition of prolactin. Decreased prolactin concentrations are a main physiological aspect in the pathogenesis of the absence of milk production (agalactia) and decreased mammary gland development in mares [144].

Another effect of exposure of these toxins is the abnormal production by the placenta of P4 that becomes depressed during the last 30 or 40 days of gestation. It was suggested that the reason for this is lower placental production of P4, which inhibits adrenocorticotropic hormone (ACTH) secretion in the fetus[140].

Additional effects of fescue toxicity on placental function are related to vasoconstriction [145]. This effect is principally important due to the nature of the fetal and maternal placenta, of being an extensive vascular interface between them. Several placental lesions have been reported in fescue toxicity, including edema, fibrosis, and mucoid degeneration of arteries. The incidence of retained placentas is 62% in mares consuming fescue pasture grasses. The primary clinical signs of ergot alkaloid poisoning in the late gestation include an extended gestation length from 11 to 12 months; dystocia, with mares trying to foal for many hours; agalactia with poor quality colostrum; "red bag" placentas from premature separation; thick edematous placentas with weights that exceed normal; and weak or dead foals with aspiration pneumonia, as consequence of a thickening of the placenta [146].

1.4.4. Mare reproductive loss syndrome

Mare reproductive loss syndrome or MRS was identified in early fetal losses (40–100 day) plus late-term abortions and the birth of weak foals, many of which died, with no immediate explanation for the cause [147].

Based on pathological examination, the cause of MRLS is not always identifiable. However, a number of disease conditions can be eliminated as possible causes of the syndrome. The main pathological findings in MRLS fetuses were the inflammation of the umbilical cord (funisitis), pneumonia, bacterial infection, and hemorrhages. The bacterial infection in aborted fetuses represents an ante mortem event, and most of the pathological lesions could be attributed to this origin. According to the literature, it could not be determined whether the bacteria are the primary cause of abortion or just represent a secondary opportunistic infection[148].

Pericarditis is another pathological finding associated with MRLS. *Actinobacillus* spp. are the most commonly reported isolates from pericardial fluid of horses with bacterial pericarditis. In other reports unrelated to MRLS, *Streptococcus* spp., *Pasteurella multocida, Staphylococcus aureus, Pseudomonas* spp., *Acinetobacter,* and *Enterococcus faecalis* were isolated in some cases [149].

MRLS caused abortion in early pregnancy, and even though the abortion happened with 2 months remaining in the breeding season, only rarely were these mares able to get back in foal. The primary reason for these mares not becoming pregnant is due to the presence of eCG (equine chorionic gonadotrophin) in their circulation implying that mares not cycle normally. The eCG levels are maintained due to the presence of endometrial cups produced by the placenta before the pregnancy loss [150].

In case of parturition, the delivery was characterized as "red bag" in 32% of the cases, indicating that the allantochorion was presented and passed concurrently with the fetus. This high incidence of red bag delivery indicates a possible premature placental separation, suggesting placental injury or problem with placentation. There are no pathognomonic findings or individual diagnostic tests that allow diagnosis of abortion by MRLS. Diagnosis of abortion or stillbirth related to MRLS is based on a combination of several factors, such as history, time of year, bacteriologic results, and the above-described pathological findings[147].

Author details

K. Satué[1*] and J.C. Gardon[2]

*Address all correspondence to: ksatue@uchceu.es

1 Department of Animal Medicine and Surgery, Faculty of Veterinary, CEU-Cardenal Herrera University, Alfara del Patriarca, Valencia, Spain

2 Department of Animal Medicine and Surgery, Faculty of Veterinary and Experimental Sciences, Catholic University of Valencia "San Vicente Mártir", Valencia, Spain

References

[1] Mizushima C. Late-term abortion associated with umbilical cord torsion in the mare: Case report. J Equine Vet Sci 2005;25(4):162–163.

[2] Schlafer DH. Examination of the placenta. In: McKinnon AO, EL Squires, WE Vaala, DD Varner, editors. Equine Reproduction, 2nd edition. Ames, Iowa: Wiley-Blackwell; 2011. pp. 99–110.

[3] Smith KC, Blunden AS, Whitwell KE, Dunn KA, Wales AD. A survey of equine abortion, stillbirth and neonatal death in the UK from 1988 to 1997. Equine Vet J 2003;35:496–501.

[4] Laugier C, Foucher N, Sevin C, Leon A, Tapprest J. A 24-year retrospective study of equine abortion in Normandy (France). J Equine Vet Sci 2011;31:116–123.

[5] Ball BA, Woods GL. Embryonic loss and early pregnancy loss in the mare. Compend Contin Educ Pract Vet 1987;9:459–470.

[6] Ginther OJ, editor. Reproductive Biology of the Mare: Basic and Applied Aspects, 2nd edition. Cross Plains, WI: Equiservices; 1992.

[7] Tibary A, Pearson LK, Fite CL. Reproductive tract infections. In: Sellon DC, Long MT editors. Equine Infectious Diseases, 2nd edition. St. Louis, Missouri: Saunders Elsevier; 2014. pp. 84–105.

[8] Woods GL, Baker CB, Baldwin JO, Ball BA, Bilinski JL, Cooper WL, Ley WB, Mank EC, Erb HN. Early pregnancy loss in broodmares. J Reprod Fertil Suppl 1987;35:455–459.

[9] Vanderwall DK. Early embryonic loss in the mare. J Equine Vet Sci 2008;28:691–702.

[10] Ball BA, Little TV, Hillman RB, Woods GL. Pregnancy rates at days 2 and 14 and estimated embryonic loss rates prior to Day 14 in normal and subfertile mares. Theriogenology 1986;26:611–619.

[11] Ball BA, Little TV, Weber JA, Woods GL. Viability of Day-4 embryos from young, normal mares and aged, subfertile mares after transfer to normal recipient mares. J Reprod Fertil 1989;85:187–194.

[12] Brinsko SP, Ball BA, Miller PG, Thomas PGA, Ellington JE. In vitro development of day two embryos obtained from young, fertile mares and aged, subfertile mares. J Reprod Fertil 1994;102:371–378.

[13] Woods GL, Hillman RB, Schlafer DH. Recovery and evaluation of embryos from normal and infertile mares. Cornell Vet 1986;76:386–394.

[14] Vogelsang SG, Vogelsang MM. Influence of donor parity and age on the success of commercial equine embryo transfer. Equine Vet J Suppl 1989;8:71–72.

[15] Brinsko SP, Ball BA, Ellington JE. In vitro maturation of equine oocytes obtained from different age groups of sexually mature mares. Theriogenology 1995;44:461–469

[16] McKinnon AO, Pycock JF. Maintenance of pregnancy. In: Samper JC, Pycock JF, McKinnon AO editors. Current Therapy in Equine Reproduction. St Louis: Saunders Elsevier; 2007. pp. 389–409.

[17] Carnevale EM, Ginther OJ. Defective oocytes as a cause of subfertility in old mares. Biol Reprod 1995;1:209–214.

[18] Torner H, Alm H, Kanitz W, Goellnitz K, Becker F, Poehland R, Bruessow KP, Tuchscherer A. Effect of initial cumulus morphology on meiotic dynamic and status of mitochondria in horse oocytes during IVM. Reprod Dom Anim 2007;42:176–183.

[19] Carnevale EM, Bergfelt DR, Ginther OJ. Follicular activity and concentrations of FSH and LH associated with senescence in mares. Anim Reprod Sci 1994;35:231–246.

[20] Woods JA, Bergfelt DR, Ginther OJ. Effects of time of insemination relative to ovulation on pregnancy rate and embryonic loss rate in mares. Equine Vet J 1990;22:410–415.

[21] Huhtinen M, Koskinen E, Skidmore JA, Allen WR. Recovery rate and quality of embryos from mares inseminated after ovulation. Theriogenology 1996;45:719–726.

[22] Ball BA, Daels PF. Early pregnancy loss in mares: applications for progestin therapy. In: Robinson NE, editors. Current Therapy in Equine Medicine, 4th edition. Philadelphia, PA: WB Saunders; 1997. pp. 531–534.

[23] Gutierrez CV, Riddle WT, Bramlage LR. Serum thyroxine concentrations and pregnancy rates 15 to 16 days after ovulation in broodmares. J Am Vet Med Assoc 2002;220:64–66.

[24] Meredith TB, Dobrinski I. Thyroid function and pregnancy status in broodmares. J Am Vet Med Assoc 2004;224:892–894.

[25] Bergfelt DR, Adams GP. Luteal Development. In: McKinnon AO, Squires EL, Vaala WE, Varner DD editors. Equine Reproduction, 2nd edition. United Kingdom: Blackwell Publishing; 2011. pp. 2056–2064.

[26] McKinnon AO, Squires EL, Carnevale EM, Hermenet MJ. Ovariectomized steroid-treated mares as embryo transfer recipients and as a model to study the role of progestins in pregnancy maintenance. Theriogenology 1988;29(5):1055–1063.

[27] Sharp DC, Thatcher MJ, Salute ME, Fuchs AR. Relationship between endometrial oxytocin receptors and oxytocininduced prostaglandin F2a release during the oestrous cycle and early pregnancy in pony mares. J Reprod Fertil 1997;109:137–144.

[28] Ababneh MM, Troedsson MH, Michelson J, Seguin BE. Partial characterization of an equine conceptus prostaglandin inhibitory factor. J Reprod Fertil Suppl 2000;56:607–613.

[29] McDowell KJ, Williams NM, Donahue JM, Poole L, Barney WE, Coe B, Deborde S, Ennis L, Newman KE, Lindemann M, Lynn B, Webb BA. Deductive investigations of the role of eastern tent caterpillars in mare reproductive loss syndrome. Proceedings of a Workshop on the Equine Placenta, University of Kentucky; 2003. pp. 99–102.

[30] Daels PF, Stabenfeldt GH, Hughes JP, Odensvik K, Kindahl H. Effects of flunixin meglumine on endotoxininduced prostaglandin F2a secretion during early pregnancy in mares. Am J Vet Res 1991;52:276–278.

[31] Bergfelt DR, Woods JA, Ginther OJ. Role of the embryonic vesicle and progesterone in embryonic loss in mares. J Reprod Fertil 1992;95:339–347.

[32] Ball BA. Embryonic death in mares. In McKinnon AO, Voss JL, editors. Equine Reproduction. Philadelphia: Lea & Febiger; 1993. pp. 517–531.

[33] Wolfsdorf KE, Rodgerson D, Holder R. How to manually reduce twins between 60 and 120 days gestation using cranio-cervical dislocation. In: Proceedings of the 51st Annual Convention of the American Association of Equine Practitioners, Seattle, Washington, USA; 2005. pp. 284–287.

[34] Whitwell KE. Abortions and stillbirths: A pathologists overview. In: McKinnon AO, Squires EL, Vaala WE, Varner DD editors. Equine Reproduction, 2nd edition. United Kingdom: Blackwell Publishing; 2011. pp. 2339–2349.

[35] McEwen B, Carman S. Equine abortion 2003–2004. AHL Newsletter 2004;8(2):22.

[36] Timoney JF, Kalimuthusamy N, Velinani S, Donahueb JM, Artiushina SC, Fettingera M. A unique genotype of Leptospira interrogans serovar Pomona type kennewicki is associated with equine abortion. Vet Microbiol 2011;150:349.

[37] Bitsch V. Cases of equine coital exanthema in Denmark. Acta Vetm Scand 1972;13:281–283.

[38] Pascoe RR. The effect of equine coital exanthema on the fertility of mares covered by stallions exhibiting the clinical disease. Aust Vet J 1981;57:111–114.

[39] Burrell MH, Whitwell KE, Wood JL, Mumford JA. Pyrexia associated with respiratory disease in young thoroughbred horses. Vet Rec 1994;134:219–220.

[40] Collinson PN, O'Rielly JL, Ficorilli N, Studdert MJ. Isolation of equine herpesvirus type 2 (equine gammaherpesvirus 2) from foals with keratoconjunctivitis. J AmVet Med Assoc 1994; 205:329–331.

[41] Studdert MJ. Equine herpesvirus 2 and disease. Equine Vet J 1996;28(6):426–428.

[42] Ostlund EN. The equine herpesviruses. Vet Clin N Am Equine Pract 1993;9:283–294.

[43] Allen GP, Bryans JT. Molecular epizootiology, pathogenesis, and prophylaxis of equine herpesvirus-1 infections. Prog Vet Microbiol Immunol 1986;2:78–144.

[44] Awan AR, Chong YC, Field HJ. The pathogenesis of equine herpesvirus type 1 in the mouse: A new model for studying host responses to the infection. J Gen Virol 1990;71:1131–1140.

[45] Rebhun WC, Jenkins DH, Riis RC, Dill SG, Dubovi EJ, Torres A. An epizootic of blindness and encephalitis associated with a herpesvirus indistinguishable from equine herpesvirus I in a herd of alpacas and llamas. J Am Vet Med Assoc 1988;192:953–956.

[46] Henninger RW, Reed SM, Saville WJ, Allen GP, Hass GF, Kohn CW, Sofaly C. Outbreak of neurologic disease caused by equine herpesvirus-1 at a university equestrian center. J Vet Intern Med 2007;21:157–165.

[47] Del Piero F, Wilkins PA. Pulmonary vasculotropic EHV-1 infection in equids. Vet Pathol 2001;38:474–475.

[48] Allen GP. Equine rhinopneumonitis. Control of abortigenic herpesviral infections. Curr Ther Theriogenol 1986;2:711–714.

[49] Edington N, Smyth B, Griffiths L. The role of endothelial cell infection in the endometrium, placenta and foetus of equid herpesvirus 1 (EHV-1) abortions. J Comp Pathol 1991;104:379–387.

[50] Allen GP, Kydd IK, Slater ID, Smith KC. Advances in understanding of the epidemiology, pathogenesis and immunological control of equid herpesvirus-1 abortion. In: Wernery U, Wade J, Mumford J, Kaaden OR, editors. Equine Infectious Diseases VIII. Newmarket (Suffolk): R & W Publications; 1999. pp. 129–146.

[51] Smith KC, Whitwell KE, Binns MM, Dolby CA, Hannant D, Mumford JA. Abortion of virologically negative foetuses following experimental challenge of pregnant pony mares with equid herpesvirus 1. Equine Vet J 1992;24:256–259.

[52] Smith KC, Mumford JA, Lakhani K. A comparison of equid herpesvirus-1 (EHV-1) vascular lesions in the early versus late pregnant equine uterus. J Comp Pathol 1996;114:231–247.

[53] Bryans JT. On immunity to disease caused by equine herpesvirus 1. J Am Vet Med Assoc 1969;155:294–300.

[54] Bryans JT, Allen GP. Control of abortigenic herpesviral infections. Curr Ther Theriogenol 1986;2:711–714.

[55] Timoney PJ, McCollum WH. Equine viral arteritis. Vet Clin North Am Equine Pract 1993;9:295–309.

[56] Siddell SG, Ziebuhr J, Snijder EJ. Coronaviruses, toroviruses and arteriviruses. In: Mahy BW, Ter Meulen V, editors. Topley and Wilson's Microbiology and Microbial Infections: Virology. London: Hodder Arnold; 2005. pp. 823–856.

[57] Gorbalenya AE, Enjuanes L, Ziebuhr J, Snijdera J. Nidovirales: evolving the largest RNA virus genome. Virus Res 2006;117:17–37.

[58] Bryans JT, Crowe ME, Doll ER, Mccollum WH. Isolation of a filterable agent causing arteritis of horses and abortion by mares; its differentiation from the equine abortion (influenza) virus. Cornell Vet 1957;47:3–41.

[59] Doll ER, Knappenberger RE, Bryans JT. An outbreak of abortion caused by the equine arteritis virus. Cornell Vet 1957;47:69–75.

[60] Jones TC, Doll ER, Bryans JT. The lesions of equine viral arteritis. Cornell Vet 1957;47:52–68.

[61] McCollum WH, Timoney PJ, Lee Jr JW. Habacker PL, Balasuriya UBR, MacLachlan NJ. Features of an outbreak of equine viral arteritis on a breeding farm associated with abortion and fatal interstitial pneumonia in neonatal foals. Equine Infectious Diseases VIII. In: Proceeding of the 8th International Conference, Dubai; 1998. pp. 559–560.

[62] MacLachlan NJ, Balasuriya UB, Rossitto PV, Hullinger PA. Patton JF. Wilson WD. Fatal experimental equine arteritis virus infection of a pregnant mare: immunohistochemical staining of viral antigens. J Vet Diagn Invest 1996;8:367–374.

[63] McCollum WH, Timoney PJ. The pathogenic qualities of the 1984 strain of equine arteritis virus. In Proceedings of the Grayson Foundation International Conference of Thoroughbred Breeders Organizations, Ireland; 1984. p. 34–44.

[64] Cole JR, Hall RF, Gosser HS, Hendricks, JB, Pursell AR, Senne DA, Pearson JE, Gipson CA. Transmissibility and abortogenic effect of equine viral arteritis in mares. J Am Vet Med Assoc 1986;189:769–771.

[65] Neu SM, Timoney PJ, Lowry SR. Changes in semen quality following experimental equine arteritis virus infection in the stallion. Theriogenology 37:407–431, 1992.

[66] Balasuriya UBR, MacLachlan NJ. Equine Viral Arteritis. In Debra C. Sellon, Maureen T. Long editors. Equine Infectious Diseases, 2nd edition. St. Louis, Missouri: Sounders; 2014. pp. 302–310.

[67] Guthrie AJ, Howell PG, Hedges JF, Bosman AM, Balasuriya UBR, McCollum WH, Timoney PJ, MacLachlan, NJ. Lateral transmission of equine arteritis virus among Lipizzaner stallions in South Africa. Equine Vet J 2003;35:596–600.

[68] Timoney PJ, McCollum WH, Murphy TW, Roberts AW, Willard JG, Carswell GD. The carrier state in equine arteritis virus infection in the stallion with specific emphasis on the venereal mode of virus transmission. J Reprod Fertil Suppl 1987;35:95–102.

[69] Balasuriya UB, Evermann JF, Hedges JF, McKeirnan AJ, Mitten JQ, Beyer JC, McCollum WH, Timoney PJ, MacLachlan NJ. Serologic and molecular characterization of an abortigenic strain of equine arteritis virus isolated from infective frozen semen and an aborted equine fetus. J Am Vet Med Assoc 1998;213:1586–1589.

[70] Broaddus CC, Balasuriya UB, Timoney PJ, White JLR, C. Makloski C, Torrisi K, Payton M, Holyoak GR. Infection of embryos following insemination of donor mares with equine arteritis virus infective semen. Theriogenology 2011;76:47–60.

[71] Vaala WE, Hamir AN, Dubovi EJ, Timoney PJ, Ruiz B. Fatal, congenitally acquired infection with equine arteritis virus in a neonatal Thoroughbred. Equine Vet J 1992;24:155–158.

[72] Del Piero F, Wilkins PA, Lopez JW, Glaser AL, Dubovi EJ, Schlafer, DH, Lein DH. Equine viral arteritis in newborn foals: clinical, pathological, serological, microbiological and immunohistochemical observations. Equine Vet J 1997;29:178–185.

[73] Neu SM, Timoney PJ, McCollum WH. Persistent infection of the reproductive tract in stallions experimentally infected with equine arteritis virus. In: Equine Infectious Diseases V. Proceedings of the 5th International Conference, Kentucky, 1987. pp. 149–154.

[74] Balasuriya UB, Hedges JF, Smalley VL, Navarrette A, McCollum WH, Timoney PJ, Snijder EJ, MacLachlan JN. Genetic characterization of equine arteritis virus during persistent infection of stallions. J Gen Virol 2004;85:379–390.

[75] Timoney JF. The pathogenic equine streptococci. Vet Res 2004;35:397–409.

[76] Timothy AS. Reproductive disorders in horses. Vet Clin Equine 2015;31:389–405.

[77] Waller AS, Sellon DC, Sweeney CR, Timoney PJ, Newton JR, Hines MT. Streptococcal Infections In: Debra C. Sellon, Maureen T. Long editors. Equine Infectious Diseases, 2nd edition. St. Louis, Missouri: Sounders; 2014; pp. 265–277.

[78] Galán JE, Timoney JF. Mucosal nasopharyngeal immune response of the horse to protein antigens of Streptococcus equi, Infect Immun 1985;47:623–628.

[79] Newton JR, Wood JLN, Dunn KA, De Brauwere MN, Chanter N. Naturally occurring persistent and asymptomatic infection of the guttural pouches of horses with *Streptococcus equi*. Vet Rec 1997;140:84–90.

[80] Chanter N, Newton JR, Wood JLN, Verhezen K, Hannant D. Detection of strangles carriers. Vet Rec 1998;142:496.

[81] Hamlen HJ, Timoney JF, Bell RJ, Epidemiologic and immunologic characteristics of Streptococcus equi infection in foals. J Am Vet Med Assoc 1994;204:768–775.

[82] Ricketts SW. Uterine and clitoral cultures. In: McKinnon AO, Squires EL, Vaala WE, Varner DD editors. Equine Reproduction, 2nd edition. United Kingdom: Wiley-Blackwell; 2011. pp. 1963–1978.

[83] Hinrichs K, Cummings MR, Sertich PL, Kenney RM. Clinical significance of aerobic bacterial flora of the uterus, vagina, vestibule, and clitoral fossa of clinically normal mares. J Am Vet Med Assoc 1988;193:72–75.

[84] Causey RC. Making sense of equine uterine infections: the many faces of physical clearance. Vet J 2006;172:405–421.

[85] Wittenbrink MM, Hoelzle K, Hoelzle LE: What's new in bacteriology of the mare's genital tract. Pferdeheilkunde 2008;24:53–55.

[86] LeBlanc MM, McKinnon AO. Breeding the problem mare. In: McKinnon AO, Squires EL, Vaala WE, Varner DD editors. Equine Reproduction, 2nd edition. United Kingdom: Blackwell Publishing; 2011. pp. 2620–2642.

[87] Lindmark H, Jacobsson K, Frykberg L, Guss B. Fibronectin-binding protein of streptococcus equi subsp. Zooepidemicus. Infect Immun 1996;64:3993–3999.

[88] Wibawan IW, Pasaribu FH, Utama IH, Abdulmawjood A, Lammler C. The role of hyaluronic acid capsular material of *Streptococcus equi subsp. zooepidemicus* in mediating adherence to HeLa cells and in resisting phagocytosis. Res Vet Sci 1999;67:129–133.

[89] Timoney JF, Mukhtar MM. The protective M proteins of the equine group C streptococci. Vet Microbiol 1993;37:389–395.

[90] Jonsson H, Lindmark H, Guss B. A protein G-related cell surface protein in *Streptococcus zooepidemicus*. Infect Immun 1995;63:2968–2975.

[91] Rasmussen CD, Haugaard MM, Petersen MR, Nielsen JM, Pedersen HG, Bojesen AM. *Streptococcus equi subsp. zooepidemicus* isolates from equine infectious endometritis belong to a distinct genetic group. Vet Res 2013;44(1):26.

[92] Erol E, Locke SJ, Donahoe JK, Mackin MA, Carter CN. Beta-hemolytic *Streptococcus spp.* from horses: a retrospective study (2000–2010) J Vet Diagn Invest 2012;24:142–147.

[93] Acland HM. Abortion in mares. In: McKinnon AO, Voss JL, editors. Equine Reproduction. Philadelphia: Lea & Febiger; 1993. p. 554–562.

[94] Roberts SJ. Abortion and other gestational diseases in mares. In: Morrow DA editor. Current Therapy in Theriogenology. Philadelphia: WB Saunders Co., 1986. pp. 705–710.

[95] LeBlanc MM, Giguere S, Brauer K, Paccamonti DL, Horohov DW, Lester GD, O'Donnell LJ, Sheerin BR, Pablo I, Rodgerson DH. Premature delivery in ascending placentitis is associated with increased expression of placental cytokines and allantoic fluid prostaglandins E2 and F2α. Theriogenology 2002;58:841–844.

[96] Gravett MG, Hitti J, Hess DL, Eschenbach DA. Intrauterine infection and preterm delivery: evidence for activation of the fetal hypothalamic-pituitary-adrenal axis. Am J Obstet Gynecol 2000;182: 404–1410.

[97] Renaudin CD, Troedsson MHT, Gillis CL. Transrectal ultrasonographic evaluation of the normal equine placenta. Equine Vet Educ 1999a;11:75–76.

[98] Renaudin CD, Liu IKM, Troedsson MHT. Transrectal ultrasonographic diagnosis of ascending placentitis in the mare: a report of two cases. Equine Vet Ed 1999b;11(2): 69–74.

[99] Macpherson CS, Bailey CS. A clinical approach to managing the mare with placentitis. Theriogenology 2008;70:435–440.

[100] Reef VB, Vaala WE, Worth LT, Sertich PL, Spencer PA. Ultrasonographic assessment of fetal well-being during late gestation: development of an equine biophysical profile. Equine Vet J 1996;28:200–208.

[101] Hong CB, Donahue JM, Giles RC, Jr, Petrites-Murphy MB, Poonacha KW, AW, Smith BJ, Tramontin RR, Tuttle PA, Swerczek TW. Etiology and pathology of equine placentitis. J Vet Diagn Invest 1993;5:56–63.

[102] Rebello SA, Macpherson ML, Murchie TA, LeBlanc MM, Vickroy TW. The detection of placental drug transfer in equine allantoic fluid. Theriogenology 2005;64:776–777.

[103] Troedsson MHT, Zent WW. Clinical ultrasonogaphic evaluation of the equine placenta as a method to successfully identify and treat mares with placentitis. In: Proceeding of Workshop on the Equine Placenta. Agricultural Experimental Station, UK; 2004. pp. 66–67.

[104] Renaudin CD, Troedsson MH, Gillis CL, King VL, Bodena A. Ultrasonographic evaluation of the equine placenta by transrectal and transabdominal approach in the normal pregnant mare. Theriogenology 1997;47:559–573.

[105] Bucca S, Fogarty U, Collins A, Small V. Assessment of feto-placental well-being in the mare from mid-gestation to term: transrectal and transabdominal ultrasonographic features. Theriogenology 2005;64:542–557.

[106] Bucca S. Diagnosis of the compromised equine pregnancy. Vet Clin North Am Equine Pract 2006;22:749–761.

[107] LeBlanc MM, Macpherson ML, Sheerin PC. Ascending placentitis: what we know about pathophysiology, diagnosis, and treatment. In: Proceedings of the 50th Annual Convention of American Association of Equine Practitioners, Denver, Colorado; 2004; p. 127–143.

[108] LeBlanc MM. Ascending placentitis in the mare: en update. Reprod Dom Anim 2010; 45(2):28–34.

[109] Ousey JC, Houghton E, Grainger L, Rossdale PD, Fowden AL. Progestagen profiles during the last trimester of gestation in Thoroughbred mares with normal or compromised pregnancies. Theriogenology 2005;63:1844–1856.

[110] Morris S, Kelleman AA, Stawicki RJ, Hansen PJ, Sheerin PC, Sheerin BR, Paccamenonti DL, LeBlanc MM. Transrectal ultrasonography and plasmaprogestin profiles identifies feto-placental compromise in mares with experimentally induced placentitis. Theriogenology 2007;67:681–691.

[111] Ryan P, Vaala W, Bagnell C. Evidence that equine relaxin is a good indicator of placental insufficiency in the mare. In: Proceeding of the 44th Annual Convention

http://dx.doi.org/10.5772/63742

American Association Equine Practitioner, Baltimore, Maryland. Ithaca: International Veterinary Information Service; 1998.

[112] Troedsson MHT. High risk pregnant mare. Acta Vet Scand 2007;49(1):1–8.

[113] Giles RC, Donahue JM, Hong CB, Tuttle PA, Petrites-Murphy MB, Poonacha KB, Roberts AW, Tramontin RR, Smith B, Swerczek TW. Causes of abortion, stillbirth, and perinatal death in horses: 3,527 cases (1986–1991). J Am Vet Med Assoc 1993;203:1170–1175.

[114] Christiansen D, Crouch J, Hopper R, Moulton K, LeBlanc MM, Ryan PL. Experimentally induced placentitis in late gestation mares with *Streptococcus equi zooepidemicus*: therapeutic prevention of preterm birth. Clin Theriogenol 2009;1:239.

[115] Murchie TA, Macpherson ML, LeBlanc MM, Luznar S, Vickroy TW. Continuous monitoring of penicillin G and gentamicin in allantoic fluid of pregnant pony mares by in vivo microdialysis. Equine Vet J 2006;38:520–525.

[116] Ousey JC, Kolling M, Allen WR. The effects of maternal dexamethasone treatment on gestation length and foal maturation in Thoroughbred mares. Anim Reprod Sci 2006;94:436–438.

[117] Gilger BC. Equine recurrent uveitis: the viewpoint from the USA. Equine Vet J Suppl 2010;37:57.

[118] Pinna AE, Martins G, Hamond C, Lilenbaum W. Molecular diagnostics of leptospirosis in horses is becoming increasingly important. Vet Microbiol 2011;153:413.

[119] Tappero JW, Ashford DA, Perkins BA. Leptospira species (leptospirosis). In: Mandell GL, Bennett JE, Dolin R, editors. Principles and Practice of Infectious Diseases, 5th edition. Elsevier Health Sciences, Philadelphia; 2000.

[120] Quinn PJ, Markey BK, Carter ME, Donnelly WJ, Leonard FC. Spirochaetes. Veterinary Microbiology and Microbial Disease. Malden: Blackwell Science; 2002.

[121] Bolin CA. Clinical signs, diagnosis and prevention of Leptospirosis in cattle. Cattle Pract 2001;9(4):267–273

[122] Whitwell KE, Blunden AS, Miller J, Errington J. Two cases of equine pregnancy loss associated with Leptospira infection in England. Vet Rec 2009;165:377.

[123] Williams DM, Smith BJ, Donahue JM, Poonacha KB. Serological and microbiological findings on 3 farms with equine leptospiral abortions. Equine Vet J 1994;26:105.

[124] Donahue JM, Smith BJ, Donahoe JK, Rigsby CL, Tramontin RR, Poonacha KB, Wilson MA. Prevalence and serovars of leptospira involved in equine abortions in central Kentucky during the 1990 foaling season. J Vet Diagn Invest 1992;4:279.

[125] Donahue JM, Smith BJ, Poonacha KB, Donahoe JK, Rigsby CL. Prevalence and serovars of leptospira involved in equine abortions in central Kentucky during the 1991–1993 foaling seasons. J Vet Diagn Invest 1995;7:87.

[126] Verma A, Stevenson B, Adler B. Leptospirosis in horses. Vet Microbiol 2013;67:61–66.

[127] Kinde H, Hietala SK, Bolin CA, Dowe JT. Leptospiral abortion in horses following a flooding incident. Equine Vet J 1996;28:327.

[128] Sebastian M, Giles R, Roberts J, Poonacha K, Harrison L, Donahue J, Benirschke K. Funisitis associated with Leptospiral abortion in an equine placenta. Vet Pathol 2005;42:659–662.

[129] Szerdi L, Haake DA. Immunohistochemical identification and pathologic findings in natural cases of equine abortion caused by leptospiral infection. Vet Pathol 2006,43:755.

[130] Hines MT. Leptospirosis. In: Sellon DC, Long MT editors. Equine Infectious Diseases, 2nd edition. St. Louis, Missouri: Sounders; 2014; pp. 302–310.

[131] Ginther OJ. Twinning in mares: a review of recent studies. J Equine Vet Sci 1982;2:127–135.

[132] Nath LC, Anderson GA, McKinnon AO. Reproductive efficiency of Thoroughbred and Standardbred horses in northeast Victoria. Aust Vet J 2010;88:169–175.

[133] Deskur S. Twinning in Thoroughbred mares in Poland. Theriogenology 1985;23:711–718.

[134] Veronesi MC, Battocchio M, Faustini M, Gandini M, Cairoli F. Relationship between pharmacological induction of estrous and/or ovulation and twin pregnancy in the Thoroughbred mares. Domest Anim Endocrinol 2003;25(1):133–140.

[135] McKinnon AO. Origin and outcome of twin pregnancies. In: McKinnon AO, Squires EL, Vaala WE, Varner DD editors. Equine Reproduction, 2nd edition. United Kingdom: Blackwell Publishing; 2011. pp. 2350–2358.

[136] Ginther OJ. The nature of embryo reduction in mares with twin conceptuses: Deprivation hypothesis. Am J Vet Res 1989;50:45–53.

[137] Morehead JP, Blanchard TL, Thompson JA, Brinsko SP. Evaluation of early fetal losses on four equine farms in central Kentucky: 73 cases. J Am Vet Med Assoc 2001;220:1828 1830.

[138] Ginther OJ. Equine pregnancy: physical interactions between the uterus and conceptus. In: Proceeding of the 44th Annual Convention American Association Equine Practitioner, Baltimore, Maryland. Ithaca: International Veterinary Information Service; 1998. pp. 73–104.

[139] Ricketts SW, Barralet A, Whitwell KE. A review of the causes of abortion in UK mares and means of diagnosis used in an equine studfarm practice in Newmarket. Equine Vet Educ Manual 2003;6:18–21.

[140] Brendemuehl JP, Williams MA, Boosinger TR, Ruffin DC. Plasma progestagen, tri-iodothyronine, and cortisol concentrations in postdate gestation foals exposed in utero to the tall fescue endophyte Acremonium coenophialum. Biol Reprod Mono; 1995; 1:53–59.

[141] Blodgett DJ. Fescue toxicosis. Vet Clin North Am Equine Pract 2001;17(3):567–577.

[142] Schultz CL, Bush LP. The potential role of ergot alkaloids in mare reproductive loss syndrome. In: Proceedings of the 5th Workshop on Mare Reproductive Loss Syndrome. Kentucky Agricultural Experiment Station, University of Kentucky, Lexington; 2002.

[143] Garrett LW, Heimann ED, Pfander WH, Wilson LL. Reproductive problems of pregnant mares grazing fescue pastures. J Anim Sci 1980;51(1):237.

[144] Cross DL. Fescue toxicosis in horses. In: Bacon CW, Hill NS, editors. Neotyphodium/ Grass Interactions. New York, London: Plenum Press; 1997. pp. 289–309.

[145] Riet-Correa F, Mendez MC, Schild AL, Bergamo PN, Flores WN. Agalactia, reproductive problems and neonatal mortality in horses associated with the ingestion of Claviceps purpurea. Aust Vet J 1988;65(6):192–193.

[146] Poppenga RH, Mostrom MS, Haschek WM, Lock TF, Buck WB, Beasley VR. Mare agalactia, placental thickening, and high foal mortality associated with the grazing of tall fescue: a case report. In: Proceedings of the Annual Meeting of the American Association of Veterinary Laboratory Diagnosticians; 1984. pp. 325–336.

[147] Powell DG. Mare reproductive loss syndrome. In: McKinnon AO, Squires EL, Vaala WE, Varner DD, editors; Equine Reproduction, 2nd edition. United Kingdom: Blackwell Publishing; 201. pp. 2410–2417.

[148] Williams NM, Bolin DC, Donahue JM, Giles RC, Harrison LR, Hong CB, Poonacha KB, Roberts JF, Sebastian MM, Smith BJ, Smith RA, Swerczek TW, Tramontin RR, Vickers ML. Gross and histopathological correlates of Mare Reproductive Loss Syndrome. In: Powell D, Troppman A, Tobin T editors. Proceedings of the First Workshop on Mare Reproductive Loss Syndrome. Lexington, KY: College of Agriculture, University of Kentucky, 2003. pp. 24–25.

[149] Slovis N. Pericarditis: a clinical perspective during an epidemic of fibrinous pericarditis in central Kentucky. Equine Vet Educ 2011;23(2):69–72.

[150] Zent WW. An overview of reproductive system changes during and after mare reproductive loss syndrome. In: Proceedings of the First Workshop on Mare Reproductive Loss Syndrome, 2003. pp. 30–31.